LYME DISEASE
in Australia

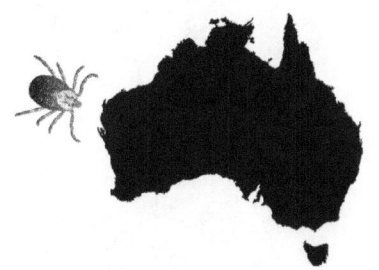

LYME DISEASE
in Australia

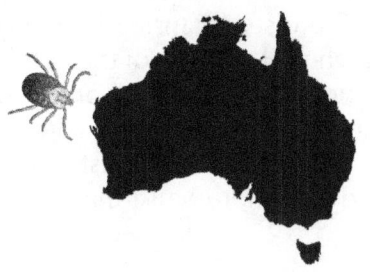

Fundamentals of an
Emerging Epidemic

NICOLA MCFADZEAN, N.D.
Naturopathic Physician

BioMed Publishing Group

P.O. Box 550531

South Lake Tahoe, CA 96155

www.LymeBook.com

Copyright 2012 by Nicola McFadzean, N.D.

ISBN: 978-0-9882437-0-5

All rights reserved. No part of this book may be copied, transmitted, or stored in a database without permission.

For related books and DVDs, visit us online at www.LymeBook.com.

DISCLAIMER

This book is not intended as medical advice. It is also not intended to prevent, diagnose, treat or cure disease. Instead, the book is intended only to share the unofficial research and opinion of the author. The book is provided for informational and educational purposes only, not as treatment instructions for any disease. Much of the book is a statement of opinion in areas where the facts are controversial or do not exist. The information in this book should not be considered any more valid than any other type of informal opinion.

The book was not written to replace the advice or care of a qualified health care professional. Be sure to check with your own qualified health care provider before beginning any protocols or procedures discussed in this book, or before stopping or altering any diet, lifestyle, or other therapies previously recommended to you by your health care provider. The treatments described in this book may have side effects and carry other known and unknown risks and health hazards.

Lyme disease is a controversial topic and this book should not be seen as the final word regarding Lyme disease medical care. The statements in this book have not been evaluated by the United States FDA.

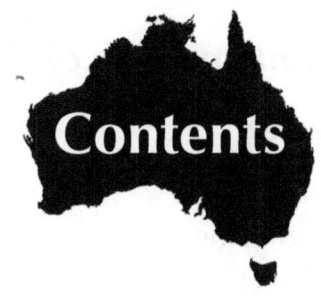

Contents

Acknowledgements	ix
Foreword	xiii
Preface	xix

SECTION ONE: *Setting the Stage*   xxi

1	**Introduction**	1
	The Purpose of the Book	2
2	**The Scope of the Problem**	5
3	**The Global Perspective**	9
4	**A Historical Perspective on Lyme Disease**	17
5	**Political Issues in Lyme Disease**	21
	CDC Surveillance Criteria	21
	IDSA Treatment Guidelines	24
	Scientific Studies Proving the Existence of Chronic Lyme Disease	30
	▸ Studies Outside the United States	30
	▸ Studies Within the United States	33
6	**Lyme Disease in Australia: Denial and Evidence**	43
7	**The Situation in Australia Today**	57
8	**Significant Case Studies and Personal Stories**	65
9	**The Keys to Change**	69

SECTION TWO: *Fundamentals of Lyme Disease* 73

10 What is Lyme Disease? 75
- Early Localized Lyme 76
- Early Disseminated Lyme 76
- Chronic Lyme Disease 77

11 How is Lyme Disease Transmitted? 79
- Is Lyme Disease Sexually Transmitted? 81
- Congenital Lyme Disease 82

12 Factors Adding to the Complexity of Lyme Disease 86
- Bacterial Strains 87
- Bacterial Forms 89
- Co-infections 91
- Biofilm 93

13 Signs and Symptoms of Lyme Disease 97
- Lyme Disease, the Great Imitator 97
- Can You Guess the Disease? 103
- Symptoms of Co-infections 105
  - *Borrelia* 106
  - *Bartonella* 106
  - *Babesia* 107
  - *Ehrlichia/ Anaplasma* 107
  - *Rickettsia* 108

14 Testing for Lyme Disease 109
- Direct Tests 111
  - *PCR* 111
  - *Culture* 111
  - *Biopsy* 112
  - *Lyme Direct Antigen Test* 112

Indirect Tests	113
▸ ELISA Test	113
▸ IFA Test	116
▸ Western Blot Test	117
Testing for Co-infections	119
▸ Antibody Tests	120
▸ FISH Tests	121
▸ PCR Tests	121
Other Tests That Might Be Useful	123
▸ CD-57	123
▸ Fry Labs Advanced Stain for Biofilm	124
▸ Elispot-LTT (Lymphocyte Transformation Test)	125
Inherent Challenges in Lyme Disease Testing in Australia	126
Getting the Most Out of Lab Testing for Lyme Disease	127

SECTION THREE:
Treatment Guidelines for Lyme Disease   131

15 Treatment Considerations	135
16 Suggested Medication Protocols	143
Acute, or Early-Stage, Lyme Disease	143
Chronic Lyme Treatment	145
▸ *Borrelia*	145
• Spirochete Forms of Borrelia	145
• Cell-wall Deficient Forms of Borrelia	147
• Cyst Forms of Borrelia	150
17 Medication Protocols for Co-infections and Related Topics	153
Babesia	153
Bartonella	156

Ehrlichia/Anaplasma and Rickettsia	157
Mycoplasma	158
Candida	158
Intravenous Versus Oral Administration of Antibiotics	159
Cautions with All Antibiotic Therapy	161
Antibiotic Therapy During Pregnancy and Breastfeeding	162
Antibiotic Therapy for Children	163
Practical Application	163
Medication Summary	164
Common Dosages	165
Sample Medication Protocols	166

18 Fundamentals of Natural Medicine in Lyme Disease   169

The Role of Natural Therapies with Antibiotic Protocols	170
General Naturopathic Principles	176
Detoxification	176
Inflammation	179
Immune function	180
Natural Antimicrobials	183
▶ *Borrelia*	183
▶ *Babesia*	184
▶ *Bartonella*	185
▶ *Candida/Yeast*	185
▶ *Viruses*	186
Biofilm	187
Digestive Health	188
▶ *Gastrointestinal Infections*	188
▶ *Side Effects of Antibiotics*	189
▶ *Leaky Gut*	190
Energy	191

- *Adrenal Fatigue* — 191
- *Mitochondrial Dysfunction* — 194
- *Methylation Defects* — 194

Hormone Health — 195

Pain Management — 197
- *Joint and Muscle Pain* — 197
- *Nerve Pain* — 198

Sleep — 199

Mood — 199

Heavy Metal Toxicity — 200
- *Testing for Heavy Metals* — 201
  - Blood Test — 202
  - Unprovoked Urine Test — 202
  - Provoked Urine Test — 202
  - Hair Analysis — 203
- *Addressing Heavy Metals* — 204

Sample Naturopathic Protocols — 206

19 Nutrition and Lyme Disease — 211

Inflammation — 211

Immunity — 215

Digestion — 216

Detoxification — 218

Summary of Nutritional Principles — 219

Drinks — 221

Lifestyle Factors — 223
- *Exercise* — 223
- *Sleep* — 226

20 Can Natural Therapies Alone Treat Lyme Disease? — 229

SECTION FOUR: *Putting It All Together* — 233

21 What Doctors Should Know About Lyme Disease — 235
22 The Emotional Challenges of Lyme Disease — 239
23 Coping Strategies — 245
24 Stories of Hope and Recovery — 251

Conclusion — 285

Appendices — 287

   A Burrascano's Treatment Guidelines 2008 — 288
   B Summary of IGeneX Australian Panels — 325
   C Healthy Fats to Take with Mepron and Malarone — 329
   D Summary of Medications and Common Dosages — 331
   E Coping with Herx Reactions — 333
   F Castor Oil Pack Instructions — 335
   G Dry Skin Brushing Instructions — 337
   H Summary of Biofilm Protocols — 339
   I Sample Naturopathic Protocols — 341

ACKNOWLEDGEMENTS

FIRST, I WANT TO THANK MY PUBLISHER BRYAN ROSNER FOR HIS motivation, guidance and amazing partnership in this project. Thank you for the time you poured into the manuscript, for the knowledge and experience you brought to it, and the sense of support and camaraderie that you provided for me along the way. Thank you to Kim Junker, best friend extraordinaire, for your amazing editing contribution, and also for your friendship and encouragement—we make a great team! To Adriana Covell, thank you for keeping my practice running while I was focused on writing, and for understanding when I wasn't available for other projects. Thank you also for what you provide to my Australian patients and the help that you give them on a daily basis. To Scott Forsgren and Connie Strasheim, thank you for the time you generously spent on the manuscript and the helpful suggestions you made.

Thank you to Nikki Coleman – the work you do is incredible! Thank you for being so committed to the Lyme community in Australia. Your contribution to this book was invaluable. I so appreciate the time you spent on it and your guidance along the way. I'm grateful to my mother, Julie McFadzean for being my Sydney liaison – for being the bearer of the test kits and for helping me with my Sydney clinics. Who would have thought that the house I grew up in would become my Sydney office all these years later?! I appreciate Mualla McManus for her contribution to this manuscript, and for her determined and unwavering commitment to changing the environment of Lyme disease in Australia; and Ann Mitrovic for providing me with great research studies that would have been hard to find from afar.

Finally, thank you to all my patients, for allowing me to love the work I do every single day, for the gratitude and appreciation you give me and for allowing me to contribute to you. Your strength and determination to keep moving forward in the face of hardship is inspirational, and it makes me love and respect you all the more.

FOREWORD

I AM THE WOMAN WHO WOULDN'T DIE. IN FACT I DIDN'T GET an invitation to my 25-year high school reunion because the organising committee had heard that I had passed away several years ago. Instead I had spent many years chronically ill. For eight years I was unable to wash or dress myself, often unable to feed myself, had trouble swallowing and was either stuck in bed, in my electric wheelchair, or if I was having a REALLY good day and was exceptionally determined, used a walking stick. Today, following correct treatment for Lyme disease I drive, have returned to work part time, wash, dress and feed myself, and am learning to ride a unicycle - I'm not very good at it, but I'm giving it a go and having fun doing it.

In 1987 my life changed forever. I was a fit, very healthy, exceptionally active 18-year old. I had been chosen among hundreds of applicants to go to Japan as a Rotary Exchange Student for a year, and I was having a ball. I threw myself into learning new things and having new experiences, including going on my school's Shugaku Ryoko (a trip for senior students to explore another city). We planned it for months, and one of the things that I looked forward to was patting the deer in Nara. I spent a long time playing with the cute deer, feeding them and patting them. It was only many hours later that I discovered a tick on my neck in the hairline, so I got a friend to pull it out (without tweezers, which I now know led to me getting Lyme disease and Babesiosis, but I didn't know correct tick bite first aid back then). A few days later I had an embarrassing red rash on my neck that looked like ringworm, so I pulled my long hair down to cover it and waited for it to go away. Little did I know how much that tick bite would change the course of my life, and that of the people that I love.

According to the surveys done by the Lyme Disease Association of Australia (and mirrored in research in the US & Europe) only 30% of people with Lyme disease remember a tick bite – this is because the tick injects you with a local anaesthetic so that it can be attached for longer. I didn't get suddenly seriously sick after my tick bite – I slowly got sicker and sicker until I could no longer function. Initially I came down with chronic fatigue syndrome-like symptoms, and that was what I was diagnosed with. More symptoms appeared over the years and as they did, I started to collect new (incorrect) diagnoses – severe irritable bowel syndrome (I spent years unable to leave my house unless I knew exactly where the toilets were along my route and at my destination, and at my worst I was also bowel incontinent and haemorrhaging from the bowel) which then was changed into inflammatory bowel disease when the pathology came back with inflammation in my bowel, gastroparesis (because my stomach wouldn't empty), trouble swallowing (I had a reconstruction of part of my oesophagus to try and fix this, but spent many years on liquid food as it was what was easiest to swallow – I still have an aversion to soup and smoothies), fibromyalgia (because I had severe muscle and nerve pain) which changed into reflex sympathetic neuropathy, sero-negative lupus, and finally when I was unable to dress, wash or feed myself anymore the doctors started exploring Motor Neurone Disease (MND) as a diagnosis.

I refused to even go and see a specialist about MND as a potential diagnosis because I knew it was a death sentence, and so my very kind local General Practitioner (GP) did some research with me – as soon as we found Lyme disease we knew that was what I had. Along the way there had been many mad dashes to the hospital, and if I ever hear the phrase "Oh, we've never seen that before" I will scream. Ironically I discovered later that I was one of the lucky ones – I remember my tick

Foreword

bite and had the classic EM rash that only 30% of Lyme patients get. In 2005, despite the fact that my blood test was negative[1], I was clinically diagnosed with Lyme disease (my Babesiosis diagnosis would follow a few years later) by a Professor of Immunology in Sydney. Unfortunately he was unable to treat me, and my GP and I were left to work it out for ourselves.

My treatment followed the Burrascano guidelines for treating Lyme disease (included as an Appendix in this book), and though the treatment prevented me from dying, without the guidance of an experienced medical practitioner to help us (and diagnose my Babesiosis co-infection), it didn't make me well. In 2009 I was lucky enough to meet Dr. Nicola McFadzean and she began treating me. Having someone who knew the nuances of Lyme disease treatment take on my care made a massive difference and within two years I was able to return to work, dress, wash and feed myself, and start on trying to ride that unicycle. Dr. McFadzean gave me my life back.

Unfortunately I passed on my Lyme disease and Babesiosis to my beautiful twin daughters through the placenta before they were born – it mildly affected one daughter, but severely affected the other. She was unlucky enough to be bitten by a tick on a camp in Sydney, and this extra exposure to the bacteria that cause Lyme disease overwhelmed her body. She has been in a wheelchair for the past 2½ years. At one point she was completely paralysed, unable to swallow and had trouble breathing, but because she had Lyme disease, doctors in our local hospital refused to treat her. In fact, at her worst, they handed her over to us, and told us to bring her back when she stopped breathing.

Many well-meaning, very good doctors have treated my family and me over the years, and have tried desperately to make me well. For that I am incredibly grateful, but their ignorance of Lyme disease ultimately led to

---

1   My Australian blood tests were negative, but my blood was sent to the USA in 2009 and I returned a weak positive test.

the loss of my ability to swallow, walk, use my arms, drive, wash or dress myself, and at 33 I had to medically retire. It is not the fault of the doctors at all. They only know what our health department tells them – and most of the health departments in Australia continue to push the myth that there is no Lyme disease in Australia (despite the large amount of evidence to the contrary) - and so doctors are not aware of it as a potential diagnosis. Even people like me who acquire Lyme disease overseas are unable to access adequate treatment. This leads to thousands of people suffering the way that I did, and has led to the death of some (for example Karl McManus who died from Lyme disease in 2010). No other disease in Australia has patients treated with such contempt – if I acquired leprosy or HIV overseas I would be able to access treatment back in Australia, but because I came back from my year in Japan with Lyme disease I have been largely unable to access treatment in Australia – which is why this book by Dr. McFadzean is so ground breaking, as it will allow local doctors to treat Lyme disease patients with confidence. Dr. McFadzean has treated close to one thousand patients with Lyme disease and many of them have been able to return to their old lives following years of disabling symptoms of undiagnosed Lyme disease and associated co-infections. Many of us owe our lives to Dr. McFadzean, and for that we are all incredibly grateful.

Currently I am the President of the Lyme Disease Association of Australia (LDAA). The Lyme Disease Association of Australia works to provide information and support to people who have Lyme disease (or suspect they have Lyme disease). The LDAA also lobbies the government, businesses and community groups on behalf of people with Lyme disease to change public health policy around Lyme disease in Australia and to work towards ending discrimination for people suffering from Lyme disease (this is a very looooooooooooooooooong process). I took over the presidency of the LDAA in 2010, which was founded in 2009 by Dr. Mualla McManus (who now runs the Karl McManus Foundation). The LDAA draws on the work of the Tick Advisory Group in Sydney (TAGS) in the 1990's, whose tireless work in Lyme disease and tick education saved many lives.

Foreword

I tell you my story, not because I am anything special, in fact my story is reflected in the story of the thousands of people who contact the Lyme Disease Association of Australia every year for help. I tell you my story to let you know that there is hope. With correct treatment, people who have been suffering for decades with a "mystery illness" that is in fact Lyme disease and its associated co-infections, can get well and return to doing the things that they love with the people whom they love.

Nikki Coleman
President, Lyme Disease Association of Australia
ACT, Australia
www.lymedisease.org.au

PREFACE

I STARTED TREATING LYME DISEASE SEVERAL YEARS AGO THROUGH my practice in San Diego, California. I was treating autistic children at the time, and started consulting with some of the children's mothers who were in their 30's and struggling with chronic fatigue and fibromyalgia-type syndromes. It seemed odd to me that so many women were feeling so poorly, but they attributed it to caring for special needs kids and soldiered on. As I worked with them and assessed them for Lyme disease (among other things), I realized how prevalent the illness was, even in California, which is not considered a key region for Lyme disease. Over the next few years, my Lyme disease practice grew and it became my major area of focus.

The connection to Australia is natural for me given that I grew up in Sydney and still consider myself to be Australian. I trained as a naturopath in Australia in the mid-90's but moved to the United States in 1998 and pursued my Doctorate in Naturopathic Medicine, a four-year post graduate program leading to board certification and licensure as a primary care physician in the state of California.

With these dual backgrounds, I feel uniquely positioned to help bridge the gap between the knowledge and experience of the United States, and the ever-increasing need for care for Lyme disease patients in Australia. As a licensed doctor in California, I can legally prescribe antibiotics, and I am familiar with, and can advise on, those regimens. My training as a naturopath means that I view the body holistically, and see how imperative it is to support the body using natural modalities and nutrition.

It is such an honour and privilege for me to work with my fellow Aussies doing what I love. My goal is to be a resource for you, to bridge the gap between knowledge and application of that knowledge in order to advise you, and to provide the understanding you might not receive from the medical community there.

My passion comes from seeing a large and ever-growing group of people suffer, and suffer unnecessarily; and out of that comes my commitment to make a difference and a contribution to the world of Lyme disease in Australia.

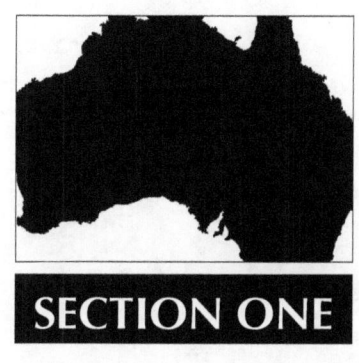

SETTING THE STAGE

1. INTRODUCTION

IF YOU ARE NEWLY DIAGNOSED, HAVE A FAMILY MEMBER WHO HAS been diagnosed, or have recently heard of Lyme disease and are wondering if it might relate to you, chances are, you are experiencing a pretty steep learning curve right now.

On first hearing the words 'Lyme disease', you might have rushed to look up Lyme on the internet, scanned a few sites, gathered some facts and read some fallacies (the differences between them barely discernible), and sat motionless, stunned, overwhelmed, and devastated. If you are a woman, you may have placed three calls in quick succession to various girlfriends, devoured a box of cookies - the empty container lying on the table next to you - and drank a couple of glasses of your favourite shiraz. If you are a man, you may have decided that your health issues were all in your head, and figured that on the back nine this weekend, it wouldn't look so bad. Unfortunately, as is often the case with the severe nature of this illness, you may already be flat out in bed, unable to do any of these things, wondering what on earth is going to happen next and what it all means for you and your family.

If you are further along the learning curve and already living in the world of chronic Lyme disease, you will know that it can be a complex, confusing, and bewildering place. The complexity of the illness makes navigating its pathways difficult, and the lack of awareness and acceptance of it by the Australian medical community certainly create massive stumbling blocks.

There is a bright side though - at least now you have a diagnosis, something you can wrap your mind around, a known entity that you can tackle, and a path to pursue towards wellness. Years of misdiagnosis and unending doctor visits with no beneficial results may have left you weary of the whole process, but I encourage you to rally your optimism, appreciate that this is a new road - a road full of new hope and new possibilities - and that even though it may be long and not particularly smooth, it does, at least, provide a renewed path of action and the potential for significant improvement, if not full recovery.

The Purpose of This Book

My hope is that this book will be a tool for you, a resource guide to help you sort through all the information being presented to you so you will feel more empowered to actively participate in your own care. I will share the historical and political context of Lyme, and give a clear description of what Lyme disease actually is, as well as guidance on evaluation and testing, and a wide range of treatment options.

In addition to being written for patients, this book is also written for health practitioners who may be new to Lyme and are trying to get up to speed to help these very sick patients with whom they are consulting, but have not found solutions by following the traditional medical algorithms. Australian GP's have not been trained to consider Lyme disease on the list of possible diagnoses, and while that may be frustrating for the many affected people who struggle to find answers and information, the GP's are not to blame. They are following what the health authorities tell them. We need to change that. We need to enhance their knowledge. We need to help them become aware, educated, and willing to address the problem alongside their patients. Clearly we need many more health professionals to be familiar with Lyme disease, so that they recognize it when they see it, and if nothing else, are able to refer out appropriately.

In this book I will also present some of the difficult challenges and complexities of Lyme disease – being realistic while remaining positive

Introduction

about the world of Lyme, and staying aware and therefore armed with knowledge. Knowledge, after all, is power. This illness is disempowering, so now is the time to take a bit of that power back, gather whatever information we have and put it to good use.

I hope to provide a resource that you can refer back to again and again. Please note though, that there is no one course of treatment that will work for everyone; some people may do well on natural treatments while others need hefty doses of antibiotics; some people may improve quite quickly while others may take months or even years. There is no set, clearly defined path that is true for everyone. In trying to present as much practical information as possible, please understand that this book does not substitute for medical advice that is specific to you. The book contains ideas and protocols, not prescriptions.

With that disclaimer in mind, I hope you find it to be a beneficial tool from which you can draw useful information. Many Australian patients have been stumbling alone in the dark, self-diagnosing, self-treating, and propping one another up emotionally, and that takes its toll. It is time to change that, bring this problem into the light, raise awareness and start Lyme sufferers in Australia on the road to recovery.

2. THE SCOPE OF THE PROBLEM

ALTHOUGH MANY PEOPLE HAVE NEVER HEARD OF LYME DISEASE, it is actually the fastest growing infectious disease, and the most common vector-borne illness, in the United States.[1]

In 1991, Lyme disease became a "notifiable" disease requiring health authorities to report confirmed cases, and the recorded numbers have risen ever since. In 2000, there were 17,730 confirmed reported cases of Lyme disease. In 2009, that number had nearly doubled to 29,959.[2] The highest reporting rates come from the north-eastern, mid-Atlantic, and north-central states, are among persons aged 5-14 years and 45-54 years, and are highest in the summer. According to the Centres for Disease Control (CDC), there are approximately 20,000 newly reported cases every year.[3]

The statistics above reflect only those cases that have been "counted" according to CDC diagnostic criteria. Who knows what the real numbers are? Who knows how many cases of Lyme disease go undiagnosed and unreported, either because they do not meet the official diagnostic criteria which we will see later are quite narrow and an inaccurate representation of real numbers of Lyme sufferers, or because they are never recognized as being caused by Lyme disease and are misdiagnosed as something else. *The Townsend Letter for Doctors and Patients*, a prestigious and respected periodical, has estimated that the actual number of new Lyme disease cases in the United States may be ten times higher than the numbers the CDC is reporting; that is, closer to 200,000 cases per year!

LYME DISEASE in Australia

The CDC itself suggests a similar likelihood.[4] Even with that under-estimation, in 2009 Lyme was still the 5th most common nationally notifiable disease. The following table shows the age and gender spread of Lyme disease cases between 2001 and 2010 in the United States.[5] How sad that the highest incidence rates were in males between five and ten years of age! The second highest group is the group that I see the most clinically – men and women between 35 and 55 years of age.

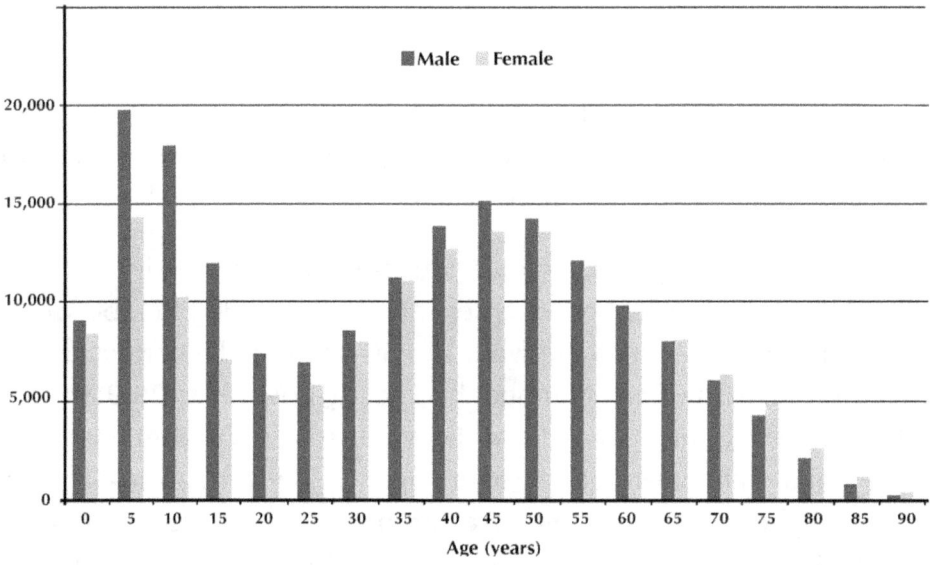

(http://www.cdc.gov/lyme/stats/chartstables/incidencebyagesex.html)

REFERENCES

1. CDC: Centers for Disease Control and Prevention [Internet]. Georgia: Centers for Disease Control and Prevention; Lyme disease data: Fast facts; 2012 Apr 12 [cited 2012 Jun 24]; [about 3 screens]. Available from: http://www.cdc.gov/lyme/stats/index.html

2. CDC: Centers for Disease Control and Prevention [Internet]. Georgia: Centers for Disease Control and Prevention; Lyme disease data: Fast facts; 2012 Apr 12 [cited 2012 Jun 24]; [about 4 screens]. Available from: http://www.cdc.gov/lyme/stats/chartstables/reportedcases_statelocality.html

3. CDC: Centers for Disease Control and Prevention [Internet]. Georgia: Centres for Disease Control and Prevention; MMWR: Lyme disease---United States, 2003—2005; 2007 Jun 15 [cited 2012 Jun 24]; [about 5 screens]. Available from: http://www.cdc.gov/mmwr/preview/mmwrhtml/mm5623a1.htm

4. Roberts DM, Carlyon JA, Theisen M, Marconi RT. The bdr Gene Families of the Lyme Disease and Relapsing Fever Spirochetes: Potential Influence on Biology, Pathogenesis, and Evolution. Emerg Infect Dis [serial on the Internet]. 2000 Apr;6(2) [cited 2012 Jun]. Available from http://wwwnc.cdc.gov/eid/article/6/2/00-0203.htm

5. CDC: Centers for Disease Control and Prevention [Internet]. Georgia: Centers for Disease Control and Prevention; Lyme disease: Confirmed Lyme disease cases by age and sex—United States, 2001-2012; updated 2012 Apr 9 [cited 2012 Jun]; [about 4 screens]. Available from: http://www.cdc.gov/lyme/stats/chartstables/incidencebyagesex.html

3. THE GLOBAL PERSPECTIVE

LYME DISEASE IS ALSO A GLOBAL PROBLEM – IT KNOWS NO INTERnational borders, nor borders of race, colour, politics, religion or socio-economic status. As people travel and birds and insects migrate, the bacteria are carried far and wide. Strains of Borrelia, the bacteria that causes Lyme disease, have been found in supposedly unaffected areas, and similarly the co-infections of Lyme (again, more on those later) are far-reaching also. And while Lyme disease is recognized in one state or province, a neighbouring state or province might authoritatively state, "We don't have Lyme disease here!" Such logic is fallacious and contrary to the way in which Lyme disease moves and spreads across geographic regions.

Global deforestation has broken down the delineation between humans and tick-dense areas. Human expansion has also resulted in the reduction of predators that hunt deer as well as mice, chipmunks and other small rodents – the primary reservoirs for Lyme disease. Researchers are also investigating the role of global warming in the spread of vector-borne diseases such as Lyme disease.

Following is a summary of some of the nations affected by Lyme disease. (Excerpted from Bryan Rosner's *Lyme disease Annual Report*):[1]

England
The British public has been warned by the Health Protection Agency (HPA) to carefully protect themselves from tick bites due to a "sharp rise in

the number of the blood-sucking parasites and increased cases of Lyme disease in Hampshire, Dorset, and Berkshire." The increase in tick population has been blamed on a "particularly wet and mild summer." According to the HPA, "Lyme disease is a highly infectious disease which is transmitted through tick bites and can lead to blindness, paralysis, and even death if left undiagnosed." Britons are advised to protect themselves by "wearing trousers, using insect repellent and checking their skin for ticks" after visits to the countryside. The HPA also notes that "incidents of Lyme disease have increased by 90% since 2006 across the UK, and New Forest, South Downs, Dorset, and Berkshire have now been named as tick hot-spots."

Sweden and Norway

The Department of Molecular Biology at Umeå University, Umeå, Sweden, released a study in 2007 that stated: "The reported geographical distribution of Lyme disease is constantly increasing in Sweden." The report cites findings, which show that birds play a key role in the spread of Lyme disease due to their long distance dispersal and their role as reservoir hosts for Borrelia. In addition to Lyme disease in Sweden, Swedish researchers also discovered that sea birds in the Arctic region of Norway carry Ixodes uria ticks infected with Lyme disease, specifically the Borrelia garinii strain. It has long been known that Borrelia garinii is one of the more common forms of Lyme disease on the European continent, and this information shows the spread of this strain to new geographical areas.

Russia

In collaboration with U.S. Centres for Disease Control (CDC) researchers, Russian scientists set out to determine which types of bacterial agents are found in the North Western region of Russia. The type of tick examined was Ixodes persulcatus. Researchers discovered the following:

Altogether, 27.7% of ticks were infected with at least one organism, while the DNA of two or more bacteria was found in 11.8% of ticks tested. The highest average prevalence of Anaplasma (20.8%) was detected in ticks

The Global Perspective

from Arkhangel'sk province, while the prevalence in ticks from Novgorod province and St. Petersburg, respectively, was 7.3% and 12.2%. Only Ehrlichia muris DNA was identified by DNA sequencing. In comparison, the prevalence of B. burgdorferi DNA was 16.6%, 5.8%, and 24.5% in the respective locations.

The Russian researchers conclude with this statement: "Since Ixodes persulcatus is so commonly infected with multiple agents that may cause human diseases, exposure to these ticks poses significant risk to human health in this region."

Germany

Researchers in Germany studied the influence of preventative measures on the risk of being bitten by a tick and suffering from Lyme disease in children attending kindergarten in forested regions of Germany. Fifty-three schools were studied, encompassing 1,707 children. Researchers concluded that "children in forest kindergartens are at a considerable risk of tick bites and Lyme disease."

Poland

Department of Occupational Biohazards investigated the prevalence of Lyme disease bacteria in ticks collected from wooded areas. 1,813 ticks from six districts were examined by polymerase chain reaction (PCR). Not only did researchers discover that a significant portion of the ticks were infected, they also were surprised to find that many ticks were infected with multiple strains of Lyme disease bacteria, including Borrelia afzelii, Borrelia garinii, and a new yet-unnamed strain, "Borrelia b.s.1."

Portugal

A Portuguese University, in a study of climate change, discovered that warmer and increasingly variable weather may result in an increased incidence of vector-borne diseases, including malaria, schistosomiasis, leishmaniasis, Lyme disease, and Mediterranean spotted fever.

Scotland

A fascinating report from the microbiology department at Raigmore Hospital in Scotland states that at least nine different strains of Borrelia have been documented in Scotland, including Borrelia afzelii and Borrelia sensu stricto. Additionally, a report appeared on September 15, 2007, in the *North Scotland Press and Journal*, entitled "Bloodsucking Ticks Blamed as Lethal Lyme Disease Cases Soar." This newspaper article not only documents the dramatic increase of Lyme disease cases in Scotland, it also provides evidence that Lyme disease can be fatal if not treated adequately. The article uses the word "rocketed" to describe the dramatic increase in cases over the past decade. Dr. Ken Oates of Health Protection Scotland observes that "There has been a genuine rise. Nobody can really say why. I would guess a summer like this, which is warm and wet, provides favourable conditions. Up to one in five ticks can carry Lyme disease in Scotland."

Croatia

As far away as Croatia, researchers are finding Lyme disease. Amazingly, 3,317 cases were reported from 1987 to 2003 in Croatia. North-western Croatia showed the highest incidence. According to a report published by the Department of Public Health, "the clinical picture of Lyme Borreliosis in Croatia is dominated by erythema migrans, followed by neurological manifestations."

Switzerland

In Switzerland, according to researchers, "the incidence of tick-borne encephalitis has been clearly increasing since 2004, and this is caused mostly by Lyme disease."

Canada

The Canadian Centre for Disease Control states "the black-legged tick, Ixodes scapularis, has a wide geographical distribution in Ontario, Canada, with a detected range extending at least as far north as the 50th parallel, and four out of five regions of Ontario affected." Additionally, "The Lyme

The Global Perspective

disease spirochete was detected in 12.9% of I. scapularis adult ticks." Also according to Canadian authorities, "characterization of B. burgdorferi in Canada displays a connecting link to common strains of Lyme disease found in the north-eastern United States." According to the Vector-Borne Disease Laboratory in British Columbia, "In 1994, British Columbia was declared an endemic region for Lyme Borreliosis." In Alberta, Lyme disease has been found to be common in rabbit ticks. The Department of Medicine at McGill University, Montreal, notes in a recent report that "Lyme disease is an expanding community health issue."

The poor recognition of Lyme disease by the medical establishment is not a phenomena limited to the United States: On September 17, 2007, CBS News Canada reported the story of approximately 100 Lyme disease sufferers who gathered on Parliament Hill in Canada to get the attention of Canadian physicians. The aim of the gathering was to get better testing for the disease and more federal money devoted to research—many in the group say they were misdiagnosed by their physicians. Amazingly, according to the CBS report, "Lyme disease is not a nationally reportable disease in Canada, according to the Public Health Agency of Canada (PHAC), meaning there are no statistics available on its prevalence." Yet, although not reportable, CBS goes on to state that "Borrelia burgdorferi is predominantly found in parts of British Columbia, southern and eastern Ontario, south-eastern Manitoba, and parts of Nova Scotia."

Try to figure out that contradiction: not reportable yet found practically everywhere. The CBS article concludes with the story of a Canadian professor who, after suspecting Lyme disease, was forced to travel to the United States and pay more than $15,000 out-of-pocket for treatment. Now, with unrelenting persecution of Lyme doctors in the United States, appropriate Lyme disease treatment may be harder and harder to find... anywhere in the world. The research identifying Lyme disease in Canada goes on and on, with over 83 official, published studies on Lyme disease in Canada. The Canadian Lyme Disease Association can be visited at www.canlyme.org.

Africa

A report published in Africa notes that "Lyme disease is now the most common vector-borne disease in Europe and North America, but there is also evidence that the disease is in Africa as well." Researchers found various strains of Borrelia in ticks located in Tunisia and Morocco, including the strains B. garinii, B. burgdorferi ss, and B. lusitaniae. More than 40 published studies have been released chronicling Lyme disease in Africa. On September 24, 2007, Afriqu' Echos Magazine, one of the larger news magazines in Africa, reported on a team of researchers who, from 1990 to 2003, studied the disease in Dielmo, a Senegalese village. They found that over 11% of Africans in the village had suffered from Borreliosis at one point in their lives. The same article in Afriqu' Echos Magazine also quotes the French Institute of Research and Development (the IRD): "Lyme disease is the most frequent bacterial disease in Africa, but it is also an affliction that is completely unknown to health professionals." The IRD evaluated a rural African area of Dakar and found that "Lyme Borreliosis was the most frequent reason for dispensary consultations after Malaria." The article in Afriqu' Echos Magazine further states that:

> "Researchers also discovered that this disease caused recurrent fever in the long term which could result in serious meningoencephalitis, which was sometimes fatal—symptoms exactly similar to those of malaria. The disease is thus systematically confused with malaria, which explains, of course, why there has been so much failure in terms of treatment since treatment for malaria is not effective against Borreliosis. Only tetracycline antibiotics produce results. Diagnosis is also made difficult by the problem of detecting Borrelia crocidurae [note this new strain of Lyme disease], the bacteria responsible for the disease. It is not detectable in the blood except during attacks of fever, and laboratory examinations are rarely possible in tropical Africa, in particular in rural areas."

Imagine the complexity now in Africa of untangling the diagnosis and treatment of two diseases, Lyme disease and malaria, which have similar symptoms and are presently ravaging Africa, but which health care practitioners are not trained to differentiate.

South America

South America is not immune either. Chile, Brazil, Argentina, Costa Rica, and other countries have reported isolated, although increasing, incidences of the Lyme disease infection. Numerous studies document Lyme disease in South America.

■ ■ ■ ■

The above information only scratches the surface. Many more pages would be needed to report all the available studies and articles. It is no great surprise that Lyme disease is emerging as a global epidemic. Geographical borders are simply imaginary lines used to differentiate political systems, allocation of land, leadership organizations, financial infrastructures and other man-made tenets. While some boundaries are physical, in the case of rivers or oceans, there is still migration of birds and animals across borders. Indeed, in many cases borders between countries hold no ecological significance, and thus do not contain microbes or disease processes. So it is with the spread of Lyme disease to Australia and other nations of the world.

REFERENCES

1. Rosner B, et al. 2008 Lyme disease annual report. South Lake Tahoe (CA): BioMed Publishing Group; 2008 [cited 2012 Apr]. Available from: http://www.lymebook.com/lyme-annual-report.

4. A HISTORICAL PERSPECTIVE ON LYME DISEASE

TO UNDERSTAND THE STRUGGLE INHERENT IN THE RECOGNITION, diagnosis and acceptance of Lyme as a valid disease in Australia, it is important to look at the history of Lyme disease, which is quite fascinating, and may date back further than we think.

It is often cited that the first cases of Lyme disease originated in a specific region in Connecticut in 1975, including the towns of Lyme and Old Lyme. However, descriptions of the illness that is now known as Lyme disease date as far back as 1764. Reverend John Walker was visiting an island off the coast of Scotland, and documented an illness with severe pain in the limbs that he related to a tick vector.[1] Many people from this area of Great Britain immigrated to North America between 1717 and the end of the 18th century, which could have perpetuated the spread between continents.

In the 19th century, the examination of preserved museum specimens found Borrelia DNA in an infected Ixodes ricinus tick from Germany that dated back to 1884, and from an infected mouse from Cape Cod that died in 1894.[2]

Early European studies reflect the skin manifestations of Lyme disease. Swedish dermatologist Arvid Afzelius presented a study at a 1909 research conference about an expanding, ring-like lesion he had observed in an older woman who had been bitten by a sheep tick. He named the lesion *erythema migrans (EM)*, which is now a primary characteristic of Lyme disease.[3]

Neurological problems following tick bites were recognized starting in the 1920s. French physicians Garin and Bujadoux described a farmer with a painful nerve inflammation accompanied by mild meningitis (swelling around the brain) following a tick bite. A large, ring-shaped rash was also noted, although the doctors did not relate it to the other symptoms. In 1930, the Swedish dermatologist Sven Hellerström linked the erythema migrans rash and neurological symptoms following a tick bite.[4]

Incredibly, in 2010, the autopsy of Ötzi the Iceman, a 5,300-year-old mummy discovered in the Italian Alps, revealed the presence of the DNA sequence of Borrelia burgdorferi. This fascinating discovery would make him the earliest known human with Lyme disease![5]

The outbreak of Lyme disease in Connecticut in the mid-70s may not have been the first cases of Lyme in the nation, but those cases certainly drew attention to a symptom cluster that did not fit with traditional and well-recognized diagnoses. A group of children in the town of Old Lyme who were affected displayed joint and muscle pain, which may have been in keeping with the diagnosis they were given of juvenile rheumatoid arthritis. However, what linked their symptoms with the possibility of Lyme disease was the presence of neurological symptoms, and the EM rash recognized from European cases.

In 1980, the New York State Health Department provided Willy Burgdorfer, a researcher at the Rocky Mountain Biological Laboratory, with collections of ticks named Ixodes dammini [scapularis] from Shelter Island, NY, a known Lyme-endemic area, as part of an ongoing investigation of Rocky Mountain spotted fever. In examining the ticks for rickettsiae, Burgdorfer noticed spirochetes - spiral-shaped bacteria - in 60% of the ticks. Burgdorfer, familiar with European literature on spirochetes, put two and two together and realized that they might be the cause of Lyme disease. The health department supplied him with more ticks from Shelter

A Historical Perspective on Lyme Disease

Island, and blood samples from patients diagnosed with Lyme disease, and with the assistance of Alan Barbour from the University of Texas Health Sciences Center, he confirmed his discovery by isolating spirochetes identical to those found in ticks from patients with Lyme disease.[6]

In June 1982, he published his findings in the journal *Science*, and the spirochete was named *Borrelia burgdorferi* in his honour.[7]

An intriguing part of the story is the conspiracy theory that Lyme disease was introduced into the north-eastern region of the U.S. by a man-made strain of Borrelia burgdorferi that escaped from a high-security biological warfare laboratory on Plum Island, which sits in Long Island Sound. In 1952, the facility was managed by the U.S. Army Chemical Corps as a component of its biological warfare program. Some claim that the bacteria were "leaked" to the island, made their home in the ticks, which then latched on to the deer, which then swam across Long Island Sound to nearby Connecticut and infected a group of teenagers who were then the first recorded cases of Lyme disease in the United States. The book *Lab 257: The Disturbing Story of the Government's Secret Plum Island Germ Laboratory*[8] by Michael Carroll presents interesting evidence in regards to that view.

While I do not claim to have enough information to be able to sort fact from fiction in this regard, there seems to be ample evidence of the existence of Borrelia burgdorferi long before the 1970's in both the United States and the rest of the world. In fact, in the United States, recent studies revealed that Ixodes ticks and B. burgdorferi were present in the north-eastern and mid-western regions in pre-colonial times and many years before European settlements were established in the U.S.

As you can see, many people think Lyme disease is a new, American disease, but clearly evidence supports its existence in various countries dating back a couple of centuries, and perhaps even thousands of years! This is important to keep in mind for Australian Lyme disease, considering the immigration patterns of Europeans to Australia and the possible transport of both the vectors (carriers) and the bacteria themselves.

REFERENCES

1. Merton N. Lyme disease in the eighteenth century. British Medical Journal. 1995;311:1478.
2. Rymon MM. Disguised as the Devil: How Lyme disease created witches and changed history. USA: Wythe Avenue Press; 2008. 52 p.
3. Afzelius A. Verhandlungen der dermatologischen gesellshaft zu Stockholm [German]. Archives of Dermatology and Syphilis. 1910;101:100–02.
4. Hellerström S. Erythema chronicum migrans Afzelii [German]. Archiv Dermatologie and Venereologie [Stockholm]. 1930;11:315–21.
5. Hall SS. Iceman autopsy: unfrozen. National Geographic. 2011 Nov.
6. Burgdorfer W. Discovery of the Lyme disease spirochete and its relation to tick vectors. Yale J Biol Med. 1984;57(4):515–20.
7. Burgdorfer W, Barbour AG, Hayes SF, Benach JL, Grunwaldt E, Davis JP. Lyme disease: a tick-borne spirochetosis? Science. 1982;216(4552):1317–19.
8. Carroll MC. Lab 257: the disturbing story of the government's secret Plum Island germ laboratory. New York: HarpersCollins; 2004. 289 p.

5. POLITICAL ISSUES IN LYME DISEASE

LYME DISEASE IS FRAUGHT WITH POLITICAL DIVISION AND CONtroversy, perhaps more so than any other disease. While this largely stems from within the United States, it unfortunately spills over into nations such as Australia and greatly shapes the recognition and acceptance of Lyme, as well as the policies and standards of care that are enforced.

CDC Surveillance Criteria

What has become clear is that being "notifiable" and being "accurately assessed" are two different things. The CDC's surveillance criteria, adopted in 1994, pose a great problem for the accurate assessment of Lyme disease, firstly because these criteria are so narrowly defined (for the purpose of having a high degree of specificity and confidence in the diagnosis); and secondly, because those criteria were simply never designed to be used for clinical diagnosis.

Even the CDC acknowledges, "This surveillance case definition was developed for the national reporting of Lyme disease: it is NOT appropriate for clinical diagnosis". Yet, the definition is repeatedly misused as a standard of care for healthcare reimbursement, product development, medical licensing hearings, and other legal cases.

Prior to 1994, Lyme disease *was* diagnosed based on certain clinical findings along with certain general laboratory findings. The criteria were as follows:

Clinical Criteria:

1. Erythema migrans rash.

2. At least one late manifestation of musculoskeletal, nervous or cardiovascular system disorders; and laboratory confirmation.

Laboratory Criteria:

1. Isolation of B. burgdorferi from clinical specimens; *or*

2. Demonstration of diagnostic levels of IgG and IgM antibodies to the spirochete in serum or CSF (could be by ELISA, Western blot or IFA); *or*

3. Significant changes in IgG and IgM antibody response to B. burgdorferi in paired acute- and convalescent phase samples.

While this criteria did have limitations - mainly that there was a strong emphasis placed on the EM rash which only a small subset of patients actually exhibited - it did have broad enough parameters to catch a wider range of cases, and it had more emphasis on clinical criteria. The lab criteria was *either* the first *or* the second *or* the third option, not necessarily all three.

The new CDC surveillance criteria are more oriented to the detection of early Lyme, and rheumatologic manifestations of Lyme, whereas we know that in reality Lyme has many diverse systemic manifestations, and that the guidelines leave out a host of other symptoms indicative of Lyme. One example is the cognitive dysfunction and neuropsychiatric manifestations associated with Lyme disease. If a patient has a positive Lyme test with symptoms of late neurological Lyme such as memory loss, difficulty concentrating and "brain fog", they would not be diagnosed as a Lyme disease case by the CDC. Why? Because cognitive dysfunction is not part of the CDC's "surveillance criteria" even though they recognize that these symptoms may be attributable to Lyme disease. Their criteria are centred more on the erythema migrans rash, arthritis, Bell's palsy, or early neurological Lyme symptoms involving meningitis or encephalitis (inflammation of the brain and surrounding tissues). The criteria that supposedly aim to achieve accurate assessment and tracking of Lyme disease may actually be preventing many people from getting the diagnosis and treatment they need – and in cases of early Lyme, this may ironically turn a treatable, acute disease into a much more difficult to treat, chronic one.

The CDC surveillance criteria also impact the laboratory testing for Lyme disease by dictating which tests are to be ordered, and what constitutes a positive test result, both to receive a positive diagnosis of Lyme disease, and to meet the criteria to be reportable to health authorities (hence influencing how many cases of Lyme disease are actually recorded).

A two-tiered approach to testing was adopted. The requirement dictated that a positive sensitive ELISA or IFA must be followed by a positive Western Blot with a defined number of approved antibody bands to be considered positive. This created a much more stringent set of criteria, and while those criteria were not intended to be adopted for clinical diagnostics, they were. In particular, they became the standard for insurance companies, for whom a stricter diagnostic criterion means fewer official diagnoses and consequently, less money paid out for patients' medical care.

While the CDC was encouraged to correct the misuse of the surveillance criteria, to date, not much has been done to rectify the problem. Even the passing of Public Law 107-116, signed by President Bush, who himself has had his own experiences with Lyme disease, in 2002, has not had a major impact. That law clearly states that the CDC case surveillance definition is unacceptable as a diagnostic tool. Unfortunately it continues to be used and this, combined with the unreliability of laboratory testing for Lyme, has led to misdiagnosis and delayed therapy. Yet 99% of practicing physicians are completely unaware of the law and still misuse the surveillance case definition.[1] Part of the necessary education for physicians is to learn the clinical presentations of Lyme disease and make diagnostic decisions based on those, as opposed to following the strict and unrealistic CDC surveillance case definition.

IDSA Treatment Guidelines

Another major barrier to adequate treatment of Lyme disease and a hugely divisive, political phenomenon is the Infectious Disease Society of America (IDSA) stance on acute versus chronic Lyme disease. Where the CDC surveillance criteria are more involved with the diagnosis of Lyme disease, the IDSA guidelines, published in 2006, provide information on the treatment of Lyme disease, including medication dosages and duration of treatment. Those guidelines recognize acute Lyme disease but more or less deny the existence of a chronic Lyme infection, speaking only of "post-Lyme syndrome". According to the IDSA, it is not possible to have the actual infection beyond the acute stage. Any symptoms that exist beyond this stage are just residual symptoms (known as post-Lyme syndrome) that, according to them, are not caused by persistent infection and will resolve themselves over time.

Not only have these guidelines severely restricted the care available to Lyme patients, they have also been used to prosecute doctors who prescribe outside the limits of their recommendations.

Given the IDSA's thinking that Lyme disease (per their standards) is only an acute and short-term infection, their treatment protocol entails only a short course of antibiotics – between 14 and 21 days. This becomes a significant issue in the world of chronic Lyme disease treatment. If the IDSA publishes guidelines limiting the treatment of Lyme to a maximum of 21 days, then that is what doctors learn and assume to be correct. Furthermore, any doctor who treats outside of those guidelines or standards of care, is subjecting him- or herself to scrutiny, censure, and even disciplinary action by the medical boards.

Following are some of the treatment recommendations given by the IDSA, according to the stage of illness:

For early Lyme disease (which by IDSA standards is necessarily associated with erythema migrans "bull's eye" rash, even though in 50% or more of Lyme disease cases this rash never occurs or is not memorable by the patient):

- Simple erythema migrans – doxycycline, amoxicillin or cefuroxime taken orally for 10-21 days.
- For Lyme meningitis and early neurological Lyme disease – ceftriaxone given intravenously for 14 days (up to maximum 21 days).
- For Lyme carditis – oral or parenteral (via intravenous route or intramuscular injection) antibiotic therapy for 14 days (up to maximum 21 days).

For late Lyme disease (which they do not consider to be "chronic" Lyme disease):

- Lyme arthritis without neurological involvement – doxycycline, amoxicillin or cefuroxime for 28 days.
- Neurological Lyme disease – ceftriaxone via IV for 2-4 weeks.

It is clear that none of the recommendations go beyond a maximum one-month course of antibiotics, with most of them suggesting 14 days only. Yet, according to extensive clinical experience by physicians who have treated thousands of cases of chronic Lyme disease, a four-week course of antibiotics will barely even scratch the surface. Most patients require several months up to a couple of years of treatment to get significant improvements in symptoms. These faulty IDSA recommendations are the key to the disparity between treatment that is needed, and treatment that is being provided.

Furthermore, IDSA guidelines also restrict other treatment approaches that might be attempted, outside of the four or five antibiotics they support.

"Because of a lack of biologic plausibility, lack of efficacy, absence of supporting data, or the potential for harm to the patient, the following are not recommended for treatment of patients with any manifestation of Lyme disease: first-generation cephalosporins, fluoroquinolones, carbapenems, vancomycin, metronidazole, tinidazole, amantadine, ketolides, isoniazid, trimethoprim-sulfamethoxazole, fluconazole, benzathine penicillin G, combinations of antimicrobials, pulsed-dosing (i.e., dosing on some days but not others), long-term antibiotic therapy, anti-Bartonella therapies, hyperbaric oxygen, ozone, fever therapy, intravenous immunoglobulin, cholestyramine, intravenous hydrogen peroxide, specific nutritional supplements, and others." (p.1094)

That's really quite a list of things *not* to do. How can the IDSA possibly verify the "lack of efficacy" for this huge, all-inclusive list of treatments, which even includes "specific nutritional supplements"? It does not seem reasonable that they can categorically dismiss such a range of modalities that have not been individually studied, and yet this broad list was included in their treatment guidelines, which became medical standard of care.

■ ■ ■ ■

Let us look now at the IDSA view on acute Lyme, post-Lyme syndrome and chronic Lyme disease.

The IDSA talks about post-Lyme syndrome, but there is no recognition of chronic Lyme disease in their treatment guidelines. In fact, they vehemently oppose the possibility of it (page numbers below are in reference to the IDSA guidelines publication, available through their website www.idsociety.org/lyme):

> "There is no convincing biologic evidence for the existence of symptomatic chronic B. burgdorferi infection among patients after receipt of recommended treatment regimens for Lyme disease. Antibiotic therapy has not proven to be useful and is not recommended for patients with chronic (> 6 months) subjective symptoms after recommended treatment regimens for Lyme disease." (p.1094).

So to clarify – the guidelines recognize a continuation of symptoms beyond the treatment regimen, which they term post-Lyme syndrome. They just deny that the symptoms are due to the presence of continued infection in the body.

"The response to treatment of late manifestations may be slow, and weeks to months may be required for improvement or resolution of symptoms after treatment. However, appropriate treatment [their 14 day protocols] leads to recovery in most patients." (p. 1110). They claim that "more indolent forms of neurological Lyme disease are actually quite rare" (p.1110). The reasons given for the persistence of symptoms include ongoing inflammatory processes, residual/irreversible neurological damage or co-infection with other agents such as Babesia (p.1115). At one point, where a tiny window seems to have been opened to the suggestion of persistent infection, somehow those particular microbes seem to be harmless:

> "Even if a few residual B. burgdorferi spirochetes or their DNA debris persist after antibiotic treatment in animal systems, they no longer appear to be capable of causing disease" (p.1119).

My favourites, though, are the implications that ongoing symptomatology is related to the emotional state of the patient, or that the symptoms are in line with what other healthy people experience.

"In many patients, post-treatment symptoms appear to be more related to the aches and pains of daily living rather than to either Lyme disease or a tick-borne co-infection. Put simply, there is a relatively high frequency of the same kinds of symptoms in "healthy" people" (p.1115).

"Previous studies of various infectious diseases have suggested that delayed convalescence can be related to the emotional state of the patient before onset of the illness. In those studies, fatigue was often a persistent symptom. Consistent with these observations, one study of patients with Lyme disease found that poor outcome was associated with prior traumatic psychological events and/or past treatment with psychotropic medications" (p.1116). So ongoing Lyme symptoms correlate with emotional instability prior to the onset of illness. Does this also mean that emotionally unstable people are more likely to attract, and get bitten by, a tick? While I do believe that psycho-emotional elements can contribute to illness, and impact recovery, it is somewhat ridiculous to postulate that the people who are reporting ongoing Lyme symptoms beyond standard 21-day courses of antibiotics are simply manifesting emotional imbalances and prior traumas rather than true infectious processes.

"To summarize, it can be expected that a minority of patients with Lyme disease will be symptomatic following a recommended course of antibiotic treatment as a result of the slow resolution of symptoms over the course of weeks to months or as a result of a variety of other factors, such as the high frequency of identical complaints in the general population" (p.1116). This argument completely fails to acknowledge the thousands of Lyme patients who were completely healthy, or at least asymptomatic, before their tick bite, and now have ongoing and continuous debilitating symptoms despite "appropriate" antibiotic therapy.

Clearly the IDSA is very specific in their diagnostic parameters and treatment protocols and very definite about the acute nature of Borrelia burgdorferi. Their position is happily enforced by medical insurance providers in the United States, who resist covering the costs of long-term medications and care needed for patients.

Of course, the elephant in the room is the thousands of people who have positive lab results for Lyme and/or co-infections and experience health issues following a tick bite; those who have been treated with short courses of antibiotics and still experience symptoms; as well as the thousands who may not necessarily have (for reasons discussed later) positive test results but have the history and symptomatology indicative of chronic Lyme/tick-borne illness.

How can we possibly explain the suffering that is caused by these infectious agents, disabling many, robbing people of quality of life, taking away their feelings of being smart, productive, happy, healthy individuals – saying that the very thing that is becoming a global epidemic does not exist beyond an acute phase, and is "cured" with 14 days of a single antibiotic?

Unfortunately, the misinformation produced by the IDSA guidelines was driven even deeper into traditional medical circles by way of a journal article published in the New England Journal of Medicine (NEJM), one of the most well-respected and credible medical publications in the world.

Political Issues in Lyme Disease

The article entitled *A Critical Appraisal of "Chronic Lyme Disease"*[2], written by a group of doctors and researchers affiliated with the Infectious Disease Society of America, acknowledges that Lyme disease is the most common tick-borne illness in the Northern Hemisphere, and that it is a serious public health problem. But it's grounding in reality stops there.

The authors recognize that "...after antibiotic treatment, a minority of patients have fatigue, musculoskeletal pain, difficulties with concentration or short-term memory, or all of these symptoms." But, instead of attributing these symptoms to an active bacterial infection, the article states: "Data from controlled trials have shown that there is substantial risk, with little or no benefit, associated with additional antibiotic treatment for patients who have long-standing subjective symptoms after appropriate initial treatment for an episode of Lyme disease." Furthermore, the article dismisses the improvements attained by patients who have received benefit from long-term antibiotic treatment: "Although anecdotal evidence and findings from uncontrolled studies have been used to provide support for long-term treatment of chronic Lyme disease, a response to treatment alone is neither a reliable indicator that the diagnosis is accurate nor proof of an antimicrobial effect of treatment."

Finally, the article concludes by stating that "It is highly unlikely that post–Lyme disease syndrome is a consequence of occult infection of the central nervous system." The following advice is offered to clinicians who see patients claiming to have chronic Lyme disease:

> "How should clinicians handle the referral of symptomatic patients who are purported to have chronic Lyme disease? The scientific evidence against the concept of chronic Lyme disease should be discussed and the patient should be advised about the risks of unnecessary antibiotic therapy. The patient should be thoroughly evaluated for medical conditions that could explain the symptoms. If a diagnosis for which there is a specific treatment cannot be made, the goal should be to provide emotional support and management of pain, fatigue, or other symptoms as required.

> Explaining that there is no medication, such as an antibiotic, to cure the condition is one of the most difficult aspects of caring for such patients. Nevertheless, failure to do so in clear and empathetic language leaves the patient susceptible to those who would offer unproven and potentially dangerous therapies."

It is not difficult to imagine the damaging and completely counterproductive effects this published article had on sufferers of chronic Lyme disease. This report raised the stakes considerably and rendered an already red-hot, hostile environment, even more perilous.

It is not true and it is not fair, but the big kids in the playground have set the rules, and now hundreds of thousands, or even more, people suffer—through denial of treatment, ridicule, rejection within the medical community, and even rejection by their friends and family members who do not understand the depth and complexity of the illness.

■ ■ ■ ■

Scientific Studies Proving the Existence of Chronic Lyme Disease

In examining the science, it becomes crystal clear that chronic Lyme disease is a true and valid condition. Although much of the research comes from other countries, especially Europe, the following studies show that standard, short courses of antibiotics lead to many treatment failures and relapses, reflecting the chronic nature of the illness.

Some of the following information was excerpted from Bryan Rosner's *Lyme disease Annual Report*.[5]

Studies Outside the United States

The Institute of Rheumatology, in Prague, Czech Republic reported a case of a female patient suffering from Lyme disease. Her case was confirmed by detection of Borrelia garinii DNA present in her blood and synovial fluid. After treatment with antibiotics, symptoms persisted and six months later, Borrelia garinii DNA was "repeatedly detected in the synovial fluid and the tissue of the patient." Additionally, even after antibiotic therapy, antigens and parts of spirochetes were detected by electron microscopy in the synovial fluid, tissue, and blood.

A similar discovery was made in Germany at the University Hospital of Frankfurt. Researchers described Lyme disease as a "disorder of potentially chronic proportions." They also noted that "therapeutic failures have been reported for almost every suitable antimicrobial agent currently available and resistance to treatment...continues to pose problems for clinicians in the management of patients suffering from chronic Lyme disease."

Another University in Germany, Ludwig-Maximilians-University, located in Munich, reported that "failures in the antibiotic therapy of Lyme disease have repeatedly been demonstrated by post-treatment isolations of the infecting Borreliae." One of the most interesting German studies, completed at Ludwig-Maximilians-Universitat Munich, attributed the clinical persistence of Lyme disease after antibiotic therapy to the presence of variants and atypical forms of B. burgdorferi. German researchers concluded that "B. burgdorferi produce spheroplast-L-form variants... these forms without cell walls can be a possible reason why Borrelia survive in the organism for a long time."

Researchers at the University of Dermatologische Privatpraxis, Munich, Germany, agreed with their German peers in a 1996 study, which noted that patients with erythema migrans failed to respond to antibiotic therapy. "Persistent or recurrent erythema migrans, major sequelae such as meningitis and arthritis, survival of Borrelia burgdorferi and significant and persistent increase of antibody titres against B. burgdorferi after antibiotic therapy are strong indications of a treatment failure."

In Austria, in 2001, the Lainz Municipal Hospital in Vienna admitted a 64-year-old woman who presented with various systemic symptoms hinting of Lyme disease. When spirochetes were detected in samples of her skin lesions, a diagnosis of Lyme disease was made. According to doctors, "Despite treatment with four courses of intravenous ceftriaxone for up to 20 days, progression of [Lyme symptoms] was only stopped for a maximum of one year."

Researchers at the Turku University Central Hospital, Finland, conducted a study in which 165 patients with disseminated Lyme disease were followed after antibiotic treatment. Approximately 10% of the patients experienced a clinical relapse with positive PCR tests and spirochetes successfully cultured from the blood of the patients. In this case, the Lyme disease relapse was evidenced not only by continuing symptoms, but also by two independent testing methods: both PCR testing and blood culture. This single study, even without aid from the numerous other studies presented in this chapter, should be enough to call into question the IDSA's staunch and dogmatic stance on chronic Lyme disease.

Italy also has experience with chronic Lyme disease. In 1992, the Universita di Genova, located in Genoa, Italy, reported on two patients with "chronic Lyme arthritis resistant to the recommended antibiotic regimens." These patients were eventually cured by long-term treatment with benzathine penicillin. The Italian researchers who conducted this study offered two possible reasons why antibiotic therapy finally worked, and both of these reasons involve active, persistent infection: "the sustained therapeutic levels of penicillin were effective either by the inhibition of germ replication or by lysis of the spirochetes when they were leaving their sanctuaries."

Moving across the globe to Thailand, scientists at KhonKaen University wrote that "Electron microscopy adds further evidence for persistence of spirochetal antigens in the joint in chronic Lyme disease. Locations of spirochetes or spirochetal antigens both intracellulary and extracellulary in deep synovial connective tissue as reported here suggest sites at which spirochetes may elude host immune response and antibiotic treatment."

In France, a study was published in the Journal of Antimicrobial Agents and Chemotherapy in 1996, conducted by the University of Marseille.

The study notes that "despite appropriate antibiotic treatment, Lyme disease patients may develop chronic manifestations."

■ ■ ■ ■

Studies Within The United States

It would be understandable for the IDSA to neglect, or at least take less seriously, research conducted outside the borders of the United States, since the IDSA is an organization that operates inside, and is accountable to, U.S. citizens and the U.S. government. However, when we examine studies conducted in the United States, you will see that a significant portion of the evidence in favour of chronic Lyme disease actually originated on American soil.

In 1996, the Fox Chase Cancer Centre in Philadelphia, Pennsylvania, conducted a study in which it was discovered that urine samples from 97 patients clinically diagnosed with chronic Lyme disease contained Borrelia burgdorferi DNA. The interesting aspect of this finding is that most of these patients had previously been treated with extended courses of antibiotics, the implications of which are simply that antibiotic therapy (even an extended course) does not always eradicate the infection. The study concluded that "a sizeable group of patients diagnosed on clinical grounds as having chronic Lyme disease may still excrete Borrelia DNA, and may do so in spite of intensive antibiotic treatment."

While the IDSA was releasing their guidelines in which it concluded that chronic Lyme disease was not a medical condition that justified extended antibiotic therapy, researchers at the New York State Psychiatric Institute were discovering just the opposite. The authors of a report produced at that institution described a case of fatal neuropsychiatric Lyme disease that was "expressed clinically by progressive frontal lobe dementia and pathologically by severe subcortical degeneration." Doctors noted that "antibiotic treatment resulted in transient improvement, but the patient relapsed after the antibiotics were discontinued...prolonged antibiotic therapy may be necessary [in some cases]."

LYME DISEASE in Australia

In Boston, Massachusetts, researchers at Tufts University School of Medicine conducted a study to investigate neurologic abnormalities found in chronic Lyme disease sufferers; 27 patients were followed. Six months after a two-week course of intravenous ceftriaxone (2 g daily), 17 patients showed improvement, 6 had improvement but then relapsed, and 4 had no change in their condition. Researchers concluded that "months to years after the initial infection with B. burgdorferi, patients with Lyme disease may have chronic encephalopathy, polyneuropathy, or less commonly, leukoencephalitis." With regard to the cause of chronic Lyme disease, Tufts University in their closing statement in the study implies a bacterial origin: "These chronic neurologic abnormalities usually improve with antibiotic therapy."

At Thomas Jefferson University, Philadelphia, Pennsylvania, urologists who treated seven patients with Lyme disease found that "neurological and urological symptoms in all patients were slow to resolve and convalescence was protracted...relapses of active Lyme disease and residual neurological deficits were common."

In direct opposition to IDSA statements, researchers at the Department of Pathology, Southampton Hospital, New York, noted that active cases of Lyme disease may show clinical relapse following antibiotic therapy. It is noted that "the latency and relapse phenomena suggest that the Lyme disease spirochete is capable of survival in the host for prolonged periods of time." In their studies of 63 patients with Lyme disease, the researchers concluded that "some patients with Lyme Borreliosis may require more than the currently recommended two to three week course of antibiotic therapy..."

Also in the State of New York, the New York University School of Medicine conducted a study, which evaluated antibiotic treatment of 215 patients between the years 1981 and 1987. Of those with "major" Lyme disease manifestations, a relapse rate of over 20% was observed.

This next study is even more interesting for several reasons, as we will see. The Albert Einstein College of Medicine, New York, reported in 1995 an "unusual" case of Lyme disease in which the patient experienced repeated neurologic relapses despite aggressive antibiotic therapy. What makes this study interesting is that each subsequent course of antibiotics given after the relapses was followed by Jarisch-Herxheimer reactions, which are known to occur only when active bacteria are dying. This implies that active bacteria were still present in the body after multiple courses of antibiotics. Additionally, subsequent to the various courses of antibiotics, the patient's cerebral spinal fluid tested positive "on multiple occasions" for not only complex anti-Borrelia antibodies, but also Borrelia nucleic acids and free antigen proteins. This study demonstrates persistent infection via two separate indicators: repeated Jarisch-Herxheimer reactions, and repeated observation of antibodies and antigens. Both indicators were found after not just one, but multiple courses of "adequate antibiotic therapy" had been administered!

Another similar case observed in Bethesda, Maryland, further calls into question the statement that chronic, persistent Lyme disease infection is "unusual." Doctors in Maryland working with the National Institute of Arthritis and Musculoskeletal and Skin Diseases, a part of the National Institutes of Health (NIH), reported that a 40-year-old white man who developed clinical Lyme disease after being bitten by a tick was treated with oral tetracycline, after which his symptoms were resolved. However, at a later date, the man was re-tested and Borrelia was detected by PCR in his peripheral blood leukocytes. After being re-treated with a longer course of ampicillin, probenecid, and concurrent cytotoxic therapy, symptoms improved significantly. This individual's case of Lyme disease illustrates two important points: First, ongoing symptoms that occurred after antibiotic therapy were confirmed by PCR testing to be caused by active bacteria. Second, re-treatment with antibiotics resulted in significant clinical improvement.

A study published in 2012 demonstrated persistence of Borrelia in monkeys despite antibiotic therapy. Rhesus macaques were infected with B. burgdorferi and a subset of them received aggressive antibiotic therapy four to six months later (antibiotic regimens being doxycycline and/

or ceftriaxone). Note that this study was done four to six months post-infection, not immediately, so the infection would have been more disseminated by that point. Subsequent studies via PCR and several other means of testing demonstrated persistence of infection despite antibiotic therapy. This implication of this is recognition that the standard antibiotic protocols suggested by the IDSA are inadequate to eradicate Borreliosis especially once disseminated, and that persistence of infection is possible despite antibiotic therapy.

The other finding of this study is that C6 peptides went down in all treated animals (C6 peptide is an immune marker sometimes used in Lyme disease diagnostics), even though the spirochetes persisted. This demonstrates that chronic infection can be present even with negative antibody tests.[3]

What does the literature tell us? If you take the time to read it and think about its implications, you'll find that the existence of chronic Lyme disease (as caused by an active bacterial infection) is quite obvious and established. Numerous scientific studies conducted across the globe by interdisciplinary scientists have plainly shown this to be the case. The controversy is one of political and dogmatic origin, not of scientific origin. The IDSA denies an active bacterial infection as the cause of chronic Lyme disease not as a result of scientific observation, but instead, because of various inefficiencies and shortcomings inherent in the bureaucratic procedures through which the IDSA operates. The process by which bureaucratic entities accept new truths and grow in knowledge has always been painfully slow and inefficient—and such is the case with the IDSA. Because chronic Lyme disease is in fact real, I am confident that it will be recognized as such sooner or later. Unfortunately, in the meantime, patients are left to dangle in the gap between two sides of an ideological debate.

■ ■ ■ ■

Another falsity that originates from the IDSA guidelines is the limited routes by which Borrelia burgdorferi (and its friends, the co-infections) can be transmitted. The guidelines state that "there is little evidence that a congenital Lyme syndrome occurs" (p. 1098) so that rules out mother-to-baby transmission. Also, "unengorged nymphal or adult Ixodes ticks also pose little or no risk of transmission of B. burgdorferi" (p. 1098), so that rules out ticks that have been attached less than 36 hours. "Many different tick species bite humans, and some "ticks" removed from humans are actually spiders, scabs, lice, or dirt, and, thus, post no risk of Lyme disease" (p. 1099), so that rules out a high likelihood of transmission based on confusion between a tick and a piece of dirt, and also rules out the possibility of transmission by other bugs such as lice or spiders. The guidelines cite the only route of transmission in fact, of any type of Borrelia, is Ixodes species ticks - Ixodes scapularis and Ixodes pacificus. All other ticks are supposedly safe and irrelevant to the conversation. In section two we will examine the evidence that clearly disproves these claims.

■ ■ ■ ■

The IDSA's slow-turning wheels and "selective filtering of information" are not the only hindrances to its production of accurate and relevant information. In 2006, its entire legitimacy was called into question when an antitrust investigation was launched to investigate its political and ethical motivations.

Former Connecticut Attorney General (now Connecticut State Senator), Richard Blumenthal, announced an antitrust investigation into the IDSA writing of the 2006 Lyme disease guidelines, which are considered the authoritative guidelines on the diagnosis and treatment of Lyme disease. He recognized that the guidelines had sweeping and significant impacts on Lyme disease medical care; that they were commonly applied by insurance companies in restricting coverage for long-term antibiotic treatment or other medical care; and that they strongly influenced physicians' treatment decisions. He also recognized that there were serious flaws in the production of the guidelines:

"My office uncovered undisclosed financial interests held by several of the most powerful IDSA panellists. The IDSA's guideline panel improperly ignored or minimized consideration of alternative medical opinion and evidence regarding chronic Lyme disease, potentially raising serious questions about whether the recommendations reflected all relevant science".

Blumenthal's findings, as cited on the official State of Connecticut Office of the Attorney General website[4], include the following:

- The IDSA failed to conduct a conflicts of interest review for any of the panellists prior to their appointment to the 2006 Lyme disease guideline panel
- Subsequent disclosures demonstrate that several of the 2006 Lyme disease panellists had conflicts of interest
- The IDSA failed to follow its own procedures for appointing the 2006 panel chairman and members, enabling the chairman, who held a bias regarding the existence of chronic Lyme, to handpick a like-minded panel without scrutiny by, or formal approval of, the IDSA's oversight committee
- The IDSA's 2000 and 2006 Lyme disease panels refused to accept or meaningfully consider information regarding the existence of chronic Lyme disease, once removing a panellist from the 2000 panel who dissented from the group's position on chronic Lyme disease to achieve "consensus"
- The IDSA blocked appointment of scientists and physicians with divergent views on chronic Lyme who sought to serve on the 2006 guidelines panel by informing them that the panel was fully staffed, even though it was later expanded
- The IDSA portrayed another medical association's Lyme disease guidelines as corroborating its own when it knew that the two panels shared several authors, including the chairmen of both groups, and were working on guidelines at the same time. In allowing its panellists to serve on both groups at the same time, IDSA violated its own conflicts of interest policy

Blumenthal added, "The IDSA's 2006 Lyme disease guideline panel undercut its credibility by allowing individuals with financial interests -- in drug companies, Lyme disease diagnostic tests, patents and consulting arrangements with insurance companies -- to exclude divergent medical evidence and opinion. In today's healthcare system, clinical practice guidelines have tremendous influence on the marketing of medical services and products, insurance reimbursements and treatment decisions."

It is clear that the very guidelines that drive decisions affecting thousands of people and their day-to-day lives were created by a group that had conflicts of interest, excluded significant medical opinion that did not support its agenda, and were driven by commercial and financial interests.

■ ■ ■ ■

As much as this kind of ignorance seems like a problem that might relate only to the United States, there is a trickle-down effect that impacts other countries including Australia, and the opinions of the medical professions there. After all, shouldn't the Infectious Disease Society of America know everything there is to know about an infectious illness like Lyme disease? And shouldn't they be right about it? One would think so; subsequently many doctors look to them for information, read their guidelines, and simply assume that they are accurate and appropriate.

This highlights one of the fundamental issues we face – trying to get chronic Lyme disease recognized in a world where denial by the medical establishment of the very problem that so many people are living with everyday has become the status quo.

On a happier note, the International Lyme and Associated Disease Society (ILADS, www.ilads.org) is a body of clinicians and researchers who have actually studied the science and recognize that chronic Lyme disease is a valid medical problem. ILADS is a non-profit, multinational, interdisciplinary medical society aimed at increasing awareness of tick-borne illness; educating within and outside of the medical community; training physicians and other health care professionals; and sharing guidelines of its own as to testing and treatment protocols for Lyme disease. ILADS is one of the most important resources available for patients and practitioners dealing with chronic Lyme disease, and this organization is growing exponentially as dozens of physicians abandon their old ways of thinking to join ILADS and take their place in the ranks of the growing number of doctors who know how to help people with chronic Lyme disease.

Lyme disease is possibly the greatest medical controversy in history. The political debate between the two sides – the IDSA on one and ILADS on the other, continues. But ILADS is working hard to present the scientific facts of the case – it has published treatment guidelines of its own, and its membership increases every year as more doctors get on board with the reality of chronic Lyme disease.

I will end this chapter by mentioning a pioneering doctor who was actually one of the Founding Members of the IDSA, Dr. Burton Waisbren. Dr. Waisbren has great influence in the medical community due to his current membership in IDSA and his status as one of it's Founding Members. In early 2012, Dr. Waisbren published a book entitled, *Treatment of Chronic Lyme Disease: 51 Case Reports and Essays in Their Regard*.[6] In this book, Dr. Waisbren describes how he now believes that chronic Lyme disease is in fact a real medical condition, and he presents 51 case reports of Lyme disease which he himself has treated, as well as the therapies he used to help these patients. Dr. Waisbren's abandonment of the IDSA Lyme disease treatment guidelines might be seen as a foreshadowing of what is to come, as more and more physicians follow suit in choosing science over entrenched dogma.

REFERENCES

1. Unknown. Federal Law and a disconnect. In: Lyme MD Blog [Internet]. Montgomery: Montgomery County, MD. 2008 May – [cited 2008 Jun 18]. Available from: http://lymemd.blogspot.com/2008/06/federal-law-and-disconnect.html.

2. Feder Jr HM, Johnson B, O'Connell S, Shapiro ED, Steere AC, Wormser GP; Ad Hoc International Lyme disease Group. A critical appraisal of chronic Lyme disease. N Engl J Med. 2007 Oct 4;357:1422-30.

3. Embers ME, Barthold SW, Borda JT, Bowers L, Doyle L, Hodzic E, Jacobs MB, Hasenkampf NR, Martin DS, Narasimhan S, Phillippi-Falkenstein KM, Purcell JE, Ratterree MS, Philipp MT. Persistence of Borrelia burgdorferi in rhesus macaques following antibiotic treatment of disseminated infection. PLoS One. 2012;7(1):e29914. Epub 2012 Jan 11. Erratum in: PLoS One. 2012;7(4):10.1371/annotation/4cafed66-fb84-4589-a001-131d9c50aea6

4. Blumenthal R. Attorney General's investigation reveals flawed Lyme disease guideline process, IDSA agrees to reassess guidelines, install independent arbiter [Internet]. Hartford (CT): Connecticut Attorney General's Office; 2002 [released 2008 May 1; cited 2012 Jun 5]. Available from: http://www.ct.gov/AG/cwp/view.asp?a=2795&q=414284

5. Rosner B, et al. 2008 Lyme disease annual report . South Lake Tahoe (CA): BioMed Publishing Group; 2008 [cited 2012 Apr]. Available from: http://www.lymebook.com/lyme-annual-report.

6. Waisbren, Burton, Treatment of Chronic Lyme Disease. South Lake Tahoe (CA): BioMed Publishing Group; 2012. Available from: http://www.lymebook.com/

6. LYME DISEASE IN AUSTRALIA: DENIAL AND EVIDENCE

WITH THE BACKDROP OF THE AMERICAN SITUATION AND THE CHALlenges faced there, one can see the context from which the experience of Lyme disease in Australia arises. But even more dire is the unsurprising fact that the health authorities still deny any existence of Lyme disease in Australia.

In spite of historical precedence and current evidence indicating otherwise, Australian health authorities continue to deny the possibility of locally acquired Lyme disease. They claim that only those who have travelled outside the country can contract Lyme since neither Borrelia burgdorferi nor the co-infections responsible for Lyme are found in Australian ticks.

As of the time of writing, the situation is still one of denial. The Fact Sheet on Lyme disease issued by the NSW Health Department[1] states:

"While locally acquired Lyme disease cannot be ruled out, there is little evidence that it occurs in Australia. There is a continuing risk of overseas-acquired Lyme disease being imported into NSW."

These conclusions were reached by an "expert" panel in April 2011, composed of specialists in public health, epidemiology, infectious diseases, rickettsial diseases and entomology. So although officials do not completely rule out the acquisition of Lyme in Australia, they certainly seem loath to admit it occurs.

LYME DISEASE in Australia

The Fact Sheet also states:

> "Only some species of ticks are capable of being infected by the Borrelia bacteria and only these infected ticks can pass the infection on to humans. This group of ticks is found in Asia, Europe and North America, but not in Australia."

The fact sheet does agree, however, that ticks can transmit infections, and that "while there is little evidence that Lyme disease is caused by Australian ticks, there may be other infections carried by Australian ticks which may cause an infection which is similar to Lyme disease. These infections are poorly characterized." That sounds conveniently vague, although it does imply that the Australian authorities are actually aware of a Lyme-like syndrome that *does* occur in Australia.

The NSW Government statement also discusses testing. While it does recognize that the diagnosis of Lyme is based on symptoms, physical findings and the possibility of exposure to infected ticks (rather than strictly on laboratory findings), it goes on to say that lab tests are rarely definitive (which I agree with), and that when testing is done in places where disease is rare or absent ("for example", their website states, "Lyme disease in Australia"), many positive test results will be false positives. This indicates to me that the government is not even open to being proven wrong. Even if an individual has a positive lab test for Lyme, it may be written off as a false positive. Further, Lyme disease is not reportable in NSW, so the health departments do not gather data on the incidence and growth rates of Lyme disease. Why should we believe that positive test results are false positives just because the Health Department does not like to think of Lyme disease as an Australian problem? This position is highly illogical.

Much of the denial of Lyme disease in Australia comes from a study by Russell and Doggett published in 1994.[2]

Russell and Doggett were given a National Health and Medical Research Council (NHMRC) grant to investigate whether Australian ticks carry the Borrelia bacteria. Although they reported that they were unable to isolate any Borrelia DNA from the 12,000 common Australian ticks collected from the Eastern seaboard, there are great limitations to that study. First, only 1,038 of those 12,000 ticks were tested by PCR (a very specific kind of testing). Second, during the study, Russell and Doggett assumed that only the B. burgdorferi strain could cause Lyme disease, and only tested the ticks for these strains. Studies in Europe, which had identified at least two other strains (B. garinii and B. afzelii) as causative factors in Borreliosis, were not acknowledged. Third, they used both fed and unfed ticks. Unfed ticks that have not had a blood meal are far less likely to contain spirochetes and other infectious agents than those that are full of blood.

Ironically, they did isolate "spirochete-like objects" in the fed ticks, but decided that they were artefacts (bacteria-like objects under the microscope but not actual bacteria) and did not include them as significant findings. In summary, the study concluded that ticks in Australia did not carry spirochetal bacteria.

Slightly misleading and somewhat confusing in the light of Russell and Doggett's published results is an article by James Alpers.[3] In this article, Alpers claims that Doggett *had* made over 70 isolates of spirochete-like organisms from more than 30 separate coastal areas stretching from Southern Queensland to northern Victoria. Richard Russell, one of the primary authors on the "there are no spirochetes in Australian ticks" study is quoted in this article:

"A number of different tick species have been found to harbour the [spirochete-like] organisms, although Ixodes holocyclus, the 'paralysis tick', has yielded more isolates than other species. We are undertaking various investigations, including molecular studies, to characterize our isolates, and if the organisms being recovered from ticks are responsible for the human infection, then the widespread origin of our many isolates indicates the disease may be quite extensive on the coast of south-east Australia."

Just two years later, Russell and Doggett published research stating that the aforementioned isolates were simply "artefact", and not spirochetal

LYME DISEASE in Australia

bacteria with potential clinical significance. And from that time the widespread denial of Lyme disease in Australia was solidified.

Before we take that one study and use it to deny an emerging health crisis, let us take a look at some of the other evidence. Even prior to that Russell and Doggett study, Borrelia had already been identified in Australia.

A publication by Carley and Pope[4] identified an Australian strain of Borrelia, which they named *Borrelia queenslandica*. They described this strain of Borrelia being isolated from wild rats called Rattus villosissimus. These rats flourish during plagues, this one centered in Queensland. When the rats died off in large numbers, an assessment of infectious agents causing the eradicating was done and three agents were found – Streptobacillus moniliformis, Hemobartonella muris and a spirochete with the characteristics of Borrelia. These characteristics, according to Carley and Pope, matched in morphology, size, restricted host range, type of infection and sensitivity to antibiotics, to Borrelia spirochetes described in other research. Antibiotics found to be effective in this mouse study included penicillin, a tetracycline (chlortetracycline), streptomycin and chloramphenicol.

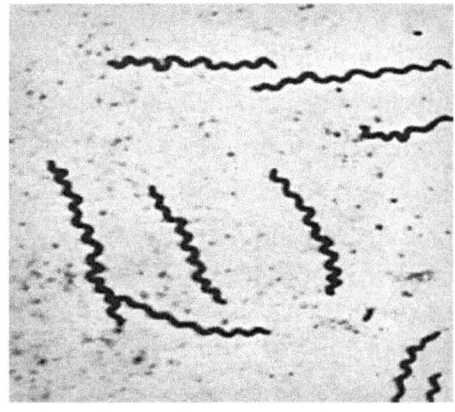

Borrelia queenslandica spirochetes as detected by Carley and Pope in 1962

The authors cited ticks of the genus Ornithodoros, in particular Ornithodoros gurneyi in inland Australia including northwestern Queensland, as significant vectors. They named the spirochetes Borrelia queenslandica because of the location of the rat plague that housed them.

Mackerras (1959) also reported the isolation of Borrelia from Australian fauna including kangaroos, wallabies and bandicoots.[5]

Of course, Russell and Doggett (1994) did not acknowledge either of these two publications in their study.

Lyme Disease In Australia: Denial and Evidence

Case reports of Lyme disease in Australia date back to the early 1980's. Three of them are reported in case reports and letters to the editor in the Medical Journal of Australia. All three meet the diagnostic criteria for Lyme disease.

In 1982, Stewart et al. described the case of a 21-year-old labourer from Branxton near the lower Hunter Valley.[6] His bite occurred in 1980, and gave rise to a red rash that spread outwards from a lump at the site of the bite, with a central clearing in the middle. The authors described it as a lesion typical of ECM (erythema chronicum migrans).

The authors stated: "This patient's clinical course presented the classical features of Lyme arthritis", which meant it was migratory, moving from joint to joint, and relapsing, coming and going. But there were two other complicating factors indicative of Lyme disease - cognitive deficits including behavioural change and memory loss; and also tachycardia (rapid heart rate).

Between the EM rash, the arthritis, the cardiovascular symptoms and neurological issues, the authors describe this patient's presentation as part of the "classic syndrome" of Lyme disease. They also mentioned that there had been six cases of EM rash diagnosed by Hunter Valley dermatologists over the prior 12 months (1981-82), "which indicates that the etiologic agent (the Ixodes tick) is well established in that area".

Another notable case report was in 1986.[7] This one was on the south coast of New South Wales (NSW), in Guerilla Bay near Moruya. A 34-year-old gardener reported to his doctor in March 1985 after insect bites on his arm and back. He had a red rash that spread out from the site of the bite, which was assessed as an EM rash. He was given antibiotics and the rash resolved only to reappear at a later date and require a second course of antibiotics.

Another, 60-year-old female patient from Bendalong, between Nowra and Ulladulla, NSW, presented with headaches, fatigue and joint pain that were associated with a rash on her chest wall and left thigh that the author reported to be consistent with an EM rash.[7] She was diagnosed with early Lyme disease and treated with doxycycline. The rash and symptoms resolved and at the time the case was written up the lady had continued to be well. That was in December 1985.

In 1986, yet another case report from the Central Coast of NSW appeared in the Medical Journal of Australia.[8] This case was a 70-year-old Sydney resident who had spent time in Gorokan on the Central Coast in December 1985. While there was no recollection of a tick bite, the patient had spent time cutting brush. In January 1986 he developed lethargy, malaise, fevers and night sweats. A few weeks later several round rashes appeared on his body, up to 5cm in diameter with central clearings, along with severe occipital headaches, a sore throat and high fevers. The rashes were consistent with the EM rashes of Lyme disease, and he was assessed as having early, uncomplicated Lyme disease based on clinical criteria and treated accordingly.

Going back now to studies looking for Borrelia in ticks - in the early to mid 1990's, at around the same time as Russell and Doggett were publishing their research claiming that no spirochetes had been identified in Australian ticks, another group at the University of Newcastle and Royal North Shore Hospital in Sydney (Professors Richard Barry, Michelle Wills and Bernie Hudson) was investigating the same question. In contrast to Russell and Doggett, Michelle Wills did isolate and grow the spirochetes from Australian ticks, and identified the spirochetes as Borrelia.

The starting point for the study, as she described in her letter to the editor published in the Medical Journal of Australia, was the notion that Australian Lyme disease is caused by a spirochete similar, but not necessarily closely related antigenically, to B. burgdorferi, and that the spirochete cycles through native fauna and domestic animals, transmitted by a tick with a wide range of hosts.

Wills et al. cultured the gut contents of a large number of ticks. 70 of 167 (42%) were culture-positive for Borrelia-like spirochetes. These spirochetes were described as indistinguishable from the reference strain of B. burgdorferi, being large, coiled, motile bacteria with an irregular rotational movement. In other words, the spirochetes they found in Australian ticks could not be differentiated from the B. burgdorferi they were comparing them to.

In a letter to the editor published in the Medical Journal of Australia in 1991, Michelle Wills B.Sc. concluded:

"These findings indicate that some species of tick often responsible for human and animal tick bites in this country commonly harbour Borrelia species spirochetes. On structural and antigenic grounds these microbes are likely to be the aetiological agents of Lyme disease in Australia."[9]

That was in 1991. Imagine how the situation today could be different if the Australian government had accepted and acted on the results of this study and not the Russell and Doggett study.

In the early 90's groups from the Royal North Shore (including Hudson) and Newcastle University (including Wills) joined forces to "define the incidence and prevalence of Lyme Borreliosis in Australia, develop screening and confirmatory laboratory tests for the disease, and to educate the medical community about Lyme disease". They had suspected that Lyme disease was more common than had been currently recognized, with an increasing number of suspected cases from the hospital's catchment area in recent years. This had actually led to the creation of a phone line where people could call in if they had suspected Lyme disease, so that they could collect samples for study. At that time Bernard Hudson, M.D. is quoted as saying "there is no doubt that Lyme disease is around on the south coast and the northern beaches of Sydney. Numerous suspected cases have come to my attention through clinicians in these areas. Now we just have to find out how common the disease actually is."

In 1994 these researchers (including Michelle Wills of the 1991 study, and Bernie Hudson M.D. of the Department of Microbiology at Royal North Shore Hospital in Sydney), published in the Journal of Spirochetal and Tick-Borne Diseases.

They proposed the existence of an indigenous form of Lyme disease in Australia based on the data they had collected since 1991. They describe the clinical presentations of erythema migrans rash arthritis and radiculopathy in candidate Lyme Borreliosis cases in Australia. When they tested the blood of these candidate patients, they discovered antibodies to European strains of Borrelia - Borrelia garinii and Borrelia afzelii, while antibodies to Borrelia burgdorferi were uncommon.

1,024 people were tested and approximately 20% tested positive on a Western Blot against the American strain B. burgdorferi, the European strain B. garinii, or B. afzelii. 56% of the positive results were due to B. garinii, 34% to B. afzelii and only 10% to B. burgdorferi (Wills, PhD, 1995).

Russell and Doggett only tested for Borrelia burgdorferi, not the European strains garinii and afzelii. From that research the authorities denied the existence of *any* Borrelia causing disease in Australia. Yet evidence seems clear that strains of Borrelia do exist – they are just more closely related to the European variants B. garinii and B. afzelii. This is a major disconnect in the available research and the significance of this is profound for the recognition of Lyme disease today.

This team of researchers and clinicians seem to have no doubt that Lyme disease exists in Australia; in fact, the publication clearly states: "One of us (Bernie J Hudson) regularly sees clinical cases of Lyme Borreliosis acquired in Australia."

The Medical Journal of Australia article goes on to discuss the case definitions of Lyme disease. It recognizes that the initial case definition in Australia has been based on the United States CDC criteria, which the authors admit to be problematic. Part of the reason they find the use of the U.S. case definitions problematic is that the clinical manifestations of Borreliosis are so different with different species of Borreliae from different parts of the world. If Australian patients are more likely to be infected with European strains, which the research certainly suggests, they are not necessarily going to present with manifestations that the United States CDC has deemed characteristic of Lyme disease. They also discuss limitations of testing, and that they have chosen to use the Western Blot over either an IFA or ELISA method of testing, because of lack of sensitivity of the latter tests.

They also offer that the European strains should be used in immunoblotting as part of their testing methodology and not the American strains, to get more accurate results. "Recombinant proteins from well-characterized North American strains may be of little use for immunoblotting [Western Blotting] in Australian LB cases." In simple terms, this means that using European strains as part of the testing methodology instead of American strains will yield more accurate results.

Dr. Hudson collated a group of 23 patients with an assumption of Lyme Borreliosis (LB) based on clinical presentation. Of them 21/23 (>90%) had Flagellin antibodies while 13/23 (55%) had antibodies to OspA (these are antigens - the different parts of the spirochete that trigger immune reactions). The control group that was clinically assessed to have a diagnosis other than Lyme Borreliosis did not manifest the same antibodies to those antigenic markers. Thus it seems that the patients who appeared to have the symptoms of Lyme disease had a high chance of finding laboratory evidence of it, *once the European strains were used*.

A telling statement in this 1995 study was that "all patients acquired their illness in Australia". But wait, I thought Lyme disease does not exist in Australia?

To summarize, Hudson et al. state:

> "Because we have detected Borrelia-specific antibodies in the serum of candidate clinical cases of LB acquired in Australia, we hypothesize that an indigenous form of Lyme Borreliosis exists in Australia. The acquisition of at least one case outside the area of distribution of I. holocyclus indicates that ticks other than this species can transmit LB in Australia."

In 1998 Hudson et al. appeared again in the Medical Journal of Australia[10], this time with a case report of Lyme Borreliosis with a positive skin biopsy for Borrelia garinii. Although the patient had traveled to Europe 17 months prior to onset of his illness, the authors stated it was more likely that the infection was acquired in Australia based on the clinical details of the case.

They deduced this for a number of reasons. Firstly the patient had no awareness of a tick bite or tick exposure during his trip to Europe; he was there only for a few days. He did not become unwell immediately after his European trip, or in the following seventeen months. He did however have a tick bite while walking in bushland in Pittwater Shire in Sydney. Sixteen days after the bite a characteristic EM rash developed; his illness commenced within a few days of the bite, starting with headache, malaise and a low-grade fever, progressing over time to include cognitive deficits, a fullness in the head, and muscle and joint pain.

What is so significant about this case is that Borrelia garinii was cultured from this patient's skin, with infection emerging after a tick bite in the Sydney region. While B. garinii is more concentrated in European countries, the authors concluded that the migratory patterns of birds from the Northern Hemisphere explains their introduction into Australia. Certainly positive polymerase chain reaction (PCR) data exist to show the presence of B. garinii in ticks in the Southern Hemisphere.[11] Unfortunately, the fact that the patient had traveled to Europe 17 months prior to onset of illness, even though he denied a tick bite or tick exposure while there, and that he was well after that trip until his Australian bite, has been used to discredit the case report and raise questions as to whether his illness might have been acquired overseas.

Given that Mackerras (1959), Carley and Pope (1962) and Wills and Barry (1994) all managed to grow and isolate Borrelia from Australian native animals but only one study has been show to the contrary; and that researchers such as Hudson et al. (1995) and Wills (1991) have described clinical presentations of Lyme disease *and* found definitive laboratory evidence to support that, it follows that perhaps the findings of Russell and Doggett should be a side note rather than the source of a national denial of a major, and growing, health crisis.

Lyme Disease In Australia: Denial and Evidence

What does become clear from an examination of the research is the major limitation of testing only for Borrelia burgdorferi, and not the European strains garinii and afzelii. This single factor made all the difference in the outcome of the Russell and Doggett study, and may well have made all the difference in the recognition of Lyme disease in Australia to the present day.

Hudson et al. in their 1995 publication even offer that if the northern European experience is anything to go on, it is probable that there will be a delay in Australia between the recognition of indigenous Lyme Borreliosis and the isolation and identification of causative spirochetes. However, not yet having identified the exact morphology and behaviour of these particular spirochetes is a very different situation than simply not looking for them at all and flatly denying the possibility of their existence in this country.

Laurie Cestnick, from the School of Behavioural Sciences at Macquarie University, NSW, in the Australian and New Zealand Journal of Public Health 1998, gives a good synopsis:[12]

> "Some people in Australia still hold the view that Lyme disease does not exist in Australia, partially because the symptoms of people infected here have been found to be slightly different to the symptoms of those infected in North America, where the spirochete, Borrelia burgdorferi, was first discovered; and also because serological evidence has been inconclusive.
>
> In European countries and Australia, there have been central nervous system (CNS) complaints of sharp, shooting pains and migraines in the absence of any rashes or arthritic pain, whereas in North America there are more peripheral arthritic complaints than direct CNS complaints, although people with both sets of complaints do exist in these areas of the world.
>
> Denial of the existence of Lyme in Australia based on different symptoms of patients here versus in America is not justifiable and may be hazardous from a treatment perspective.

LYME DISEASE in Australia

The causative agent of Lyme, the spirochete B. burgdorferi, has been detected in the cerebrospinal fluid of many persons with the symptoms of Lyme. In most cases, however, symptoms of Lyme exist in the absence of positive Borrelia serology.

Lyme researchers in Australia are of the strong opinion that the spirochete exists here, but behaviours of the spirochete and our immune systems make it difficult to detect serologically ... treatment decisions must be made based on the symptomatology of the patients and exposure to endemic areas for Lyme disease as opposed to positive serology.

In summary, given exposure to a tick, particularly in a proposed endemic area, and even one symptom of Lyme, the logical decision appears to be to offer treatment and ask more detailed questions later."

REFERENCES

1. Fact sheet: Lyme disease [Internet]. North Sydney (NSW): NSW Ministry of Health (Aus); [updated 2012 May 26; cited 2012 Jun 26]. [About 4 screens]. Available from: http://www.health.nsw.gov.au/factsheets/infectious/lyme_disease.html
2. Russell RC, Doggett SL, Munro R, Ellis J, Avery D, Hunt C, Dickeson D. Lyme disease: a search for a causative agent in ticks in south-eastern Australia. Epedemiol Infect. 1994 Apr;112(2):375-84.
3. Alpers J. Borrelia isolated from Australian ticks. Today's Life Science. 1992 Apr:40-2.
4. Carlye JG, Pope JH. A new species of Borrelia (B. Queenslandica) from Rattus villosissimus in Queensland. Aust J Exp Biol Med Sci. 1962 Aug;40:255-61 [5] Mackerras MJ. The haematazoa of Australian mammals. Aust J Zool. 1959;7(2):105-135.
5. Stewart A, Glass J, Patel A, Watts G, Cripps A, Clancy R. Lyme arthritis in the Hunter Vally. Med J of Aust. 1982;1:139
6. McCrossin I. Lyme disease on the NSW south coast. Med J of Aust. [Letter]. 1986 Jun 23;144.
7. Lawrence RH, Bradbury R, Cullen JS. Lyme disease in the NSW central coast. [Letter]. 1986 Oct 6;145:364.
8. Wills MC, Barry RD. Detecting the cause of Lyme disease in Australia. Med J of Aust. [Letter]. 1991 Aug 19;155:275.
9. Hudson B, Stewart M, Lennox V, Fukunaga M, Yabuki M, Macorison H, Kitchener-Smith J. Culture-positive Lyme Borreliosis. Med J of Aust. 1998 May 18;168:502.
10. Olsen B, Duffy CD, Jaenson TG, et al. Transhemispheric exchange of Lyme disease spirochetes by seabirds. J Clin. Microbiol. 1995 Dec;33(12):3270-74.
11. Cestnick L. Lyme disease in Australia. Aust N Z J Public Health. 1998;22(5):524.

7. THE SITUATION IN AUSTRALIA TODAY

IN THE LIGHT OF ALL THE RESEARCH PRESENTED SUPPORTING THE existence of Lyme disease in Australia, it is most surprising to see the government and health authorities still in denial. Certainly the current situation also points to a very different story than the one resulting from the health departments, the majority of Australian GP's (General Practitioners) and that isolated study discussed in the previous chapter – namely, that there is no Lyme disease in Australia. The available evidence indicates that the reality of the situation is quite the opposite – that indeed, there is plenty of Lyme disease in Australia, with more and more cases being diagnosed each week.

According to the Lyme Disease Association of Australia (LDAA – more about this organization later), there are currently at least 15,000 diagnosed cases of Lyme disease in Australia, with conservative estimates of another 200,000 people undiagnosed. Bearing in mind that Australian doctors are not trained to look for or test for Lyme disease, the numbers of official diagnoses are not likely to represent anything close to the actual number of people suffering with an incorrect diagnosis or without a diagnosis at all.[1]

These numbers may also be skewed due to misconceptions about the transmission of Lyme. In traditional medical circles, the belief continues that only four species of ticks can transmit Borrelia and related co-infections - in America, the Ixodes scapularis and Ixodes pacificus

(Black-legged Tick), commonly known as deer ticks; and in Europe and Asia, the Ixodes ricinus (Castor Bean/Sheep Tick) and the Ixodes persulcatus (Taiga Tick). This perpetuates the myth that without those four types of ticks, Australia could not possibly harbour Lyme disease. However, since those early investigations, many more species of ticks have been identified as vectors, including over a dozen more species of Ixodes ticks, some of which are definitely found in Australia.

As an example, Ixodes holocyclus, also known as the paralysis tick or grass tick, is one of the major suspects for introducing tick-borne illness into the country. This is not the exact same type of tick as the American deer tick, but it is still known to carry diseases in Australia, and is a likely vector for Borrelia.

With about 75 tick species in the country[2] including the Ixodes holocyclus and other variants of Ixodes ticks, it is no surprise that Lyme disease would exist endemically in Australia.

Another issue is the geography of Lyme disease. While health authorities may claim that most of the cases of Lyme disease have been acquired overseas, a recent study by Peter Mayne, M.D. gives definitive evidence for the existence of endemic B. burgdorferi infection and its associated co-infections – that is, infection actually acquired within Australia.[3]

In later chapters the common co-infections of Lyme disease will be discussed in more detail. For now, it is sufficient to be aware that when ticks and other vectors transmit the Borrelia bacteria, they can also transmit other bacteria and parasites along with it. Some co-infections, such as Babesia, Bartonella, Ehrlichia and Rickettsia, are commonly seen. These are referenced in Dr. Mayne's study.

In his study of 51 subjects, most patients reported symptom onset in Australia without recent overseas travel. 28 of 51 (55%) tested positive for Lyme disease. Of 41 patients tested for tick-borne co-infections, 13 (32%) were positive for Babesia species and nine (22%) were positive for Bartonella species. Twenty-five patients tested positive for Ehrlichia species and (16%) were positive for Anaplasma phagocytophilum while none were positive for Ehrlichia chaffeensis. Among the 51 patients tested for Lyme disease, 21 (41%) had evidence of more than one tick-borne infection. Positive tests for Borrelia, Babesia duncani, Babesia microti, and Bartonella henselae were demonstrated in an individual who had never left the state of Queensland. Positive testing for these pathogens was found in three others whose movements were restricted to the east coast of Australia. Interestingly, four subjects from this study had not left Australia, and still had positive lab results for Lyme and Babesia.

Dr. Mayne's study reinforces the position that tick-borne illness in Australia is possible, likely, and in fact, proven. Although larger subject groups must be studied to develop this body of knowledge and give it credibility with health authorities, this is a significant starting point for further research.

Researchers at the University of Sydney are looking into the diagnostic aspects of Lyme disease in Australia – comparing the results of testing for Borrelia done in Australia with results of tests run through a United States laboratory called IGeneX, a specialty Lyme lab. The goal of the research is to assess whether results are comparable from both, and whether the Australian testing is sensitive enough to detect Borrelia. A second goal is to evaluate whether the U.S. CDC surveillance criteria are appropriate in Australia.

Results so far show that of 148 Australian patients, 70% returned a positive IgG or IgM western blot (a specific type of antibody test), through IGeneX lab in the United States. Further 53% returned confirmation of exposure of up to 3 other tick borne pathogens (e.g. Rickettsia species, Babesia species, Bartonella species). Put simply, when tested through a specialized lab, with more sensitive diagnostic procedures, 70% of Australian patients showed a positive result while 53% of that group tested positive for co-infections.

Using the Australian standards of testing and the limitations therein, a much smaller number would test positive proving that the limitations in Lyme testing lead to undiagnosed cases of Lyme and are a major public health concern warranting immediate attention.[4]

Peter Mayne also published a study in 2012 where he examined tissue biopsies at the centre of the EM rash on four patients. PCR testing was carried out and all four samples tested positive for Borrelia. All four patients acquired their infection in Australia. Interestingly, when biopsies were performed on the outer edges of the EM rash, the PCR testing came back negative, suggesting that if a skin biopsy of a rash is to be performed, testing the central part gives a more reliable test result.[5]

Co-infections, although given less credence by authorities, may play an important role in the spread of Lyme disease in Australia.

Bartonella is one of the primary co-infections in Lyme disease. Until recently there was little formal evidence of Bartonella in Australia, although Australian Lyme sufferers have tested positive for Bartonella via IGeneX antibody testing and exhibited symptoms of Bartonellosis from a clinical standpoint.

In 2011 a study was published showing that a number of Bartonella species were found in marsupial fleas in Australia. The study stated that "the clustering of Bartonella species with their marsupial flea hosts suggests co-evolution of marsupial hosts, marsupial fleas and Bartonella species in Australia." In simple terms, researchers deduced that the bugs and the hosts were adapting to one another over time to support proliferation of the species.[6]

Babesiosis, another common co-infection, is a well-documented disease of cattle (Babesia bigemina and Babesia bovis) and dogs (Babesia canis, Babesia vogeli and Babesia gibsoni), and Babesia tick vectors have been imported to the continent since European settlement. Until recently, it was considered unlikely in Australia, at least in humans.

Then in April 2011, a 56-year-old South Coast man changed the playing field when he died from Babesiosis, the first reported case in humans in Australia. The man had been very ill for several months prior to his death, and had first been hospitalised in November 2010, following a motor vehicle accident. Over subsequent months his condition deteriorated

– he required surgery, parenteral nutrition and broad-spectrum antibiotic therapy. He developed anaemia and a severe drop in his platelet count, and his liver function worsened. In later months his white blood count also dropped. He received multiple blood transfusions. His condition continued to deteriorate, but by the time Babesia microti, the most common strain causing Babesiosis in the United States, had been identified and aggressive treatment commenced, he was already too ill, and he passed away five days later on April 18, 2011.

Although doctors originally thought blood products received via transfusion might have been a source of the parasites, later analysis showed evidence of parasitemia in his blood films before he received any transfusions. Therefore transfusion was ruled out as a primary cause.

His death did raise questions about the possible hosts for Babesia and the presence of strains in Australia that cause human illness since he had no significant history of travel, nor had he been in contact with anyone who had recently traveled from the United States. His last trip was 40 years ago to New Zealand, also a country with no known Babesiosis. He did have pre-existing health issues of diabetes, hypercholesterolemia, hypertension and depression, which restricted him from working or travelling, so he remained on his farm on the south coast of New South Wales with his son and his dog.

Researchers reporting and analysing the case concluded that it was locally acquired in 2012, and the Medical Journal of Australia supported that position when they reported the gentleman's death as the first locally-acquired case of Babesiosis in a human in Australia.[7]

■ ■ ■ ■

Aside from these research studies and papers, we can see from the sudden increase in media coverage of Lyme disease that it is a hot topic, and one that is getting more and more attention. Ranging from articles in the Sydney Morning Herald to segments on the Today Tonight program and Sunday Night program, Lyme disease is beginning to receive a lot of mainstream media coverage.

In fact, using Google Analytics and Google Trends which track the patterns of people on the internet – what they search, where they live, and so on, we see that worldwide, Australia is ranked number three in Google searches on Lyme-related topics, behind only the United States and Canada. The numbers below represent a ratio – the top-ranking search always gets 100, and the following numbers are a calculated ratio based on that.

Web Search Interest: Lyme disease
Worldwide, Last 12 months

United States	100	Canada	47
Australia	39	Ireland	23
United Kingdom	19	Philippines	9
Netherlands	4	India	3
Germany	2		

If Lyme did not actually exist in Australia, would so many people need to search for information about it? I believe that the recent media coverage of Lyme disease has led to thousands of people recognizing themselves or their loved ones in the stories they are hearing – identifying with the symptom patterns, and relating to the lack of answers they have been given by the medical profession. Media coverage and awareness are important steps, but the urgent and ultimate need is for that information to infiltrate the medical profession, in particular general practitioners who are in contact with potential Lyme patients every single day, and who either diagnose them incorrectly or tell them that "nothing is wrong", thus sending them on a wild goose chase for a phantom diagnosis which might prevent them from ever getting the help they need.

REFERENCES

1. Lyme Disease Association of Australia. [Internet]. Kaleen: Lyme Disease Association of Australia; Date unknown. About Lyme disease: what is Lyme disease? [cited 2012 Jun]; [about 1 screen]. Available from: http://lymedisease.org.au/about-lyme-disease/myths-surrounding-lyme-disease-in-australia/

2. Department of Medical Ontology. Ticks: introduction [Internet]. Wentworthville NSW (Aus): University of Sydney and Westmead Hospital; 1998 Jan 28 [updated 2010 Dec 1; cited 2012 Jun]; [about 2 screens]. Available from: http://medent.usyd.edu.au/fact/ticks.htm

3. Mayne P. Emerging incidence of Lyme borreliosis, babesiosis, bartonellosis, and granulocytic ehrlichiosis in Australia. Int J Gen Med. Epub 2005 Mar 19.

4. Herzberg G, Hudson B, Mayne P, McFadzean N, McParland B, Mitrovic A, Schloeffel, R. Lyme Borreliosis diagnostics in Australia: limitations, concerns and a way forward. Poster session presented at: The Australasian Society for Infectious Diseases; 2012 Mar; Fremantle, WA; and The Zoonosis meeting at Sydney University; 2012 Jul; Sydney, Aus.

5. Mayne P. Investigation of Borrelia burgdorferi genotypes in Australia obtained from erythema migrans tissue. Clinical, Cosmetic and Investigational Dermatology. 2012:5; 69-78.

6. Kaewmongkol G, Kaewmongkol S, McInnes L, Burmej H, Bennett MD, Adams PJ, Ryan U, Irwin PJ, Fenwick SG. Genetic characterization of flea-derived Bartonella species from native animals in Australia suggests host–parasite co-evolution. Infect Genet and Evol. 2011;11:1868-72.

7. Senanayake SN, Paparini A, Latimer M, Andriolo K, Dasilva AJ, Wilson H, Xayavong MV, Collignon PJ, Jeans P, Irwin PJ. First report of human babesiosis in Australia. Med J Aust. 2012;196(5):350-52.

8. SIGNIFICANT CASE STUDIES AND PERSONAL STORIES

THERE ARE MANY PERSONAL STORIES OF LYME PATIENTS IN AUSTRALIA, heartbreaking stories of mothers and their children sick with Lyme, whole families affected - financially ruined from medical bills, dissatisfied with a medical system that denies the problem even exists and instead sends them for psychiatric evaluations implying they are crazy - the list goes on and on. The stories I hear every day are horrendous. It is no surprise that Lyme sufferers in Australia are angry, and on a mission to correct the injustices and misinformation.

The media has begun to publicize various cases involving Lyme. In early 2012, the Today Tonight show posted a segment about a man who became ill on the job after numerous tick bites, and actually won a government workman's compensation case due to an infection with Lyme disease.

Robert Sotur was a gardener at a Coffs Harbour Resort, and had been bitten by ticks at least 500 times over ten years. He saw dozens of doctors and a neurologist who all said the same thing - the bites meant nothing. But the evidence was irrefutable. He had never left Australia, yet after numerous tick bites received on the job, he contracted, and now suffers from Lyme disease. Sotur says he is "constantly itchy, with rashes, nausea, bloating, headaches, vision loss, the cough - the list goes on and on."

This case is remarkable because Mr. Sotur received government compensation for a disability caused by a disease that the Federal Government, the Australian Medical Association, and Australian State Governments all agree does not exist in Australia.

There are those who openly disagree with the status quo, however. The Today Tonight story quotes Gull Herzberg, MD, a General Practitioner who specializes in Lyme disease: "Yes. Lyme disease is in Australia. I've seen people with symptoms, had test results that they have Lyme disease, and have responded to Lyme disease treatment. I'm using international testing, I'm using protocols that come from overseas, I'm seeing people improve."

Others fight the government's ignorance with the law. There is currently a class-action lawsuit by over fifty individuals who have never left Australia but have come down with Lyme-like symptoms. The lawyer handling the case, David Jones, states:

> "There needs to be an acceptance that there are many people within our community that are having symptoms that are Lyme or Lyme-like, and Governments need to take these people seriously. They need to commission the research, and they need to determine whether or not this disease, or a disease like it, exists here in Australia."[1]

Perhaps one of the most significant cases of Lyme disease in Australia so far was that of Karl McManus, who was bitten by a tick on the chest in July 2007 at a wildlife park on Sydney's Northern Beaches. A week later he developed flu-like symptoms but, due to a lack of knowledge about Lyme disease in Australia, did not recognize the telltale signs and the potential seriousness of the tick bite. As weeks went by Karl experienced profuse sweats, muscle twitches, mood swings and a darkening of his complexion. He became sensitive to light and noise and refused to see his friends. He began to lose dexterity in the fingers of his left hand and also started to get muscle wasting – all common signs and symptoms of Lyme disease.

In November 2007 Karl saw a neurologist who acknowledged his muscle wasting and muscle twitching but, despite inconsistent diagnostic test results, diagnosed him with multi-focal motor neuropathy (MFMN). From that point, Karl's diagnoses ranged from MFMN to motor neurone disease to multiple sclerosis.

Dissatisfied by his diagnosis, Karl and his wife, Mualla, decided to research his condition on the Internet, and came across Lyme disease. Given New South Wales (NSW) government's position as stated on their official website that there is no evidence of Lyme disease contracted within Australia, the McManus' thought Lyme disease unlikely, but pursued testing nonetheless.

Karl's blood tests in Australia by the ELISA assay came back negative. Since the treatments he had received were not working, he was put on antibiotics to test the possibility of a Lyme diagnosis, and experienced a worsening of symptoms consistent with a Herxheimer reaction (Herxheimer reactions will be explained fully in section two but suffice it to say for now that they are a worsening of symptoms at the beginning of treatment from the toxic by-products of parasites and bacteria dying off; the presence of a "Herx" supports the diagnosis of infectious illness). This alerted the McManus' that they were on the right track.

In April 2008, they sent blood samples to IGeneX in the U.S., and results came back positive not only for Borrelia, but also for Babesia duncani and Rickettsia – two of the co-infections of Lyme disease.

Karl continued his antibiotic protocol for Lyme disease and began to regain his strength, but then he got the flu and regressed. Getting the correct treatment was very difficult for him because of the denial of Australian doctors as to the causative agent, and their insistence that his true diagnosis was motor neurone disease or multiple sclerosis (MS). He chose to fly to Germany in early 2009 to pursue treatment, improved while there, and continued to get IV antibiotics on his return to Australia. He was gaining muscle strength, however, his tongue became paralysed and he could no longer ingest enough calories to sustain his weight, which started dropping. He had a feeding tube put into his stomach, and while in the hospital, was treated as a motor neurone disease patient, not a Lyme patient. Subsequently, fluids were restricted which meant he could not flush toxins out of his body (toxic build up is a big problem for Lyme patients), and he was not given adequate calories. He continued to lose weight and strength, and went from being able to walk (assisted) and talk (albeit slurred) when admitted to the hospital, to not being able to walk or talk at all – just four days later. He returned home in terrible shape, and when he got the flu not long after that, the paralysis of his tongue and the build up of mucous overwhelmed him. He passed away on July 14, 2010.

Since then, his wife Mualla Akinci McManus has dedicated her life to the cause of Lyme disease in Australia by working tirelessly to change the acceptance of Lyme disease and promote education and awareness. While Karl's story has a tragic end, Mualla is determined that others will not have to endure the same.

Karl was bitten on the northern beaches of Sydney, and subsequently tested positive for Lyme disease, Babesia duncani and Rickettsia. These infections, if treated aggressively enough, may not have been fatal, but due to medical practitioners overlooking the central role that chronic infection was playing in his health, he did not receive the appropriate treatment, and he lost his life to Lyme disease.

REFERENCES

1. Camp Other. More on Lyme disease in Australia on the Today Tonight Show Blog Entry [Internet]. 2012 Feb 21 [cited 2012 Jun]. Available from: http://campother.blogspot.com/2012/02/more-on-lyme-disease-in-australia-on.html

9. THE KEYS TO CHANGE

EDUCATION OF THE MEDICAL COMMUNITY IS THE FOUNDATION for change and progress in Australia. The government simply cannot continue to deny the existence of Lyme disease in Australia given the case reports that are emerging, especially in patients who have never left the country. Still, whether any significant paradigm shift comes from that sector is yet to be seen. On the other hand, doctors and health professionals usually enter their profession with a desire to help others, to relieve suffering, and to remain committed to that despite policy and rhetoric that might potentially mislead them. It is here that we need to focus our efforts to expand the possibilities for Lyme disease treatment in Australia.

The Lyme Disease Association of Australia (www.lymedisease.org.au) and the Karl McManus Foundation (www.karlmcmanusfoundation.org), central institutions for the advancement of education, patient advocacy and research into Lyme disease in Australia, are working to ensure that. These two non-profit groups are working tirelessly to further the cause and increase awareness.

Furthermore, the ILADS organization in the United States is also a good source of information and recognizes chronic Lyme disease as a valid and significant issue internationally. They publish treatment guidelines that doctors can refer to (http://www.ilads.org/lyme_disease/treatment_guidelines.html). These guidelines were written by a panel of Lyme disease experts, are peer-reviewed and endorsed by the national Lyme

Disease Association and the California Lyme Disease Association. ILADS is the most significant United States organization with an agenda to help chronic Lyme disease sufferers and educate physicians who wish to help these patients.

Joseph Burrascano, MD, has also written treatment guidelines that have been used extensively as a reference in the Lyme community. These are also available to the public, and have been a valuable source of information for patients. They are specific enough in medication protocols to be highly valuable to prescribing doctors. His guidelines are reprinted in Appendix A and are also available online at http://www.ilads.org/lyme_disease/B_guidelines_12_12_08.pdf.

The key to enhancing the Australian experience is to include other forms of education for doctors, nurses, and allied health professionals. One example is the ILADS physician training program, which places physicians and allied health practitioners in clinical settings with experts in Lyme disease; however it would require Australian physicians to travel to the United States. Physician and naturopathic training programs in Australia will help to facilitate the sharing of information and are currently under development.

The Australian media is starting to give Lyme disease extensive coverage, which raises awareness also. Unfortunately, though, the push to recognize Lyme disease in Australia will also require a grass roots movement since it is unlikely to come from the government, Australian health institutions, and media alone. This may not be fair, and it may be the hard way to do it, but unfortunately at this point, it is just the way it is.

I am confident that the medical environment in Australia is going to change – it is already changing. There are more doctors emerging who are willing to treat Lyme disease, some with the guidance of more experienced doctors. We are currently moving from a phase of complete denial into a phase of slight openness. Even if they do not have all the knowledge and need direction from more experienced practitioners, at least they are willing to do their part in helping people get better. This, in itself, is a big step forward.

The Keys to Change

As awareness grows, more cases will be diagnosed. As more cases are diagnosed, there will be a push towards more research studies. Solid published data cannot be ignored – and finally the government will amend its position on Lyme disease in Australia. Even the evidence gathered so far is irrefutable. It must only be a matter of time.

Meanwhile, organizations such as the Karl McManus Foundation and the Lyme Disease Association of Australia disseminate information, support and hope to Lyme sufferers who may not have had too much of any of those things so far.

Lyme disease has always been controversial, and it has always been misunderstood.

Jonathan Edlow, Professor of Medicine at Harvard Medical School, quotes the late Ed Masters (discoverer of STARI, a Lyme-like illness) in his book *Bull's-Eye*, on the history of Lyme disease. Edlow writes:

> *Masters points out that the "track record" of the "conventional wisdom" regarding Lyme disease is not very good: "First off, they said it was a new disease, which it wasn't. Then it was thought to be viral, but it isn't. Then it was thought that sero-negativity didn't exist, which it does. They thought it was easily treated by short courses of antibiotics, which sometimes it isn't. Then it was only the Ixodes dammini tick, which we now know is not even a separate valid tick species. If you look throughout the history, almost every time a major dogmatic statement has been made about what we 'know' about this disease, it was subsequently proven wrong or underwent major modifications."*[1]

And so it is in Australia.

REFERENCES

1. Edlow JA. Bull's-Eye: Unravelling the medical mystery of Lyme disease. 2nd rev. ed. New Haven: Yale University Press; 2003. 304 p.

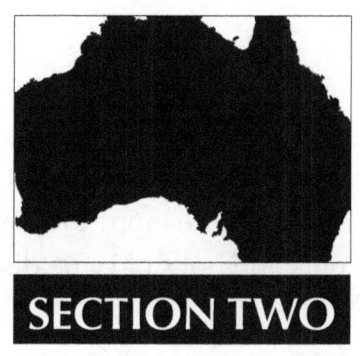

FUNDAMENTALS OF LYME DISEASE

Now that we have looked at the historical and political context of Lyme disease, let us turn to a more thorough discussion of the nuts and bolts of Lyme disease.

10. WHAT IS LYME DISEASE?

BY DEFINITION, LYME DISEASE REFERS TO THE INFECTIOUS ILLNESS caused by the bacteria Borrelia burgdorferi, along with other strains of Borrelia such as afzelii, andersonii and garinii. Borrelia is a spiral-shaped bacterium, known as a spirochete ("spi-ruh-keet"), which crosses over into the blood stream of a human during the bite of an infected tick.

Having said that, the narrow definition of Lyme disease given above, as a strictly bacterial infection caused by Borrelia, may not appropriately reflect the diversity and complexity of the illness. It is more clinically useful to expand the definition to include related co-infections that are transmitted along with Borrelia, such as Babesia, Bartonella, Rickettsia and Ehrlichia. "Tick-borne disease" is another term that may be more inclusive, however, even that limits the recognition of transmission to one vector (the tick), which may not be 100% accurate either.

There are different phases of infection in Lyme disease. Lyme disease is classified according to the longevity of infection, where it has spread in the body and how systemic it has become as well as the types of signs and symptoms it is causing. The earlier the infection can be identified, the greater the success in treatment, which is why awareness of the early forms of Lyme is crucial, including clinical presentations that are not "textbook". It is also important to note that the following phases may not necessarily occur along a linear timeline; some people experience symptoms of advanced, chronic Lyme disease shortly following their infection.

Early localized Lyme

The classic sign of early local infection with Lyme disease is a circular, outwardly expanding rash called erythema migrans (or EM rash), which may occur at the site of the tick bite three to thirty days after the bite. I say "may" because, in reality, the EM rash is absent in over 50% of Lyme disease cases.[1]

The textbook presentation of the EM rash would be a target shape – a red outer ring with a central clearing – appearing as a bull's eye, hence its nickname "bull's eye rash". Many patients have no recollection of such a rash, or if they think back to a rash they might have had, they may have not recognized it as an EM rash. This is one of the reasons that an acute Lyme infection may not be diagnosed accurately.

The "textbook" presentation of EM rash must also be put in context. One study shows that the tell-tale central clearing was absent in over half of a series of EM rashes examined.[3] Rashes can cover large parts of the body, and they may be patchy or diffuse. They can also mimic other common presentations including a spider bite, ringworm, or cellulitis. In one study, a series of eleven EM rashes were misdiagnosed and treated as cellulitis, with all eleven patients showing clinical evidence of Lyme disease progression.[4]

Along with a rash, early localized Lyme may present with flu-like illness, fevers, malaise, muscle soreness and headache. Lyme disease can progress to later stages even in patients who do not develop a rash. Therefore, Lyme disease should be considered when a flu-like illness is combined with possible exposure through activities such as camping, bushwalking or gardening.

Early disseminated Lyme

In early disseminated Lyme, the bacteria spread through the bloodstream and affect other parts of the body. Muscle, joint and tendon pain may appear, often migrating to different parts of the body. Dizziness and headaches, heart palpitations, severe fatigue and mood changes are common.

Neurological symptoms can also start to appear. These include Bell's palsy, which is the loss of muscle tone on one or both sides of the face, as well as meningitis, which involves severe headaches, stiff neck and sensitivity to light. Many people experience burning or shooting pains and unusual skin sensations such as crawling, tingling or burning. Cognitive changes are also common – brain fog, memory loss and difficulty with focus and concentration. Psychological symptoms include severe anxiety, irritability and even the development of obsessive-compulsive traits.

Chronic Lyme disease

Chronic Lyme disease is trickier to define in light of the Infectious Diseases Society of America's (IDSA) denial of its very existence (see Section 1), but this is the phase of Lyme disease that thousands of people suffer from on an ongoing basis.

Joseph Burrascano, MD, a physician at the forefront of Lyme disease treatment and research in the United States, and author of *Advanced Topics in Lyme Disease: Diagnostic Hints and Treatment Guidelines for Lyme and Other Tick-borne Illness*[5] (a set of treatment guidelines that is widely referenced in the United States, and which is included in an Appendix in this book) offered the following definition:

For a diagnosis of chronic Lyme disease, these three criteria must be present:

1. Illness present for at least one year (this is approximately when immune breakdown attains clinically significant levels).

2. Persistent major neurologic involvement (such as encephalitis/encephalopathy, meningitis, etc.) or active arthritic manifestations (active synovitis).

3. Active infection with B. burgdorferi (Bb), regardless of prior antibiotic therapy (if any).

ILADS, the USA organization that recognizes chronic Lyme disease, has adopted a set of treatment guidelines, which have been widely used in clinical practice (available at www.ilads.org). They state the following: *"Chronic Lyme disease* is inclusive of persistent symptomatologies including fatigue; cognitive dysfunction; headaches; sleep disturbance; and other neurologic features such as demyelinating disease, peripheral neuropathy and sometimes motor neurone disease; neuropsychiatric presentations; cardiac presentations including electrical conduction delays and dilated cardiomyopathy; and musculoskeletal problems".

The guidelines also introduce definitions for *persistent* Lyme disease—symptoms continuing despite 30 days of treatment; *recurrent* Lyme disease—the patient relapsing in the absence of another tick bite or EM rash; and *refractory* Lyme disease—a patient responding poorly to antibiotic therapy.

REFERENCES

1. Stricker RB, Lautin A. The Lyme wars: time to listen. Expert Opin Investig Drugs. 2003;12:1609–14.
2. Lyme Disease Wikipedia [Internet]. San Francisco: Wikimedia Foundation. Last modified 2012 Aug 2 [cited 2012 Jul]. Available from: http://en.wikipedia.org/wiki/Lyme_disease
3. Nadelman RB, Wormser GP. Erythema migrans and early Lyme disease. Am. J. Med. 1995;98(4A):S15–S24.
4. Nowakowski J, McKenna D, Nadelman RB, et al. Failure of treatment with cephalexin for Lyme disease. Arch Fam Med. 2000;9:563–7.
5. Burrascano J. Advanced topics in Lyme disease: diagnostic hints and treatment guidelines for Lyme and other tick-borne illness. 15th. rev. ed. 2005 Sep; Available from: http://www.ilads.org/files/burrascano_0905.pdf

11. HOW IS LYME TRANSMITTED?

TRADITIONALLY, LYME DISEASE HAS BEEN CONSIDERED EXCLUSIVELY a tick-borne illness, and while that is no doubt the most common route of transmission, evidence indicates that there are other routes of transmission.

There are a variety of reasons why only 50% of Lyme disease patients recall a tick bite.[1] First, ticks that most often transmit Lyme disease are in the nymph stage of their lifecycle and are about the size of a poppy seed. Therefore, even in obvious locations on the body, they are incredibly difficult to see or feel. Couple that with the tendency for ticks to gravitate towards less obvious areas of the body such as the scalp, hairline, underarms and groin, and it is easy to understand why identifying them is problematic.

Second, ticks numb the skin with an injection of local anaesthetic before they actually bite, so that they can remain undetected while attached. This means that people may not feel the bite, or the tick itself.

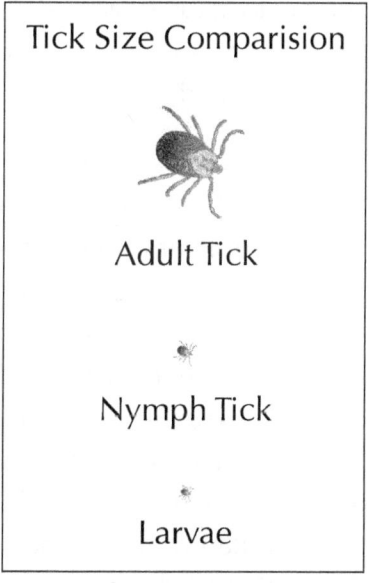

Sizes of ticks at different stages of their life cycle[2]

Third, it is possible that other insects such as fleas, mites, lice and mosquitoes may be able to transmit Borrelia spirochetes to humans and cause infection. Certainly there is clear evidence of those insects housing Borrelia species. Case reports in Australia demonstrate illness after bites with mosquitoes and bird mites.

Studies have also shown the presence of Borrelia burgdorferi-like organisms in mosquitoes, horse flies, and deer flies in areas where Lyme disease is present, however, the researchers postulated that those insects were unable to transmit the infections to humans.[3,4]

A Czech study looked for Borrelia and Anaplasma species in chigger mites collected from wild birds. They found through PCR testing that Borrelia as well as the strains of B. garinii, which are known to cause Lyme disease in humans, and B. valaisiana were present in the chiggers.[5]

Also in the Czech Republic, studies proved the presence of Borrelia burgdorferi species in mites from wild rodents, including B. afzelii (also known to cause Lyme disease in humans). Their conclusion was that Borrelia can reside in other vectors besides ticks, and that further study was warranted.[6]

Bartonella, one of the more common co-infections of Lyme disease, has been found in fleas in Australia. The authors described Bartonellosis as "an emerging or re-emerging disease in humans worldwide". In Australia the marsupial hosts included red foxes, bandicoots, rabbits, feral cats, woylies and bush rats. The authors concluded that, "The clustering of Bartonella species with their marsupial flea hosts suggests co-evolution of marsupial hosts, marsupial fleas and Bartonella species in Australia". In simple terms, Bartonella species, which were initially introduced from various hosts following the colonisation of Australia, are adapting to Australian animals and the Australian environment to optimise their survival and virulence.[7]

So, the evidence indicates that Borrelia and its co-infections exist in other vectors outside of the tick population, and that further research is needed to evaluate their ability to spread disease.

Is Lyme Disease Sexually Transmitted?

Another major point of contention and controversy is the possibility of the sexual transmission of Lyme disease.

Given that syphilis, also a spirochete bacterium, is sexually transmitted, it seems reasonable to postulate that Lyme may be sexually transmitted also. Outside of simply being spirochetes, both syphilis and Borrelia morph, or transform, into different bacterial forms (including spirochete, cell-wall deficient, and cyst forms) to evade attack by antibiotics and the immune system; they both can remain dormant in their host for years at a time; and they both gravitate to body fluids such as urine, semen, vaginal secretions and breast milk.

There is significant evidence supporting the position that Lyme disease may be sexually transmitted. Dr. Gregory Bach, D.O., O.P.C. from Pennsylvania published an abstract in 2001 that contained telling information from the analysis of his patient population. Dr. Bach had observed that the majority of partners of his Lyme patients were presenting with Lyme disease also, despite only one partner having a history of tick exposure. Further, he noticed that sexually active couples had significantly more antibiotic treatment failures, which led him to believe that one partner might have been re-infecting the other. He continued by analysing body fluids of his Lyme patients.

He found that:
- Laboratory testing of semen samples provided by male patients (positive by Western Blot and PCR in blood), and the male partners of female Lyme patients, were positive 40% of the time.
- In the semen itself, Lyme spirochetes were detected in 14 of 32 Lyme patients.
- **ALL** positive semen/ vaginal samples in patients with known sexual partners resulted in positive Lyme titres and/or PCR in their sexual partners.

With evidence of spirochetes found in both semen and vaginal secretions, Dr Bach rightly concluded that the area of sexual transmission of Lyme is desperately in need of further research.

Of course, the United States CDC (Centres for Disease Control) opposes that view and claims that there is no evidence of sexual transmission at all. They argue that the spirochetes that cause syphilis are structurally and behaviourally very different from those causing Lyme disease, and that basically, they act very differently and do not share the same routes of transmission or pathology. It seems odd that from a genetic perspective Borrelia appears to be a far more advanced pathogen than syphilis, and yet the CDC doubts its ability to be transmitted in bodily fluids.

They also argue that even though it is not uncommon for more than one member of the household to have Lyme disease, the only reason for this could be that they share the same environment so both must have had their own tick bite.

Congenital Transmission of Lyme Disease

Another point of contention is the possibility of congenital transmission – that is, mothers passing Lyme disease to their babies in utero. There are a growing number of children in Australia diagnosed with Lyme disease who have never travelled outside of Australia, and whose mothers have Lyme disease.

Once again, while the official government party line is a resounding "No!" to congenital transmission, there certainly seems to be valid evidence.

A study published in the Annals of Internal Medicine reported on a pregnant woman who developed Lyme disease during her first trimester, but did not receive antibiotic therapy. Her infant, born at 35 weeks gestational age, died of congenital heart disease during the first week of life. Histologic examination of autopsy material showed the Lyme disease spirochete in the spleen, kidneys, and bone marrow of the infant.[8]

Another case report described a 24-year-old woman with untreated Lyme disease in the first trimester of pregnancy that gave birth at term to a 2.5 kilogram stillborn. Borrelia burgdorferi was cultured from the liver, and spirochetes were seen in the heart, adrenal glands, liver, brain, and placenta of the baby.[9]

Yet another report was a 37-year old woman who received penicillin orally for one week for an erythema migrans rash during the first trimester of pregnancy, and subsequently delivered a 3.4 kilogram infant at term who died 23 hours later of what was believed to be "perinatal brain damage". Borrelia burgdorferi was identified in the newborn's brain.[10]

A publication entitled "Maternal Lyme Borreliosis and Foetal Outcome" provided a review of 95 cases of pregnant women with Lyme disease. Antibiotic treatment was administered parenterally - given via injection or intravenously - to 66 women, and orally to 19. Infection remained untreated in 10 pregnancies. Adverse outcomes were seen in 8 of 66 parenterally treated women, 6 of 19 orally treated women, and 6 of 10 untreated women. In comparison to patients treated with antibiotics, untreated women had a significantly higher risk of adverse pregnancy outcome – a full 60% of untreated women had adverse outcomes compared with 12% and 31% of treated mothers (parenteral and oral treatment, respectively). Loss of the pregnancy and cavernous hemangioma (grossly dilated blood vessels and vascular channels) were the most common adverse outcomes.

Further, in this same study when antibiotics were given to the mothers, in 17 cases the EM rashes had not resolved by the end of the course of medication. Adverse pregnancy outcome was more frequent among these mothers than the mothers where the EM rash had resolved.

A study by Alan MacDonald states clearly that transplacental transmission of the spirochete from mother to foetus is possible.[11] He also reports that the variety of manifestations of gestational Lyme Borreliosis mimic the diversity of prenatal syphilis. Among the medical problems are foetal death, hydrocephalus, cardiovascular anomalies, neonatal respiratory distress, hyperbilirubinemia, intrauterine growth retardation, cortical blindness, sudden infant death syndrome and maternal toxaemia of pregnancy.

Charles Ray Jones, MD, paediatric Lyme expert, at a presentation given at the ILADS Annual Conference in Toronto, Canada in 2011, stated his opinion that mothers with Lyme disease who were not treated with antibiotics during pregnancy had a 50% chance of passing Lyme on to their baby. In mothers treated with one antibiotic during pregnancy, that likelihood went down to 25%. In mothers treated with two antibiotics during pregnancy, the rate dropped to below 5%.

Research is unclear as to whether Lyme disease can be passed to a baby through breast milk. Certainly, spirochetes, or the DNA of the bacteria, have been detected in breast milk through PCR testing, though the rates and likelihood of transmission through the mother's milk are unknown based on a lack of research data or clinical case studies.[12] Because of this, it would seem prudent to treat a woman who is breastfeeding and has an active Lyme infection with antibiotic therapy, or to advise not to breastfeed, to minimize any risk to the baby.

REFERENCES

1. Steere AC, Broderick TF, Malawista SE. Erythema chronicum migrans and Lyme arthritis: epidemiologic evidence for a tick vector. Am J Epidemiol. 1978;108:312–21.
2. Lyme Disease Wikipedia [Internet]. San Francisco: Wikimedia Foundation. Last modified 2012 Aug 2 [cited 2012 Jul]. Available from: http://en.wikipedia.org/wiki/Lyme_disease
3. Magnarelli LA, Anderson JF, Barbour. The etiologic agent of Lyme disease in deer flies, horse flies, and mosquitoes. AGJ Infect Dis. 1986 Aug;154(2):355-8.
4. Magnarelli LA, Anderson JF. Ticks and biting insects infected with the etiologic agent of Lyme disease, Borrelia burgdorferi. J Clin Microbiol. 1988 Aug;26(8):1482–86.
5. Literak I, Stekolnikov AA, Sychra O, Dubska L, Taragelova V. Larvae of chigger mites Neotrombicula spp. (Acari: Trombiculidae) exhibited Borrelia but no Anaplasma infections: a field study including birds from

the Czech Carpathians as hosts of chiggers. Exp Appl Acarol. 2008 Apr;44(4):307-14. Epub 2008 Apr 10.

6. Netusil J, Zákovská A, Horváth R, Dendis M, Janouskovcová E. Presence of Borrelia burgdorferi sensu lato in mites parasitizing small rodents. Vector Borne Zoonotic Dis. 2005 Fall;5(3):227-32.

7. Kaewmongkol G, Kaewmongkol S, McInnes LM, Burmej H, Bennett MD, Adams PJ, Ryan U, Irwin PJ, Fenwick SG. Genetic characterization of flea-derived Bartonella species from native animals in Australia suggests host-parasite co-evolution. Infect Genet Evol. 2011 Dec;11(8):1868-72. Epub 2011 Aug 12.

8. Schlesinger PA, Duray PH, Burke BA, et al. Maternal-foetal transmission of the Lyme disease spirochete, Borrelia burgdorferi. Ann Intern Med. 1985;103:67-8.

9. MacDonald AB, Benach JL, Burgdorfer W. Stillbirth following maternal Lyme disease. NY State Med J. 1987;87:615-16.

10. (Weber K, Bratzke HJ, Neubert U, et al. Borrelia burgdorferi in a newborn despite oral penicillin for Lyme borreliosis during pregnancy. Pediatr Infect Dis J. 1988 Apr;7(4):286-9.

11. MacDonald AB. Gestational Lyme borreliosis: implications for the fetus. Rheum Dis Clin North Am. 1989 Nov;15(4):657-77.

12. Schmidt BL, Aberer E, Stockenhuber C, Klade H, Breier F, Luger A. Detection of Borrelia burgdorferi DNA by polymerase chain reaction in the urine and breast milk of patients with Lyme borreliosis. Diagn Microbiol Infect Dis. 1995 Mar;21(3):121-8.

12. FACTORS ADDING TO THE COMPLEXITY OF LYME DISEASE

THE NARROW DEFINITION OF LYME DISEASE AS A STRICTLY BACTERIAL illness caused by Borrelia burgdorferi spirochetes is somewhat outdated due to a number of other factors that complicate the issue and must be considered. These complicating factors can create layers of complexity in the realm of chronic Lyme disease.

Complicating Factor #1: Bacterial Strains

There is a great diversity among Borrelia burgdorferi subspecies – over 100 strains in the United States and 300 strains worldwide. It is unclear how many or exactly which strains exist in Australia, but it is thought that Australia may have some unique strains that are as yet unidentified.

In the game of life called "survival of the fittest", the ability of a microbe to adapt, morph, create new strains and create strains that act differently is crucial to its ability to evade the immune system, avoid any therapy that might kill it, and prosper in its ecological surroundings. That ability allows the microbe to establish a permanent domain, not just a temporary home, creating the chronicity of illness we see in Lyme disease.

Some of the strain variations of Borrelia that have been identified in various continents include:

North America: B. burgdorferi, B. americana, B. andersonii, B. bissettii, B. californiensis, B. carolinensis, B. garinii, B. kurtenbachii and B. lonestari

LYME DISEASE in Australia

<u>Canada</u>: B. burgdorferi, B. bissettii

<u>Europe</u>: B. burgdorferi, B. afzelii, B. bavariensis, B. bissettii, B. garinii, B. finlandensis, B. lusitaniae, B. spielmanii and B. valaisiana

<u>Asia</u>: B. afzelii, B. garinii, B. lusitaniae, B. sinica, B. valaisiana and B. yangtze

<u>Japan</u>: B. garinii, B. japonica, B. tanukii, B. turdi and B. valaisiana

All of these strains have been isolated from ticks and animals, but not all have been proven to cause disease in humans. The three strains most recognized to cause Lyme disease are B. burgdorferi, B. afzelii and B. garinii. B. lonestari is also reportable to the CDC in the United States as Lyme disease.

Amongst Borrelia there are currently 14 known genospecies. This diversity of strains is significant because each strain may act differently. For example, the Borrelia burgdorferi, which is responsible for much of the Lyme disease in the U.S., presents differently than B. afzelii and B. garinii, which are more common in Europe. The European strains appear clinically with more neurological symptoms than the B. burgdorferi. Since Australian Lyme is thought to originate more from European and Japanese strains, it fits that the symptoms of Australian Lyme sufferers have a strong neurological component.

This may have significance for both testing for Lyme disease in Australia and the appropriate treatment of Lyme disease in Australia. PCR testing (which we will talk more about later) looks for the actual DNA of the bacteria in the blood. If PCR testing only looks for B. burgdorferi, many cases of Lyme disease in Australia may be missed. PCR testing must be inclusive of other strains to be useful. And still, many strains may be yet unidentified, so there may actually not be an accurate test for some strains.

As for treatment, the strong neurological element of Australian Lyme must be considered. This type of Lyme typically requires more aggressive

Factors Adding to the Complexity of Lyme Disease

treatment and antibiotics that cross the blood-brain barrier to get into the neurological system. A longer duration of treatment may be required for more deep-seated neurological issues. Additionally, different strains may be more or less susceptible to different kinds of antibiotics.

The co-infections of Borrelia also represent diverse strains. In the aforementioned study of Bartonella found in fleas in Australia, many different strains were identified. Some of these strains were the same as those found in other countries, such as Bartonella henselae and Bartonella quintana, however others were strains that are now specific to Australia through their adaptation to the environment. These include B. coopersplainsensus, B. queenslandensis and B. rattaustraliani. Over 30 different strains were cited in that one particular study. Again, this may have ramifications for both the testing and treatment of Bartonella in Australia.

Bacteria adapt genetically to fit their environment. It is survival of the fittest, even at that microscopic level. Variations occur over time and in different ecosystems, giving the microbe more and more resilience. This creates a more complex situation for humans to research, study and adapt to in ways that are clinically beneficial for the person suffering from the disease.

Complicating Factor #2: Bacterial Forms

The Borrelia bacterium is a sneaky and wily bug, and it can actually morph into three distinct forms - again, with the view to evading the immune system and gaining a stronger foothold in the body. The three forms are the spirochete, the cell-wall deficient form, and the cyst form.

In very simple terms, think of them as a caterpillar, a cocoon, and a butterfly, respectively. These are three different manifestations of the same creature, according to the position in their life cycle. In each phase, the creature looks very different and acts very differently – some phases are more vulnerable to attack by outside forces than others, some are more resilient. Some impact the environment around them more than others.

So, too, the three different forms of Borrelia bacteria look and act differently from the other forms, and impact their environment differently. One of the fundamental distinctions here, however, is that the butterfly cannot really decide he wants to revert back to a caterpillar when it suits him, whereas a Lyme spirochete can go from one form to another in a non-linear fashion. A Lyme spirochete, when threatened, can morph into a cyst form, or become cell-wall deficient. It is a survival mechanism for the bacteria, but one that makes it all the more complex for us to understand and treat effectively.

These three forms are so important to us clinically because all three must be addressed for treatment success to occur, and each form has wildly different susceptibilities to the available therapeutic options.

The form of Borrelia that we hear about most is the spirochete form, or the spiral-shaped form of the bacteria. It is most often implicated in early, acute Borrelia infections. Even in chronic infection, the spirochete forms cause more of the conventionally recognized symptoms, such as flu-like illness, Bell's palsy, and the bull's eye rash. Since the spirochetes are spiral-shaped bacteria, they penetrate the tissues easily, drilling their way into tissue and bone. Their mobility contributes to the multi-systemic characteristics of Lyme disease – the spirochetes do not contain themselves to any one organ or system within the body.

The cell-wall deficient form is the form that may cause the most problems in persistent, chronic illness. They can be hard to treat, as the lack of a cell wall makes targeting by antibiotics and the immune system difficult. They can trigger autoimmune disease, and can be responsible for the numerous syndromes and conditions not typically associated with Lyme disease, such as paralysis, multiple sclerosis, psychiatric manifestations, and chronic fatigue syndrome. The cell-wall deficient forms clump together in colonies deep within the body and can be very challenging to treat effectively.

Often, antibiotic therapy is given to address a single form of the bacteria, which actually can cause more trouble down the road. If only the

Factors Adding to the Complexity of Lyme Disease

spirochete or cell-wall deficient form is treated, the bacteria may respond by morphing into a different, more defensive, cystic form. Spirochetes tend to do that when they feel threatened or are under attack. With the spirochete load reduced, the patient may feel better for a period of time, especially since cystic forms do not necessarily cause symptoms, but in this scenario, the bugs are not gone, they are just in hiding. As soon as treatment stops, the cyst forms can return to spirochete forms and the patient is back to square one. However, the patient may be in a worse situation because now, their body has been compromised by the side effects of significant antibiotic therapy. Combining different antibiotics and therapies that inhibit cyst form development is the key to a successful recovery. This will be discussed in detail in section three. Finally, to make matters even more complicated, it has been shown that a single spirochete which has converted to cyst form may re-emerge from cyst form later only to have multiplied into five spirochetes; so the bacteria can actually reproduce while at the same time undergoing transformation from one form to another.

With the three forms of Borrelia – the spirochete, the cell-wall deficient form, and the cyst form - we have a triple-layered problem, and we need a triple-layered solution. Fortunately, different classes of antibiotics have different activity according to the varying structures and traits of bacteria, so there are ways to combine them to address all three forms. This requires prescribing doctors to layer different medications, a minimum of three at a time (or two consistently plus one pulsed), and for physicians who are less familiar with the workings of the wily, Lyme bacteria, this may seem like an overly aggressive approach. I hope with a greater understanding of the various forms of the bacteria outlined in this book, and with the detailed treatment suggestions for each form, physicians will see how crucial this approach is to effectively treating chronic Lyme disease.

Complicating Factor #3 – Co-infections

Co-infections have already been mentioned and will be discussed in light of symptoms, testing and treatment later in the book. What is important here is to understand how prevalent co-infections are, and how they add complexity to the Lyme disease picture.

In that picture, we see several key co-infections which operate alongside the Borrelia. They are Bartonella, Babesia, Ehrlichia and Rickettsia. With the exception of Babesia, which is a parasite, the other microbes are bacteria.

One point to distinguish here for the purposes of this book is "co-infections of Lyme", versus "opportunistic infections that we commonly see in Lyme disease". For example, Mycoplasma species and Chlamydia pneumonia are other infections that we commonly see in Lyme patients. Epstein-Barr, Cytomegalovirus and Human Herpes Virus 6 are chronic viruses that many Lyme patients carry. Candida albicans, which is naturally occurring yeast in the gut, is often overgrown in Lyme patients (independent of antibiotic therapy). However, I will not refer to them as co-infections because they are not necessarily transmitted along with the Borrelia via an infected tick; rather they are opportunistic and are often present in Lyme patients because of the immune suppression and increased susceptibility of Lyme sufferers. Bartonella, Babesia, Rickettsia and Ehrlichia can be transmitted in the same tick bite as Borrelia, and so that is why I refer to them in this book as the co-infections of Lyme.

According to Richard Horowitz, MD, who has treated thousands of Lyme cases, when he started treating Lyme disease 20 years ago in New York, he believed that most of his patients were simple Lyme patients (without co-infections). Today, he states that over 80% of his patients carry at least one co-infection, with many having multiple co-infections.

It appears that Australian Lyme patients also reflect similar statistics. Even though testing may not accurately reflect this (again, perhaps due to strain variants, but mostly due to low numbers of patients being comprehensively tested), more often than not, the Lyme patients in Australia present with symptom pictures of co-infections. Many respond to treatment for the specific co-infections, which can involve herbs and medications that would not significantly impact the Borrelia bacteria.

One of the challenges of co-infections is identification. As with Lyme disease, diagnosis of co-infections must primarily be based on the clinical picture – that is, a patient's signs and symptoms. Reliable lab testing for most co-infections is not available in Australia, and even when testing is done through overseas labs, the results are not always definitive.

The second challenge is that the co-infections require different treatment protocols than the actual Borrelia infection. Bartonella, Ehrlichia and Rickettsia are closer in structure to Borrelia, since all of them are bacteria. Babesia, however, is an intracellular parasite. Therefore the antibiotics that work for Borrelia are not going to adequately address Babesia. Treatment durations and dosing schedules may also differ for co-infections.

It is possible to weave treatment protocols together to work on a number of different infections at once, but it requires an understanding of different medications and their interactions to create a safe and effective protocol. Many doctors feel hesitant to prescribe multiple antibiotics to cover the different forms of Borrelia as well as the co-infections that are present, but this is often necessary for recovery to occur. Sometimes a combination of antibiotics and herbal antimicrobials can be used to address co-infections concurrently.

In my opinion, missing a co-infection in diagnosis, and/ or under treating co-infections, is one of the biggest factors in Lyme disease treatment failure. Many co-infections go undiagnosed, and while addressing Borreliosis will lead to improvement, that improvement is limited without also recognizing and treating the co-infections. In fact, many Lyme disease researchers now hypothesize that some of these co-infections act to protect Borrelia, such that Borrelia treatment may be ineffective or minimally effective unless co-infection treatment is also successfully administered.

Complicating Factor #4 – Biofilm

Technically, biofilm is a polysaccharide matrix that can be produced by colonies of bacteria such as Borrelia. In simple terms, biofilm is sticky goo that the bacteria produce and subsequently hide in. There are many different types of biofilm. For example, plaque production in the mouth is the result of biofilm from oral bacteria, and there are biofilms in the gut also. Some biofilms serve a beneficial purpose in the body – not all are detrimental – however, several types of infectious microbes produce biofilm around themselves. In fact, it is postulated that up to 80% of infections involve some kind of biofilm, and this can complicate the treatment process.

Just as humans form communities to prosper and ensure survival, bacteria do also. The biofilm they create clumps them together, anchors them to tissues and gives them a protective film. This can make them harder to target by the immune system, and it gives them a shield against antibiotics and other antimicrobials. Alan MacDonald, one of the pioneers in biofilm and Lyme disease investigation, discovered that the DNA of the bacteria actually constituted part of the biofilm matrix. Elements such as calcium, magnesium and iron are also present. All forms of Borrelia (cyst, L-forms and spiral forms) have been found within biofilms.[1]

Eva Sapi, PhD, a researcher from the University of New Haven, has also been at the forefront of research on biofilms and Lyme disease. Her research showed that certain enzymes such as nattokinase and lumbrokinase are effective in breaking down the biofilm matrix. The herbs samento and banderol were also effective. This has possible implications for treatment regimens for chronic Lyme disease, and will be discussed in more detail later.

■ ■ ■ ■

It is clear that Lyme disease is not a straightforward health problem; rather it is complex and complicated. Therefore, it is important to be aware of all the different elements of Lyme disease so that it can be treated adequately. There are many other complicating factors involved in Lyme disease, such as parasitic infections, heavy metal toxicity, nutrient deficiencies, chronic inflammation, hormone dysregulation, and others.

Some of these will be covered later in this book, others can be researched in other books and resources. This chapter was written as an introduction to complicating factors, not a comprehensive list of them.

REFERENCES

1. MacDonald AB. Summation of Biofilms of Borrelia burgdorferi. Biofilms of Borrelia burgdorferi and clinical implications for chronic borreliosis. Lyme Disease Symposium; 2008 May 17; New Haven, CT; p. 71. Available at: http://www.molecularalzheimer.org/files/Biofilm_New_Haven_ppt_Read-Only_.pdf

13. SIGNS AND SYMPTOMS OF LYME DISEASE

Lyme Disease, The Great Imitator

Lyme disease is known as the "Great Imitator." Its list of symptoms is long and varied, and it can present differently in different individuals. A child with a diagnosis of autism may be showing the neurological manifestations of Lyme disease while an individual with a diagnosis of osteo- or rheumatoid arthritis may be showing more musculoskeletal manifestations.

Following is a list of illnesses that Lyme disease can mimic:

- Attention Deficit Disorder
- Autism
- Chronic Fatigue Syndrome
- Crohn's Disease
- Encephalitis
- Fibromyalgia
- Interstitial Cystitis
- Irritable Bowel Syndrome
- Juvenile Arthritis
- Lupus
- Meningitis
- Motor Neurone Disease
- Multiple Sclerosis
- Obsessive-Compulsive Disorder

LYME DISEASE in Australia

- ▸ Parkinson's Disease
- ▸ Psychiatric Disorders (depression, bipolar, OCD etc.)
- ▸ Raynaud's Syndrome
- ▸ Rheumatoid Arthritis
- ▸ Scleroderma
- ▸ Sjogren's Syndrome
- ▸ Thyroid Disorders

And that is just a sampling.

Lyme disease can trigger autoimmunity, so some people will present with rheumatoid arthritis, lupus, Sjogren's, Hashimoto's thyroiditis or any number of autoimmune diseases. It may not be that these diagnoses are incorrect; it may just be that the Lyme infection has unbalanced the immune system sufficiently to trigger the autoimmune mechanism. Where there is autoimmune disease with sufficient evidence of Lyme disease (either through lab work or clinically), treating the Lyme will often improve, if not eliminate, the autoimmunity.

The key concept to grasp here is that of underlying cause. Western medicine has somehow distanced itself from the quest for discovery of the underlying cause of illness. As is the case with fibromyalgia or chronic fatigue syndrome, the diagnosis describes a set of symptoms but does not explain why they occur. Granted, often chronic fatigue syndrome is preceded by an acute viral illness, but even patients without the acute phase will be given the diagnosis of chronic fatigue simply based on, you guessed it, their symptom of chronic fatigue. Because Western medicine only looks at symptoms, many disease pictures with varying symptoms may be thought to be different diseases because they have different symptoms, when in fact the underlying cause may be singular: Lyme disease.

Clues to Lyme disease being causative are:

1. An individual has a constellation of symptoms involving multiple body systems.

2. Traditional diagnostic tests do not lead to anything conclusive or any clear diagnosis ("Your tests came back normal. There's nothing wrong with you.").

Signs and Symptoms of Lyme Disease

3. An official diagnosis can be made (such as one of the above) but standard medical treatment does not have the expected benefit or result.

4. A therapeutic trial of anti-Lyme treatment (such as a course of antibiotics) leads to Herxheimer reactions and subsequent symptom improvement.

Since Lyme disease shows such a great variety of symptoms in every possible body system, it does not always fit any classic disease picture. Here is a fairly comprehensive list of the possible symptoms of Lyme disease (reproduced with permission from the Canadian Lyme Disease Foundation, www.canlyme.org):

Skin

- Rash at the site of the bite
- Rash on other parts of the body
- Raised rash, disappearing and recurring
- Striae (stretch marks) that may be red or purple
- Scratches on the skin (like cat scratches)
- Lumps (nodules) under the skin

Head, Face, Neck

- Unexplained hair loss
- Headaches, mild or severe
- Seizures
- Pressure in head, white matter lesions in brain (MRI)
- Twitching of facial or other muscles
- Facial paralysis (Bell's palsy)
- Tingling of the nose, tongue, or cheek
- Facial flushing
- Stiff or painful neck
- Jaw pain or stiffness
- Dental problems (unexplained), tooth pain
- Sore throat, clearing throat a lot, phlegm, hoarseness, runny nose
- Difficulty swallowing, feeling as if something is stuck in the throat

Eyes/Vision

- Double or blurry vision
- Increased floaters
- Pain in the eyes, or swelling around the eyes
- Hypersensitivity to light
- Flashing lights
- Phantom images in the periphery of vision

Ears/Hearing

- Decreased hearing in one or both ears, plugged ears
- Buzzing in the ears
- Pain in the ears, over sensitivity to sounds
- Ringing in one or both ears

Digestive and Excretory Systems

- Diarrhoea
- Constipation
- Irritable bladder (trouble starting, stopping)
- Interstitial cystitis
- Upset stomach (nausea or pain)
- GERD (gastroesophageal reflux disease)

Musculoskeletal System

- Bone pain, joint pain or swelling, carpal tunnel syndrome
- Stiffness of joints, back, neck, tennis elbow
- Muscle pain or cramps
- Fibromyalgia
- Tendonitis

Respiratory and Circulatory Systems

- Shortness of breath
- Air hunger - cannot get full/satisfying breath
- Chronic cough
- Chest pain or rib soreness
- Night sweats or unexplained chills

- Heart palpitations or extra beats
- Endocarditis
- Heart blockage

Neurological System

- Tremors or unexplained shaking
- Burning or stabbing sensations in the body
- Weakness, peripheral neuropathy or partial paralysis
- Pressure in the head
- Numbness in the body, tingling, pinpricks
- Poor balance, dizziness, difficulty walking
- Increased motion sickness
- Light-headedness, wooziness

Psychological/ Psychiatric

- Mood swings, irritability, bipolar disorder
- Unusual depression
- Disorientation (getting or feeling lost)
- Feeling as if you are losing your mind
- Over-emotional reactions, crying easily
- Too much sleep, or insomnia
- Difficulty falling or staying asleep
- Narcolepsy, sleep apnoea
- Panic attacks, anxiety
- Obsessive-compulsive traits

Cognitive

- Memory loss (short or long term)
- Confusion, difficulty in thinking
- Difficulty with concentration or reading
- Speech difficulty (slurred or slow)
- Word finding difficulty
- Stammering speech
- Forgetting how to perform simple tasks

Reproduction and Sexuality

- Loss of sex drive
- Sexual dysfunction
- Unexplained menstrual pain, irregularity
- Unexplained breast pain, discharge
- Testicular or pelvic pain
- Vulvodynia

General Well-being

- Phantom smells
- Unexplained weight gain or loss
- Extreme fatigue
- Swollen glands/lymph nodes
- Unexplained fevers (high or low grade)
- Continual infections (sinus, kidney, eye, etc.)
- Symptoms seem to change, come and go
- Pain migrates (moves) to different body parts
- Early on, experienced a "flu-like" illness, from which you have not recovered completely
- Low body temperature
- Allergies/ chemical sensitivities
- Increased effect from alcohol and possibly more intense hangovers

That is quite an impressive list for such a tiny bacteria, but it is a true representation of what Lyme sufferers experience. If asked to tick the boxes on a list, many Lyme patients would have 30 or 40 of the above ticked.

What makes it all the more devastating for Lyme sufferers is that oftentimes they do not appear as sick as they really are. Certainly, on the inside, they feel like death warmed up, but outwardly they do not have any major observable manifestations. In fact, I often hear stories of their closest family members, co-workers and friends saying, "But you look so good. Surely you're not that sick?" It is another reason why doctors miss the gravity of their situation; their outward presentation does not always match their inward experience.

Signs and Symptoms of Lyme Disease

Can You Guess the Disease?
Given what you now know about Lyme can you tell which disease is being described?

#1 Who Am I?
I could potentially put you in a wheelchair. When I produce some numbness and tingling, you'll probably go and see a neurologist. They will do an MRI and tell you that you have white lesions on your brain, but they will also tell you that there is not too much you can do about it. Or, they may find nothing, and suggest you see a counsellor for hypochondria, so you may spend years thinking you are crazy and have no real health problems.

#2 Who Am I?
I make you really, really tired. I mean really tired. It's easy to think of me as something that lingers after a more acute illness. I make it so that you just can't bounce back. The fatigue is overwhelming, and your doctors tell you that you are just doing too much. They suggest that perhaps you need a vacation, or to slow down at work. You know it's more than that, but your blood work doesn't show any real problems and I make it look like nothing is really wrong with you. Mostly you're just tired and wondering if you'll ever get your spark back.

#3 Who Am I?
Within a few months, I can take you from a healthy, happy individual, to one completely unable to care for yourself. I sap your muscle strength and ability to move. I'll impact your legs and arms, and you will require help to move around. Later, when you are lying in bed, you'll need help lifting your arms and being fed. I might seriously impact your ability to eat, and even breathe. Ultimately, I may take your life.

#4 Who Am I?
I give you headaches, and I make you tired. You are grumpy and irritable all the time. I give you night sweats. Your other female friends go through

similar things, but somehow this seems different. I work in cycles so every four weeks it seems worse, but I'm also making you sick at other times too, so it doesn't quite make sense. You see your ob-gyn and she checks your hormones, and they may be off so she gives you prescription hormones. You take them but I don't go away.

#5 Who Am I?

I make you hurt all over. Your muscles just ache and it's hard to get any relief. You are really tired, too, and proper and refreshing sleep seems to be elusive. I make you feel sick and tired, but it looks as if there's nothing wrong with you. Your doctors tell you that you're depressed and want to put you on anti-depressant medication. It helps a bit so you think that you might be on the right track, but then you start forgetting things and words are harder to put together. You wonder if it's because of the medications so you stop them, but nothing changes. Every day you wake up exhausted no matter how many hours you've slept.

#6 Who Am I?

I make your joints very sore and stiff. They are swollen, they are hot to touch, and they are red. I take the fun out of life because I stop you from being able to move around too much. Certainly sports and fitness are out of the question. I trick you because you feel well enough to be active, but your joints just won't allow it. You go to the doctor and he does some labs and says, "Yes, you have an illness." Then he tells you the treatment is immune steroids to combat the inflammation. He doesn't know you have an infection and that immune suppression will make you worse in the long run. In desperation you say yes and it helps then, but over time, things get worse. You gain 20 kilos out of nowhere, and sink into depression.

#7 Who Am I?

You have a small child, and you think your world is just perfect, but you notice your child is not hitting his milestones. Development seems delayed. It's your first child so you don't think too much of it, but then you realize that it's not quite right. You take your little guy to the paediatrician who assesses him and says that there is indeed a problem, although from that point he doesn't seem to have too many ideas for solutions. You go home devastated, thinking that this is just something you will have to live with and adapt to the best you can.

■ ■ ■ ■

Here is what these cases have been diagnosed (and possibly misdiagnosed) as:

1. Multiple sclerosis.
2. Chronic fatigue syndrome.
3. Motor neurone disease.
4. Female hormone imbalance.
5. Fibromyalgia.
6. Rheumatoid arthritis.
7. Autistic-spectrum disorder.

So how did you do? Did you recognize the above descriptions as some commonly diagnosed diseases and syndromes? What appears to be one disease may actually be Lyme disease in disguise, and so in the abovementioned cases, the patients' recovery was jeopardized by a faulty diagnosis.

Symptoms of Co-infections

We have already established that in many cases Lyme disease actually involves a range of different microbes (called "co-infections") such as Borrelia, Bartonella, Babesia, Ehrlichia and Rickettsia. While there is significant overlap between the symptoms of each one, there are also a few clues that can help determine which co-infections are present in an individual. Given that so much of the Lyme diagnosis is based on a clinical picture, health practitioners should understand the co-infections and their hallmark symptoms in order to determine which treatments will best help their patient.

Borrelia

- Gradual onset of symptoms
- Multi-system – e.g. - joint pain along with cardiac involvement; cognitive deficits with fatigue and muscle/ joint pain
- Migratory pain from joint to joint
- Fatigue and lethargy, worse in the afternoon
- Four-week cycles
- Stiff, crackly joints
- Headaches originating in the neck
- Slow response to treatment with initial flare (Herxheimer reaction), improvement over weeks with monthly symptom flare
- EM rash in 25% to 50%

Bartonella

- Gradual onset of initial illness
- Central nervous system symptoms out of proportion to musculoskeletal
- CNS irritability including muscle twitches, tremors, insomnia, seizures, agitation,
- Anxiety, severe mood swings, outbursts and antisocial behaviour; OCD traits
- Headaches – feel like ice picks in the head
- Gastritis or abdominal pain, bowel problems (IBS)
- Tender sub-cutaneous nodules along the extremities, especially the outer thigh, shins, and triceps
- Occasional lymphadenopathy (swollen, enlarged lymph nodes)
- Striae or stretch marks that are new, out of place, can be white or red/ purple in colour
- Pain in the sides and back of the ribs
- Pain in soles of the feet, painful to walk in the morning
- Tachycardia (rapid heart beat)
- Photophobia (light sensitivity)
- Rapid response to treatment but a rapid return of symptoms if treatment is stopped too early

Babesia

- Night sweats and sometimes day sweats as well
- Shortness of breath, air hunger, sighing
- Dry chronic cough
- Fullness in the throat, difficulty swallowing
- Severe headaches - dull, all over head, feels like head is in a vice
- Dizziness, light-headedness
- Capillary angiomas especially on breasts
- Vasculitis (red skin with white splotches)
- Hormone imbalance
- Easy bruising
- Burning symptoms
- Head/ tooth/ sinus/ jaw symptoms
- Bell's palsy
- Nausea
- Ear ringing
- Blurry vision
- Vivid/ violent dreams, nightmares
- Flushing
- Flare-ups every 4-6 days
- Failure to respond to Lyme treatment
- Feeling of spaciness, wooziness, and impending doom

Ehrlichia/ Anaplasma

- Rapid onset of initial illness
- Headaches - sharp, knife-like, and often behind the eyes
- Muscle pain, not joint pain, can be mild or severe
- Neurological symptoms – seizure disorders, shooting pains
- Tendon pain
- Pain in the right upper quadrant of the abdomen
- Low WBC count, elevated liver enzymes
- Rapid response to treatment

LYME DISEASE in Australia

Rickettsia

- Fever/ chills
- Headaches
- Confusion
- Aching muscles
- Gastrointestinal symptoms – nausea, loss of appetite
- Swelling of lymph nodes
- Malaise

14. TESTING FOR LYME DISEASE

TESTING FOR LYME DISEASE IS YET ANOTHER ASPECT THAT FUELS THE controversy and exacerbates the issue of misdiagnosis and under-diagnosis of Lyme. This is because many Lyme tests are not sensitive enough to catch all cases. This is truer of some types of tests than others, as we will see.

The thing to stress before we launch into a discussion on lab testing for Lyme disease is that Lyme disease is primarily a clinical diagnosis which can be made based on a person's history, symptom picture and physical examination. Laboratory findings should be used to back up, or confirm, clinical presentation. Many cases of Lyme disease are not diagnosed because of negative lab results, even in the face of a textbook presentation of signs and symptoms, or a strong enough case history to warrant the diagnosis. In many cases a therapeutic trial of an agent that would kill the Lyme bacteria, such as an antibiotic or a herbal antimicrobial, can give valuable clues into the presence of infection. Theoretically, if the person did not have Lyme disease, a course of antibiotics would not dramatically affect their symptom picture. An antibiotic trial that validates the Lyme diagnosis might give a response of either an improvement, or a worsening of symptoms consistent with a Herxheimer reaction (this will be explained in more detail in later sections). Either way, some shift in symptoms would be expected.

In Section One in our discussion of the inherent political challenges in Lyme disease, we learned that the CDC surveillance criteria were initially designed for epidemiological purposes, such as, to track prevalence of Lyme disease cases. They were never meant to be used for diagnostic purposes.

As a reminder the CDC surveillance criteria entail a two-tiered approach to testing, and dictate that a positive sensitive ELISA or IFA must be followed by a positive Western Blot with a defined number of approved antibody bands to be considered positive.

It is this system - where an ELISA test is the first test run, and Lyme disease is often ruled out when a negative result is returned - that has also been adopted in Australia. As we will see, however, that is a flawed system and leaves many people inaccurately diagnosed, and without the medical support and treatment they need.

■ ■ ■ ■

So that you know what all these tests are, let us get some definitions and descriptions out of the way.

In broad terms, tests for Lyme disease can be categorized as direct and indirect.

- ▶ Direct tests look for the bugs or parts of the bugs in various body tissues and fluids. Direct tests include PCR, FISH, cultures and biopsies, and antigen-capture tests.
- ▶ Indirect tests measure a person's immune reaction to the bugs. Indirect tests include ELISA, IFA and Western Blots for Borrelia, and IgG and IgM antibody tests for co-infections.

Lab testing efficacy is determined by sensitivity and specificity. Sensitivity is how likely the test is to find the infection if it is present. A highly sensitive test has a high probability of finding, or measuring, a particular criterion. Specificity, on the other hand, is how accurate a test is in measuring a particular organism, species, or substance. If a test is specific it will clearly define a marker, without too much variability, confusion, false positives or false negatives. In other words, a highly sensitive test will find a needle in a haystack. A highly specific test will tell you for sure that it is a needle.

■ ■ ■ ■

Direct Tests

PCR

PCR stands for Polymerase Chain Reaction. It is a test whereby the DNA, or genetic material of the bacteria, is detected in the blood, serum or other bodily fluids such as the cerebrospinal fluid (CSF) or urine. The downside of the PCR test is that the bacteria often like to hide in the tissues, not simply float around in the blood, so they are difficult to detect. The upside is that the PCR test is not dependent on immune reactions or immune function. A person with a dampened immune response is just as likely to show a positive PCR as a person with a strong immune response. This may not be true of indirect tests, which rely heavily on immune response.

A PCR test that detects a spirochete in the blood is quite specific. While there is some possibility of a false positive, a spirochete visualized is a spirochete visualized; it is specific. The test is not that sensitive, however, as spirochetes may not be easily found in the blood due to their burrowing and hiding in the tissues. If the spirochetes are not hanging out in the blood stream, looking for them there may be a futile endeavour. For this reason PCR tests may be more useful in the early stages of infection when spirochetes are more likely to be in the blood.

PCR testing is also limited by the number of Borrelia strains it can identify. Since there are several strains of Borrelia worldwide known to cause disease in humans, a PCR must assess a range of those strains to be more sensitive.

Culture

The culture test for Borrelia has not been widely used clinically to date, although a culture test is now available in the United States.

In a culture test, a small amount of the patient's blood is removed from their body and introduced into a specific medium that promotes growth of a certain type of bacteria. The bacteria that grow are identified by their cell characteristics and growth characteristics, further confirmed by immuno-staining. To go one step further, PCR testing can be run and various strains identified from the sample. In simple terms, the blood sample is put into a specific medium, allowing some time for the Borrelia to grow, then double-checked that it is Borrelia by examination of its traits and its DNA.

The Borrelia culture is a step forward in that it is deemed more reliable than the Western Blot test, and more sensitive than a PCR. Unfortunately, at the time of writing the test is not available in Australia, as the sample must reach the lab (in Pennsylvania) within 24 hours of being drawn. However, the development of the technology may well spread globally with the rising incidence and recognition of Lyme disease.

Biopsy

A biopsy is another direct test as it measures the actual microbes, not an immune response to a microbe.

Biopsies are tissue samples that are taken from almost anywhere on the body and evaluated for different infections. Although biopsies are not commonly done in the Lyme community, they can be helpful especially when there is a localized zone of infection, such as at the site of a recurring EM rash. Biopsies are also sometimes done to assess small fibre nerve degeneration, which is linked with neuropathy and progression of Lyme disease.

A biopsy is a more invasive procedure than a blood draw, and is not among the first-line lab tests performed to evaluate or diagnose Lyme disease.

Lyme Direct Antigen Test

An antigen capture test looks for Borrelia bacteria, or parts of Borrelia bacteria, in the urine. Again, it is a direct test as it is not relying on an immune response but rather looking for the microbe itself. The antigens are parts of the Borrelia bacteria – when isolated from the urine, they are combined with rabbit antibodies specifically targeted to B. burgdorferi antigens. These antigen-antibody complexes are treated with a colour developing solution, which turns blue-purple and shows the presence of the Borrelia.

The urine antigen test is often done with a "provocation". By giving antibiotics a few days prior to the collection, thus provoking the bacteria, we can accelerate their destruction making their remnants more likely to show up when measured in the urine.

The urine test is a 3-day sample and can safely be shipped from Australia to IGeneX laboratories in the United States.

Indirect Tests

ELISA test

The ELISA test, the problem child of Lyme testing and diagnostics, is the mostly widely run test in the general medical community, and also one of the least useful. Unfortunately, it is the test that is used as a first port of call for many doctors, and a negative result on the ELISA, also used as a screening test for Lyme disease, is used, often incorrectly to rule it out. The ELISA test is offered by many labs worldwide and is often covered by insurance (in fact, insurance often requires that it be the first test run, and will not cover other tests without the ELISA).

There are some fundamental problems with relying on the ELISA test to diagnose Lyme disease. First, the ELISA test does not have adequate sensitivity to fit the two-tiered approach recommended by the CDC. The group responsible for Lyme disease proficiency testing for the College of American Pathologists stated that a screening test must have at least 95% sensitivity to provide an adequate screen, and that the ELISA test simply does not have that level of sensitivity.[1]

In fact, studies have shown that in patients with culture-positive Lyme disease, only 65-70% show an antibody response. Therefore, a full 30-35% of confirmed Lyme cases would have been missed with ELISA testing alone.

To understand how indirect tests such as the ELISA work, we must understand some basic facts about the immune system.

Antibodies are immune cells, and there are two different kinds of antibodies that are evaluated in Lyme testing (and really, testing for any infection). One is the IgM antibody and the other is the IgG antibody. Typically an IgM antibody is going to present much earlier in infection, approximately two to four weeks after exposure. The IgM antibody may stay elevated, indicating an ongoing active exposure. It may also convert to an IgG response. The IgG antibody has a slightly different role. It is not a "first responder" like the IgM antibody. It comes in later, after several weeks of infection, and may stay elevated for long periods of time – months or even years after the initial infection.

Think of the IgM antibodies as the marines (M for marine). They are the first on the scene when there is a threat or invasion; they attack first and ask questions later. The IgG are the ground forces (G for ground). They let the marines suss out the situation first then come into play later, maybe several weeks or even months later. Both arms of this immune system military are necessary and have their strategic roles. The timing of each becomes relevant according to which diagnostic tests are ordered in which time frame post-infection.

Even though they are first on the scene, even the IgM antibodies take a few weeks to appear, typically within 2-4 of the initial infection. One can see then, that a patient presenting with an EM rash a few days after infection needs to be immediately evaluated and diagnosed clinically. By the time antibodies appear, the infection may already have been present for a few weeks and valuable treatment time been lost. I would go so far as to say that a flu-like illness with a known exposure to ticks, such as through camping or bush-walking, should be viewed this way.

IgG antibodies can be confusing as they can also show exposure to an infection without an active infection. An example of this might be after a vaccine, where a variant of a microbe is introduced to the immune system to force it to have an immune response. That way, IgG memory cells are formed, and if that individual encounters the infection again, the IgG memory cells recognize it right away, direct the immune system into action (quick, send in the Marines!) and mount a quicker, more efficient response to the microbe. IgG antibodies may reflect an individual being exposed to Borrelia without becoming sick with it.

One of the problems with this testing is when it measures immune response. Since Lyme disease is known for dampening (weakening) the immune response, this becomes very problematic. The bugs in this case reduce a person's capability to cause an immune reaction – the indirect tests such as ELISA are measuring an immune reaction – and so negatives arise even in the presence of disease. Further, in more chronic infections, IgG antibodies may be absent 50% of the time, posing further complications for diagnosis in chronic illness.[2,3,4] Subsequently we also evaluate IgM antibody response in persistent or recurrent disease.

The other limitation of antibody testing is that if an individual is treated with antibiotics early, to the extent that the infection is mostly eradicated, it can reduce or completely quell their antibody response. Therefore, they could test negative but still have some infectious process in their body. At a later stage, if symptoms return, most of the antibody markers may not be present.

ELISA testing is also hampered by the actual testing methodology. Testing must be developed to detect more unique and specific antigens for Borrelia. Most commercially available kits use a whole cell sample of the Borrelia microbe. More sensitive testing would recognize and use smaller, more specific pieces of the bug that are known to be reactive, not the whole thing lumped into one.

We can see a double-pronged problem with the ELISA testing. First, the test itself is not sensitive enough. Second, the Borrelia microbe curtails immune response so that the signals necessary to trigger a positive result are lower. Together, it is a profoundly unreliable system.

Let's use the analogy of sound. If a microphone recorded sound, it would need the sound to be at a certain decibel (volume) level to be able to record it, but the microphone would also need to be of good quality with a decent level of sensitivity. If either the volume was too low or the microphone was of low quality (not designed to record lower and higher notes, just the central ranges), then the sound would not register or be accurately recorded. If both were present – poor sound output *and* low microphone quality - the chances of a great recording would be doubly jeopardized.

This is how it is with ELISA testing for Lyme disease, and why it is so crucial to combine laboratory findings with the clinical picture to make an accurate diagnosis. Indirect lab tests alone, especially ELISA tests, leave a lot to be desired in terms of sensitivity, and many very ill patients will go undiagnosed. Despite CDC guidelines and their two-tiered approach, a negative ELISA test cannot rule out Lyme disease and should never be used as a stand-alone test.

IFA Test

Another indirect test is the Immuno Fluorescence Assay, or IFA test. It detects antibodies against B. burgdorferi, but it pools the various antibodies (IgG, IgM and IgA). Therefore, it is looking for an immune response but is not as variable based on time after infection in comparison with the ELISA. The IFA is typically run *in conjunction with* Western Blots. It should not be used *instead of* a Western Blot.

The IFA test is useful when run with other tests, to make up part of the picture. It is not necessarily a stand-alone test and is not necessarily diagnostic in and of itself. While concerns have arisen over time as to the specificity of the IFA for Lyme-specific antibodies and for its potential for cross-reactivity with antibodies to other spirochetes, studies have shown that with high quality testing procedures and highly experienced lab technicians, the IFA test has good specificity and sensitivity. Therefore the IFA should be run through a lab that specializes in Lyme testing to increase its validity.

Western Blot Test

The Western Blot test is one of the foremost tests used in the evaluation of Lyme disease. It is also an indirect test, as are the ELISA and IFA; however it is a more sensitive test if performed by a laboratory that looks for all the bands that are related to Borrelia. IgM and IgG antibodies are evaluated separately, with the IgM being detected as early as one week post-exposure.

Unfortunately, as has been the case with anything so far relating to CDC criteria, the CDC has also played a role in creating limitations in Western Blot testing and reporting.

A Western Blot reports certain numbers, or "bands", which can be positive, negative, or equivocal. The bands represent certain antigens, which are the parts of the bacteria that the immune system reacts to.

There is a discrepancy as to which bands are clinically significant, and how many of the bands need to be positive to get a positive result. FDA-approved, commercially available kits (such as the Mardx Marblot) are restricted from reporting all of the bands. These rules were set up in accordance with the CDC surveillance criteria. Private laboratories that are not beholden to these rules and criteria are free to produce tests that actually help people get an accurate assessment.

In IgM testing, by CDC criteria, two of the following bands must be positive to record a positive result:

23-25 kDa

39 kDa

41 kDa

IGeneX, on the other hand, a U.S. based specialty Lyme lab, recognizes the following bands as clinically significant and relevant to Lyme disease:

23-25 kDa

31 kDa

34 kDa

39 kDa

41 kDa

83-93 kDa

Their research has shown that the 31, 34 and 83-93 bands are significant and quite specific to Borrelia infection. The 41 band, on the other hand, shows a lot of cross-reactivity with other flagella-bearing organisms, so a positive 41 can be indicative of other types of infections.

Clearly, the expanded IGeneX criteria give a more rounded and inclusive view of Lyme immune recognition, and allow for a more clinically helpful assessment. Many Lyme-literate medical doctors and experts in Lyme disease believe that just one positive or even equivocal of the above bands is clinically significant.

The other benefit of IGeneX testing is that the bands are reported according to a range – from IND (indeterminate, or weak positive), +, ++, +++ all the way through to ++++. The stronger the immune response to a band, the more +'s are reported. Therefore, even if a patient's test results are negative, but they have, for example, two IND bands (an IND does not "count" as a positive band), it gives clues that the person may be affected by Borrelia. It may seem logical that the more +'s a patient has, the more aggressive and severe their infection, but in fact the opposite might be true. Because Lyme disease disables the immune system, sometimes the sickest individuals have a lower immune response and a 'less positive' looking test result; it does not mean they are any less sick.

The IgG Western Blot has even more stringent criteria than the IgM Western Blot. At least five bands must be positive (out of a possible 10) to be regarded as positive according to the CDC. The test looks for 10 bands: 18, 23-25, 28, 30, 39, 41, 45, 58, 66 and 83-93 kDa. Results showing four positive bands, or five equivocal (borderline) bands, report as negative and are completely disregarded. Bands 31 kDa and 34 kDa - both of which are significant antigens that appear later in the immune response and are highly Lyme specific - so specific, in fact, that these bands represent the antigens used in developing the Lyme vaccine - are also excluded. How ironic that these antigens were relevant enough for developing the Lyme disease vaccine, but not relevant enough to be included in the laboratory reporting for Lyme. (By the way, the Lyme vaccine is no longer available due to numerous lawsuits by people who believed that the vaccine made them sick and actually infected them with Lyme disease; the manufacturer cites "low sales" as the reason for the withdrawal in 2002).

To demonstrate this, one study showed that although 89% of patients with EM rash developed IgG antibodies as detected by Western Blot some time during their disease, only 22% were positive by the standards of the CDC.[5]

Another limitation to the Western Blot is the CDC's belief that an IgM Western Blot should only be used within the first month of infection, even though other studies have shown that the IgM Western Blot can be positive even in recurrent or persistent disease. Some patients who have been ill for many years will still show a positive IgM Western Blot and a negative IgG Western Blot. Other patients with culture-positive Lyme disease will remain seronegative on any kind of Western Blot testing (approximately 20-30% in fact). Such is the challenge of Lyme disease.

Although the most clinically useful of all indirect tests, a positive Western Blot still only suggests exposure to Lyme disease; it does not diagnose Lyme disease. Diagnosis is still done based on the clinical picture – a person's history and exposure coupled with their current symptoms.

Testing for Co-Infections

Along with testing for Borrelia, it is imperative to test for co-infections. Information gained from co-infection testing can make a significant difference to the treatment path chosen. Different microbes require different medications and different herbs to counter them. Probably the best example of this is Babesia. Babesia is a parasite, while Borrelia is a bacterium. The medications that work well for Borrelia will not work well for Babesia. The consensus among hundreds of Lyme-treating doctors is that undetected and untreated co-infections are one of the key reasons for treatment failure in Lyme disease.

There are a few different ways to test for co-infections. The main types are antibody tests, FISH tests and PCR tests. Note: At the current time, there is no comprehensive testing available in Australia for the common co-infections of Lyme disease. Australian patients are advised to send their blood to IGeneX in the United States to have co-infection testing done.

Antibody tests

The co-infections that IGeneX offers antibody testing for are:

Babesia duncani

Babesia microti

Bartonella species

Ehrlichia chafeensis (HME)

Anaplasma phagocytophila (HGA)

Rickettsia rickettsii/ typhi

Antibody testing, similar to what we discussed in the indirect tests for Borrelia, measures the immune system's reaction to these various microbes. The tests done are IgG and IgM. Remember, IgM is a marker of either a new infection or current/ active infection. IgG indicates either prior exposure or a more chronic/ longer-term infection.

In interpreting these tests, I regard an elevation in either antibody clinically significant when combined with a symptomatic patient. IGeneX criteria for all the co-infections listed above are the following:

IgM	<20	negative
IgM	20-160	may or may not indicate active infection
IgM	>160	indicates an active infection

IgG	<40	negative
IgG	40-160	may or may not indicate active infection
IgG	>160	indicates an active infection

As an example, if a patient has an IgM level of 20 for a particular infection, I would consider treating that co-infection, *especially if the symptom picture matches that of the co-infection*. Remember, for co-infections as well as Borrelia, the diagnosis is based primarily on clinical presentation.

FISH tests

The Fluorescent In-Situ Hybridization (FISH) test is a direct test - it does not rely on immune response and is a way to visualize the microbes directly - that uses a sample examined as a thin smear in order to identify and mark the ribosomal RNA. Under a microscope, the bugs, whose presence indicates an active, current infection, literally glow in the dark.

The Babesia FISH test detects both Babesia duncani and Babesia microti. It is performed on whole blood, since the parasites exist within the red blood cells themselves.

The Bartonella FISH test detects B. vinsonii, B. berkhoffii, B. henselae and B. quintana, so it can detect several different strains. The FISH test actually shows the microbes fluorescing under a microscope. Bartonella, rod-shaped bacteria, have been stained with a substance specific to mark them so a positive result will reflect the sighting of characteristic bacteria of this shape.

FISH tests have a high level of specificity so there are very few false positives. Remember though, a negative FISH does not necessarily mean that the infection is not present. It simply means that it was not detected in that particular sample.

PCR Tests

Like the FISH, PCR tests for co-infections are direct tests. DNA, or parts of the DNA of the bacteria, are evaluated in the blood sample. In my experience, FISH tests are more sensitive than PCR tests for co-infections and are more frequently utilized.

Chlamydia pneumonia, Mycoplasma pneumonia and other Mycoplasma species are other infections that often exist in chronically ill Lyme patients. Australian Biologics, a lab in NSW, offers PCR testing for these microbes as well as PCR testing for Borrelia. This panel can also help generate information on which infections are playing a role in an individual's illness.

■ ■ ■ ■

By now you may be asking why we test at all, if the tests are not 100% reliable and if Lyme disease is a clinical diagnosis anyway. The answer is that the more information we can gather, the better. Testing can give confirmation on a suspected illness, shed light on which co-infections are present and help in assessing the severity of an infection. For example, if a patient tests indeterminate on the Lyme Western Blot but has a positive FISH test for Babesia and Babesia duncani antibodies at 80 or 160, then they may have a dominant Babesia infection, and treatment should start there.

Similarly, if a patient shows a positive PCR for Borrelia, a positive IgM Western Blot, and all negative co-infection testing, and unless they have symptoms that are pathognomonic of a specific co-infection, their initial treatment should be tailored around the Borrelia. However, another person can have positive antibodies to Borrelia, Babesia, Bartonella and Rickettsia, and in that case, we know we have a complex situation that is going to require several different medications to address them all.

Lab tests are very useful and should be regarded as important pieces of the puzzle. Alone, they do not rule in or out infection, but when combined with history, symptoms, tick exposures and so on can give very useful information to help shape the big picture.

Testing for Lyme Disease

Other Tests That Might Be Useful

Not only are there tests for the infections themselves, but there are a couple of other markers and tests that can help assess an individual's health. This is not a complete list of tests as there are literally dozens of tests that may be useful in various scenarios.

CD-57

The CD-57 is not so much a test to detect Lyme disease as it is an immune marker that tends to be low in the presence of Lyme disease. CD or cluster designation markers are identifying markers on certain immune cells called T cells and NK cells. They give cells their variance in appearance and function. So far, there are approximately 200 known CD's, numbered according to their order of discovery. Any T cell or NK cell will carry many different CD markers.

If a cell expresses a certain marker, it is designated with the number of that marker and a "+" sign. So if an immune cell expresses the CD-57 marker, it is written as CD-57+. Through laboratory testing, we can measure the number of cells that carry a certain designation, either on the T cell or NK cell.

Clinically, measuring certain CD markers can help evaluate certain illnesses. Lyme disease has been associated with a low CD-57 count – specifically Borrelia infection (as opposed to co-infections). The sicker the patient, the lower the CD-57 count appears to be.

Measuring the CD-57 count can be helpful for a number of reasons. First, other illnesses such as chronic fatigue syndrome, rheumatoid arthritis or multiple sclerosis might mimic Lyme, but those illnesses will not cause a drop in the CD-57, so this marker can help in determining Lyme disease as distinct from other chronic illnesses with similar symptom pictures. Also, the CD-57 can be used to track treatment progress, as it should return towards normal levels as the infection improves. It also can give clues into co-infections. CD-57 levels are impacted by Borrelia but not significantly by co-infections, so if a patient is still symptomatic despite

Lyme treatment and has a rising CD-57 count, it can be a clue that co-infections, not the Borrelia itself, are driving the remaining symptoms.

Of course, nothing is as straightforward as it seems, especially in Lyme disease. Many chronically ill Lyme patients present with a low CD-57 count, and despite long-term treatment and a resolving symptom picture, their counts stay frustratingly low. There are sometimes discrepancies between one lab and another, and numbers can fluctuate up and down between readings in ways that do not seem to correlate with the degree of illness or recovery.

It is important to remember that the lab is running the CD-57 on the NK cells, not the T cells. T cells will express CD-57 markers, but they are not clinically relevant to Lyme in the same way that the CD-57+ NK cells are. Running the CD-57 test on the T cells may be one reason for apparent discrepancies in results.

The CD-57 test is a worthwhile test to run as a gauge of immune response to Borrelia. While it sometimes shows inconsistencies, it may provide another piece of the puzzle and more information to shed light on that person's case. In Australia the CD-57+ NK test is available domestically as well as through IGeneX.

Fry Labs Advanced Stain for Biofilm

We have already seen that the production of biofilm by colonies of bacteria can create bacterial defences that are difficult to overcome. The bacterial colonies produce biofilm then hide in it, evading antibiotic and immune attack. The colonies become quite sophisticated – they attach to other structures that allow the flow of nutrients in and toxins out of their milieu, making them very resilient.

Fry Labs (Arizona, U.S.) initially began smear testing to provide assessment of Bartonella and other protozoans in the blood of chronically ill patients. As their work progressed, they saw colonies with biofilm in many of the blood samples. They have further developed their stain techniques and can provide insight into the degree of biofilm involvement, literally giving a visual picture of it. In patients who are being treated with antibiotic therapy and making slow or minimal progress, assessing this biofilm may be of great value.

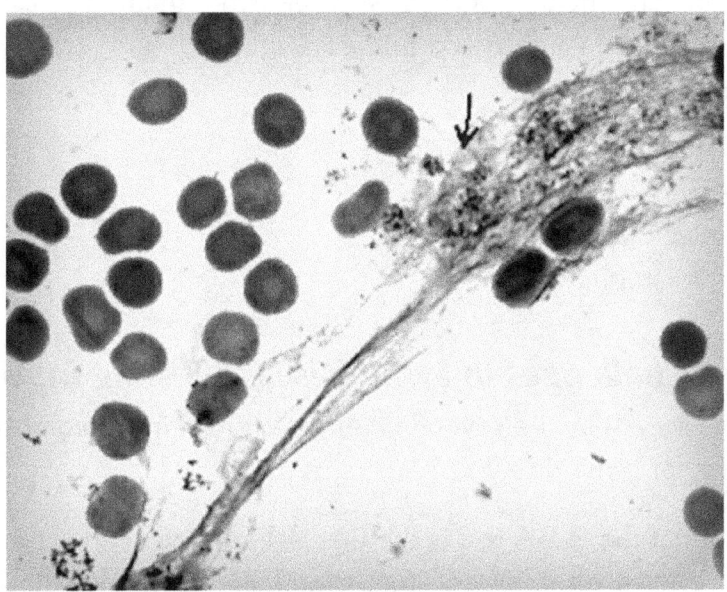

Demonstration of biofilm development on a smear test through Fry Laboratories[6]

Elispot-LTT (Lymphocyte Transformation Test)

Run by Infectolab in Augsburg, Germany, the Elispot-LTT test uses a different part of the immune system to the antibody testing. Antibodies are part of the humoral immune response; we also have a cellular immune response that involves T cells and NK cells. (The CD-57 cell marker described above is part of the cellular immune system).

A Borrelia infection will activate T cells as well as antibodies. Activation of T cells occurs immediately after infection, and stops approximately six to eight weeks after completion of effective therapy or when the infection is resolved. Therefore, measuring T cell reactivity to Borrelia might be another useful diagnostic tool, as it is not as subject to the variability of antibody responses in different patients and at different times of infection.

According to Infectolab, the Elispot-LTT will detect even a single reactive T cell, is accurate in both acute and chronic infection, and is a helpful indicator of whether infection is truly resolved at the end of therapy. The Elispot-LTT test is available for a range of infectious agents including Borrelia, Chlamydia pneumonia, Chlamydia trachomatis, Ehrlichia, Anaplasma, Yersinia and the Epstein-Barr virus.

Infectolab
49-821-4550-740 (ph)
49-821-4550-741 (fax)
service@infectolab.de (email)
www.infectolab.de (website)

Inherent Challenges in Lyme Disease Testing in Australia

As you can see, there are several challenges to getting accurate and reliable testing for Lyme disease in Australia.

The first is that the ELISA test is the first test administered if Lyme is suspected. We have already seen that the ELISA test is not a sufficiently sensitive test to be clinically useful. Unfortunately, many doctors run the ELISA test, and if the results are negative, make a definitive statement that the person does not have Lyme disease. Any discussion of Lyme disease after that meets with a cold response or a total dismissal.

In those very few cases where the ELISA test comes back positive, a follow up confirmation test would be the Western Blot. If run through larger commercial labs, the Western Blot test is not going to recognize some of the bands that are necessary to give the complete picture, such as the 31 and 34 kDa bands.

Often, if an ELISA is negative, doctors will not run Western Blots at all. They have been taught about the two-tier testing – ELISA first, then Western Blot only if ELISA is positive. That two-tiered system was designed for research and epidemiological purposes; it was never meant to be used for clinical diagnostic purposes and is simply not appropriate or adequate in the clinical setting.

Any of the indirect tests have the inherent challenge that they measure immune response. We know that Lyme can dampen immune response, so the very markers needed to diagnose infection are dampened by the infection itself, leading to a lower chance of diagnosis. It is ironic that the more profound and chronic the infection in the body, the lesser the response may be on indirect testing.

Adequate testing for co-infections is not available within Australia. Australian patients can get tested for Rickettsia and Mycoplasma quite easily, but Babesia, Bartonella and Ehrlichia are not currently available so testing done within Australia will provide an incomplete picture of a person's chronic infections and may lead to inadequacies in treatment protocols.

Getting the Most Out of Laboratory Testing for Lyme Disease

There are ways to get more reliable and comprehensive testing done. Here are some ways to maximize laboratory information:

- ▶ Make sure testing is done through a lab that has expertise in Lyme and co-infection testing, and is not restricted to CDC criteria. IGeneX Laboratory in Palo Alto, California is a specialist Lyme lab that offers the most reliable and comprehensive testing at this time. It is possible to send blood samples from Australia to IGeneX via Fedex or other international courier.
- ▶ To run IGeneX testing, contact the lab directly and request a blood kit. A doctor's signature is required on the requisition form to authorize the testing.

    1-650-424-1191 (ph)
    1-650-424-1196 (fax)
    customerservice@igenex.com (email)
    www.igenex.com (website)

- ▶ Run as many different types of tests as possible, both direct and indirect. This means doing IFA, PCR and Western Blots for Borrelia.

Australian Biologics lab based in Sydney offers a Borrelia PCR as well as PCR testing for Mycoplasma and Chlamydia, but this test alone is not sufficient for a complete evaluation of Lyme disease – the range of testing offered by IGeneX provides a far more comprehensive picture. IGeneX testing (PCR and Western Blot) also covers a variety of strains of Borrelia, including the B. afzilii, B. garinii, and B. andersonii. Even though Australian Lyme more closely represents the European strains than the American strains, the IGeneX tests are still able to detect it.

Australian Biologics
02-9283-0807 (ph)
02-9283-0910 (fax)
www.australianbiologics.com.au (website)

Based on the data that IGeneX has collected to date, a comprehensive Lyme panel will detect about 80% of all Lyme patients (this represents the sensitivity of the test). The overall specificity of this panel is greater than 95% with all three types of tests run (IFA, Western Blot and PCR). This is equivalent to Australian Panel 3 (below).

IGeneX offers three Australian Panels. The basic one contains the Borrelia Western Blots plus antibody testing for co-infections but omits the PCR tests and the FISH tests (the two direct tests). While Panel 1 is a good value and a good option if funds do not permit the more complete panels, I recommend Panels 2 or 3 for the greatest harvest of usable information. Panel 2 is the Western Blots and antibody tests, plus the PCR for Borrelia. Panel 3 is all of the above plus the Babesia and Bartonella FISH. Panel 3 is the most complete option for Lyme disease testing.

Australian Tick Borne Disease Panel 1

Test Code	Test
188	Lyme IgM Western Blot
189	Lyme IgG Western Blot
200	Babesia microti IgG & IgM antibody
720	Babesia duncani IgG & IgM antibody
206	HGE (Anaplasma phagocytophila) IgG & IgM antibody
203	HME (Human Monocytic Ehrlichia) IgG & IgM antibody
285	Bartonella henselae IgG & IgM
965	Rickettesia rickettsii/typhii IgG antibody

Australian Tick Borne Disease Panel 2

Test Code	Test
188	Lyme IgM Western Blot
189	Lyme IgG Western Blot
200	Babesia microti IgG & IgM antibody
720	Babesia duncani IgG & IgM antibody
206	HGE (Anaplasma phagocytophila) IgG & IgM antibody
203	HME (Human Monocytic Ehrlichia) IgG & IgM antibody
285	Bartonella henselae IgG & IgM
965	Rickettesi rickettsii/typhii IgG antibody
453/456	Lyme Multiplex PCR - serum & whole blood

LYME DISEASE in Australia

Australian Tick Borne Disease Panel 3

Test Code	Test
188	Lyme IgM Western Blot
189	Lyme IgG Western Blot
200	Babesia microti IgG & IgM antibody
720	Babesia duncani IgG & IgM antibody
206	HGE (Anaplasma phagocytophila) IgG & IgM antibody
203	HME (Human Monocytic Ehrlichia) IgG & IgM antibody
285	Bartonella henselae IgG & IgM
965	Rickettesii rickettsii/typhii IgG antibody
453/456	Lyme Multiplex PCR - serum & whole blood
640	Babesia FISH
289	Bartonella FISH

▶ Always do co-infection testing in conjunction with Lyme testing. Co-infections often go undiagnosed, and that can contribute significantly to treatment failures. The IGeneX panels cover Babesia, Bartonella, Ehrlichia, Anaplasma and Rickettsia. Ideally, antibody and FISH tests (available for Babesia and Bartonella only) would be run. PCR testing is also available for co-infections but is run less frequently. Rickettsia testing can also be reliably done through Australian labs.

▶ If there is poor response to antimicrobial therapy or if improvement is slow, consider that biofilm might be an issue. We will discuss ways to deal with biofilm in the treatment section, however one option for evaluation is through the Advanced Stain by Fry Laboratories.

Again, blood can be sent directly to Fry Labs from Australia. A doctor would need to sign off on the requisition form.

Fry Laboratories
1-480-292-8560 (ph)

1-480-656-4932 (fax)
info@frylabs.com (email)
www.frylabs.com (website)

- To get as complete a picture as possible, run additional immune markers such as the CD-57 NK cell count. Make sure the lab uses the NK cells, not the T cells, in their testing methodology. C4a and C3a complement are two other markers that may indicate inflammation and neurotoxicity in the system. These are also immune markers that can be run through local, commercial labs.
- Determine whether antimicrobial therapy is indicated prior to testing. There are mixed views as to whether testing should be "provoked", that is, an antimicrobial given for a few weeks before the blood is collected with the aim of killing off some microbes and stirring up the immune system to produce a louder "noise" for the test to measure. Certainly, many patients are too ill to be able to tolerate such an approach, as the Herxheimer reaction may be too great (more on Herxheimer reactions in the following section). Many patients require a gentler introduction to antimicrobial therapy, whereas a provocation can require higher doses right off the bat. Also, many patients would have a difficult time convincing their local doctor to give them such doses of antibiotics without an official diagnosis to base it on.
- Having said that, there are some cases where I have used antibiotics and/or antimicrobial herbs to try to generate a greater immune response. And there are some cases where a negative IgM Western Blot has turned into a positive Western Blot after a few weeks of antimicrobial therapy. In general, I do not use provocation for the majority of my patients prior to testing.

The most important thing to stress is that Lyme disease is still a clinical diagnosis. We use lab testing to support that diagnosis, to give information on co-infections, and to give quantitative information that we can use over the course of treatment to track progress. The best way to get accurate and reliable information is to do testing through a specialty Lyme lab such as IGeneX and to run a variety of test types (both direct and indirect) to increase the likelihood of revealing evidence of the infection. Co-infection testing is imperative to round out the picture.

Lab testing for Lyme disease in Australia is limited. The PCR from Australian Biologics may be a good starting point but is not sufficient by itself. Even with a positive PCR for Borrelia, co-infection testing must still be performed, and I still prefer to see a Western Blot as well, as I can get a sense of how active the infection is and how the immune system is coping with it.

The extra steps and cost required to ship blood to the United States are well worth it for the wealth of information it can provide, and the thousands of dollars it could possibly save from futile treatments and years of heartache from not getting an accurate assessment of the chronic infections at play in the body.

REFERENCES

1. Bakken LL, Callister SM, Wand PJ, Schell RF. Interlaboratory comparison of test results for detection of Lyme disease by 516 participants in the Wisconsin State laboratory of hygiene/College of American Pathologists proficiency testing program. J Clin Microbiol. 1997 Mar;35(3):537-43.
2. Engstrom SM, Shoop E, Johnson RC. Immunoblot interpretation criteria for serodiagnosis of early Lyme disease. J Clin Microbiol. 1995 Feb;33(2):419-27.
3. Aguero-Rosenfeld ME, Nowakowski J, McKenna DF, Carbonaro CA, Wormser GP. Serodiagnosis in early Lyme disease. J Clin Microbiol. 1993 Dec;31(12):3090-3095.
4. Aguero-Rosenfeld ME, Nowakowski J, McKenna DF, Carbonaro CA, Wormser GP. Evolution of the serologic response to Borrelia burgdorferi in treated patients with culture-confirmed erythema migrans. J Clin Microbiol. 1996 Jan;34(1):l-9.
5. Aguero-Rosenfeld ME, Nowakowski J, McKenna DF, Carbonaro CA, Wormser GP. Evolution of the serologic response to Borrelia burgdorferi in treated patients with culture-confirmed erythema migrans. J Clin Microbiol. 1996 Jan;34(1):l-9.
6. Reproduced with permission.

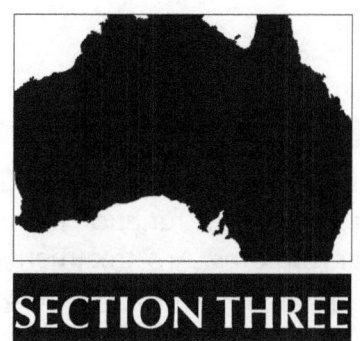

SECTION THREE

TREATMENT GUIDELINES FOR LYME DISEASE

Lyme disease is a multi-factorial and multi-system illness. It affects many different body systems, from immune function to hormones, and it creates a wide range of different symptoms. Any treatments undertaken, whether pharmaceutical or naturopathic, must address these multiple facets.

Chronic Lyme disease is not an easy illness to treat. There are several major considerations when creating treatment protocols for Lyme disease.

Please note: The treatment guidelines contained in this book are for informational purposes only; they are not intended to be prescriptions for treatment for any individual or individuals. Consult a licensed, qualified physician before attempting to use any Lyme disease treatment. Use of the treatment guidelines in this book while not under the care of a licensed physician may result in injury or death. Your own licensed physician should be the one to make final decisions about your medical care and which treatments you use.

15. TREATMENT CONSIDERATIONS

Treatment consideration #1:
Lyme disease may require hefty doses of antibiotics for a long time

The first point to know is that the bacteria and parasites in Lyme disease often require higher than typical doses of certain antibiotic and antiparasitic medications. A good example is doxycycline. Doxycycline is often dosed at 100mg twice daily but in Lyme disease, research has shown that dose to be bacteriostatic – that is, it will halt the progression of the bacteria but not fully kill it off. To be bacteriocidal, or able to fully kill the bacteria, Borrelia requires doses of 400mg per day. This is alarming to some doctors who have not prescribed doses that high in the past, and some patients have been denied treatment for this reason.

Yes, Lyme disease requires multiple antibiotics at high doses. It is part of what makes it a challenging illness to treat. I will discuss how to prevent side effects and protect the body during these long courses of antibiotics in the section on naturopathic treatments.

The duration of treatment is also a contentious one, due to the IDSA guidelines, which list 28 days as the longest duration of treatment, even in severe neurological Lyme. In reality, chronic Lyme disease requires far longer treatment times than that. The average treatment time for most patients is from 12-24 months. I rarely see a patient who can resolve their symptoms in less than 12 months. Some require 2-3 years of treatment;

and yet others fare best when they continue with some kind of antibiotic protocol indefinitely.

A rule of thumb that is followed by many Lyme-literate medical doctors operating under ILADS protocols is to treat for two months beyond resolution of a person's symptoms. That means that a person must feel like they have been back to their old self (if they can remember what that is!) for a couple of months before discontinuing antibiotics. Even then, it is sensible to continue with herbal antimicrobials for a few months beyond ceasing antibiotics, to further address any remaining infection and to prevent relapse.

Treatment consideration #2:
Treatment must be a multi-tiered, multi-layered approach

We have already seen that chronic Lyme disease involves an infection with the Borrelia bacteria, and that Borrelia can exist in three different forms – as a spirochete, a cell-wall deficient form and a cyst form. The bacteria can morph back and forth between forms to evade attack by the immune system and antimicrobial therapy.

Each form of Borrelia is susceptible to different antibiotics. *Therefore each of the three forms must be addressed for recovery to be possible*. If only one form of Borrelia is treated, it can simply morph into other forms and long-term improvement will be elusive.

Even for Borrelia in the absence of co-infections, three medications must be layered into the treatment protocol – one for spirochetes, one for cell-wall deficient forms, and one for cyst forms. In some cases, natural treatments can be substituted for medications, but by and large, three antibiotics are required.

Typically, the medications are commenced one at a time, spaced out by 2-4 weeks to allow the body time to adjust to one before adding another. This also allows time to gauge any allergic or other medication reactions without confusing which one is the culprit. Ultimately, the goal is to have coverage of the three different forms.

Treatment Considerations

We have also seen that Lyme disease often involves different microbes known as co-infections, including Bartonella, Babesia, Ehrlichia and Rickettsia. Mycoplasma is another common microbe in Lyme patients. These co-infections must also be addressed in addition to the Borrelia. When the co-infections are bacterial in nature, it is easier to do this, as there may be crossover benefit between Lyme medications and medications that will be effective for the co-infection. Examples are doxycycline and minocycline, both of which are used for Borrelia, Mycoplasma and Ehrlichia. Babesia, on the other hand, is a tougher case because it is an intra-cellular parasite. The medications that are effective for Borrelia will not be effective for Babesia since one is a bacteria and the other is a parasite. Babesia will require its own medication protocol.

Part of the challenge is deciphering where to start. This is where lab work can come in very handy. If a particular infection is registering very high antibodies, then likely it is a potent infection that requires prioritising. If a patient has a strongly positive Western Blot that shows activity in several different bands and a mild elevation of Bartonella antibodies, the Borrelia appears dominant, and I would consider starting there. Treating Lyme disease can be compared to peeling layers off an onion, and it must be determined which layer of the onion is currently the top layer, and should be dealt with first.

If Babesia is present, it moves up the priority list to number one, especially when the patient's symptoms reflect a Babesia infection because Babesia is a very disruptive infection, and progress against the other infections will most likely be out of reach until it is addressed. The symptoms I look for in Babesia include night sweats, low-grade fevers, temperature regulation problems, neck pain, head and neck symptoms such as ringing in the ears and blurry vision, spaciness and feeling "detached," and complete hormonal mayhem. Flushing in the face, mottling of the skin anywhere on the body, and tiny red dots on the skin called capillary angiomas are also clues.

A person presenting with more neurological issues such as cognitive deficits, numbness and tingling in any part of the body, Bell's palsy, along with joint and muscle pain that migrates, suggests a dominant Borrelia infection. A patient with agonizing pain in the soles of their feet, where it feels like walking on glass in the morning, rib pain, severe anxiety and weird looking scratches or stretch marks on their skin may have Bartonella.

Typically we start with what seems to be the dominant infection. Babesia, if suspected, is given high priority in treatment as an ongoing Babesia infection can hinder progress of Lyme treatment. We also adjust treatment protocols based on the patient's response. If a patient is getting treated primarily for one infection with limited benefit, it may be that a co-infection is present and creating most of that person's symptoms. In general, co-infections hinder progress against Borrelia.

Treatment consideration #3:
There might be Herxheimer reactions

The third factor to consider when shaping Lyme treatment is the possibility of Herxheimer reactions (or Jarisch-Herxheimer reaction), aka "Herxes". Adolf Jarisch, an Austrian dermatologist, and Karl Herxheimer, a German dermatologist, put their names to these reactions when they discovered the phenomena while treating syphilis with mercury back in the late 1800's and early 1900's. Today, "Herxing" has become just as valid a verb as "googling", especially in the Lyme community.

Herxing refers to a temporary worsening of symptoms, caused by the release of neurotoxins as pathogens are killed. It is the pathogens themselves that release the neurotoxins, but it becomes the task of the body to detoxify and excrete them. Herxing typically reflects a transient worsening of a person's existing symptoms, or even the onset of new symptoms.

While spirochetes are renowned for their ability to trigger Herxes, other bacteria such as Bartonella can, too. I have also observed significant Herx reactions in patients with Candida (yeast) overgrowth when it is treated, and also in the parasitic illness Babesia.

Treatment Considerations

Inherent in these die-off reactions is an elevation in cytokines, which are chemical mediators of the immune system. Some cytokines will lessen symptoms and moderate inflammation, while some will kick it up. The cytokines involved in Herxes are more inflammatory, and therefore will give the patient the experience of a worsening of symptoms, and possibly even the introduction of new symptoms.

The body works hard to clear the endotoxins that have been released, through its natural detoxification mechanisms. Variations in a patient's experience of Herxing depend greatly on their detoxification mechanisms. Many people with chronic Lyme disease have compromised detoxification systems, which makes the Herxheimer reactions more profound. Primary detoxification mechanisms include the liver, kidneys, and skin.

There are ways to assist the body in detoxifying the toxins that arise in a Herx reaction, and those will be discussed under naturopathic therapies. For now, suffice it to say that treating Lyme disease may well lead to Herxheimer reactions, and it is important to be aware of them. Different people will have different levels of sensitivity to the endotoxins released by dying organisms. For some, it is possible to push through Herxes and continue treatment. For others, the pace of treatment may be dictated by the severity of the Herxes. If Herxes get too severe, treatment will need to be slowed or even stopped for a period of time for the patient to stabilize. Herxing is not a "badge of honour" where how much they can endure proves how tough they are. There are some times where Herxing can in fact be dangerous for the individual.

Herxing is also not required for the treatment to work. Some people do not Herx significantly at all when starting treatment and still benefit from the treatment, usually those who are genetically good detoxifiers, pay attention to their nutrition, and supplement with supportive nutrients and herbs for detoxification. This may also be the case during treatment of early or uncomplicated infection.

Herxing is not limited to pharmaceutical protocols. Antibiotics and natural treatment modalities can both cause Herxes. Additionally, Rifing

- a frequency-based therapy, Hyperbaric Oxygen Therapy (HBOT), and other antibacterial treatments can all trigger the Herxheimer reaction. Effectively, anything that kills off these bugs can trigger Herxes.

It can be tricky to determine whether a patient is having a Herx reaction or an adverse reaction to a particular antibiotic, but I have two guidelines for this:

1. A medication reaction is usually quite immediate – within minutes to hours of taking the drug. A Herxheimer reaction often takes several days to appear (as the endotoxins build up gradually and reach a tipping point at which stage they make the person feel worse).

2. A medication reaction often produces new symptoms, and/or shows up as allergy-type symptoms such as nausea, headaches and rashes. A Herxheimer reaction is typically representative of the symptoms the person usually experiences, just in a more severe way, so there may be more joint pain, more cognitive deficits, more night sweats – whatever the person's usual symptoms are, but flared. Often people have an intuitive sense of whether a worsening of symptoms is a medication reaction or a Herx reaction.

It can also be tricky deciding whether to push through a Herx or slow down treatment to let the body recover and catch up. Some guidelines for this include:

1. The person's lifestyle – Do they have to work to support themselves? Do they have someone to care for them at home? How functional do they need to be in their daily lives? An example might be a college-age person who has the summer off and wants to use that time to treat aggressively. They may be willing to go through more severe Herxing to get through it within a set time frame. A single mum who has to work to support her family is more likely to need a slow and steady approach.

2. Any life-threatening aspects to the Herxes - Some patients with motor neurone disease may have breathing or swallowing difficulties so a Herx reaction could be life threatening. Severe cardiac involvement

is another questionable symptom. If a patient has major tachycardia or arrhythmia, pushing too much can be dangerous.

Herxing can be a significant phenomenon and can greatly impact the pace at which treatment progresses. Often, awareness of what Herxing is and what can be expected goes a long way towards alleviating the anxiety that may be caused by symptoms seemingly getting worse at the start of treatment. I always assure my patients that some Herx reaction is to be expected, that the "worse before better" is typical, and may even be a good sign that the treatment is working well. But I also monitor them closely and will advise people to back off or slow down a particular medication or therapy if I feel that their body is not keeping up with the die-off reactions produced. The patient's safety must always come first; then their need to be functional in their daily lives and their psycho-emotional capacity to withstand Herxing should be closely considered.

Treatment consideration #4:
What works for one might not work for another

There is a great individualization of treatment that must take place in addressing Lyme disease. An obvious factor in this is medication allergies. A person with a penicillin allergy is not going to be able to take a medication that a non-allergic person can take, and alternative medications will need to be chosen.

Medication side effects can drive treatment decisions. One of the side effects of doxycycline is sun sensitivity. Some people may experience that side effect so severely that they just cannot take doxycycline. Nausea, vomiting, headaches, tinnitus, and many other side effects may present themselves. Even within medication classes, two very slightly different drugs may give totally different side effects, for example, azithromycin and clarithromycin, both in the macrolide family. One person might tolerate one well, and the other not at all. Another patient might be the exact opposite.

Remember, medication allergies and side effects are different from Herxheimer reactions, which we often discern as a worsening of the person's usual symptoms.

In some cases, different people simply benefit more from one medication choice or combination than another. To some extent this can be predicted (especially by co-infection picture), but sometimes it appears to have no rhyme or reason. The reality is medication protocols can at times seem like trial and error. There is no guarantee that what works for one person will work equally well for another. Often, treatment decisions have to be made one at a time, step-by-step, depending on the reaction to the last step, and adjusted along the way wherever necessary. Awareness and understanding of this can make the treatment journey much less frustrating.

Treatment consideration #5:
Plateaus may occur with long-term antibiotic use

If a medication is continued for a long duration, the pathogens may become resistant to it, and the medication will lose its desired effect. To overcome this, medications should be rotated periodically. The time frame may vary – Dr. Joseph Burrascano suggests every six weeks. My rule of thumb in clinical practice is to continue medication regardless of duration of treatment as long as the patient is improving. If the patient has hit a plateau and is clearly not improving on that regimen, I will change the protocol. Typically one medication will be changed at a time so as not to overwhelm the patient's system or trigger another major Herx from too many new medications. Also, the choice of which new drugs to add into the mix should take into account which infections are currently dominant, or on the "top" layer of the onion that we are trying to "peel."

16. SUGGESTED MEDICATION PROTOCOLS

THERE IS NO COOKIE-CUTTER, ONE-SIZE-FITS-ALL PROTOCOL FOR Lyme disease treatment, but there are certain guidelines and plans that make sense. Let us now turn to the various medications that can be used to address these different infections. Please note that the following treatment protocols have been drawn from the ILADS treatment guidelines, Dr. Joseph Burrascano's Treatment Guidelines, information presented by other Lyme-literate medical doctors and experts in the field at ILADS conferences, and my own clinical experience. This information does not represent the position of the IDSA which believes only in 14-28 days of antibiotic therapy. I believe their position is flawed and not valid in the real world of Lyme disease.

Acute, or Early-Stage, Lyme Disease

Before we go through all the various medications used in chronic Lyme treatment, let us look at possible medication protocols for acute Lyme. Acute Lyme here refers to the first few weeks of infection. As we have learned, lab testing may not be reliable at that early stage as the immune system may not yet have mounted a response, so diagnosis is made based on history of tick bite, EM rash and/ or flu-like illness following a tick exposure.

If a person has had a known tick bite, it may be indicated to do prophylactic treatment even in the absence of the EM rash or symptoms. It is critical to begin treatment as quickly as possible in early Lyme disease, as early, aggressive treatment may prevent the development of chronic Lyme disease and may literally save the patient's quality of life for years to come.

A prophylactic protocol could involve four weeks of the following combination of antibiotics -

    Doxycycline 200mg – twice daily
    Tinidazole 500mg – twice daily

Western Blot testing would be done 6-8 weeks after the bite.

For a known acute Lyme illness, 6-8 weeks of treatment is required, but if treated early enough and aggressively enough, Lyme may be eradicated completely. Doxycycline is typically the medication of choice in early Lyme, not only because of its activity against Borrelia but also for its ability to eliminate Ehrlichia and some of the other co-infections.

The following is Dr. Richard Horowitz's acute Lyme protocol (presented at ILADS Conference, Toronto, 2011)[1]:

First month:

    Doxycycline 200mg – twice daily
    Hydroxychloroquine (Plaquenil) – 200mg –twice daily; *or*
    Tinidazole 500mg – twice daily

Second month:

    Cefuroxime 500mg – twice daily
    Azithromycin 500mg – once daily;
    or clarithromycin 500mg –twice daily
    Hydroxychloroquine (Plaquenil) 200mg – twice daily; *or*
    Tinidazole 500mg twice daily

I have also combined the following and prescribed a two-month protocol of –

    Doxycycline 200mg – twice daily
    Azithromycin 500mg – once daily
    Cefuroxime 500mg – three times daily
    Tinidazole 500mg – twice daily

Suggested Medication Protocols

If the person is not symptomatic at the end of the two-month protocol, it is still advised to follow with antimicrobial herbs for two more months. If no symptoms remain beyond that, Lyme disease has probably been eradicated. If symptoms persist, however, treatment would be continued per the regimens for chronic Lyme disease.

Chronic Lyme Treatment

For simplicity and organization of information, the medication protocols suggested are listed according to which phase of the Borrelia life cycle they address, and for the intended co-infection.

Borrelia

Spirochete Forms of Borrelia

The medications used for these forms act by damaging the spirochete's cell wall. The two main classes of medications are penicillins and cephalosporins, although work by Eva Sapi of University of New Haven indicates that tinidazole (listed here under cyst-form medications below) may be an effective medication for all forms of Lyme disease including spirochete forms.[2]

Penicillins

Amoxicillin:

Amoxicillin is an oral form of penicillin. It is not considered the most effective antibiotic for Borrelia, but amoxicillin is still more effective than penicillin V. High doses ranging from 3-6 grams per day must be taken to achieve benefit.

To boost the effectiveness of amoxicillin, probenecid can be given simultaneously, at a dose of 500mg every 8 hours. Another alternative is Augmentin XR, which is amoxicillin and clavulanate. 1000mg can be given every 8 hours, up to 2000mg every 12 hours. Additional amoxicillin may still have to be given separately for full benefit.

Amoxicillin is contraindicated in anyone with a penicillin allergy. It can be safely used in pregnancy and breastfeeding, and is often given to children.

Bicillin LA:

Bicillin LA is an injection into the muscle, administered 2-3 times per week. It is a long-acting penicillin so it is easier to get sustained levels of this antibiotic, which gives greater benefit. Bicillin LA is significantly more effective than oral amoxicillin due to it's good central nervous system penetration, which helps neurological symptoms. In particular, I find Bicillin LA to be very helpful in addressing the cognitive deficits that are so typical in Lyme disease, such as brain fog and memory loss. As an injectable, it bypasses the gastrointestinal tract so it does not contribute to gut issues to the same extent that oral antibiotics might.

As with oral amoxicillin, it should not be used in anyone with a penicillin allergy. Some patients find the injections themselves to be quite uncomfortable, and this can be partially offset by making sure the liquid is at room temperature before injecting (not straight out of the fridge) and by injecting it slowly, over a period of a few minutes. Heating pads afterwards can help disperse the medication through the muscle tissue, minimizing aching in the area.

Bicillin LA is readily available in Australia. I consider it to be a good compromise between oral and IV antibiotics. It comes in vials containing 0.9 million units. Most start with 1 vial injected in the gluteus muscle three times weekly, and some do two vials of 0.9 million units three times weekly.

Bicillin injections can produce significant and prolonged Herxes. Some patients will notice a Herx reaction in the first few days while others experience it around day 25-30 of their Bicillin regimen. Bicillin LA is one of my favourite medications in the treatment of chronic Lyme disease.

Cephalosporins
Ceftriaxone:
Ceftriaxone is a 3rd generation cephalosporin that is given intravenously for the treatment of Lyme disease. Theoretically it can also be given intramuscularly, however that is not a practical long-term dosing method and is not widely used.

IV ceftriaxone has historically been given in doses of two grams every day. More recently, better results have been seen with pulsed dosing of two grams twice daily, four days on with three days off each week.

(See below for more information on the merits of IV versus oral antibiotics).

Cefuroxime axetil:
Cefuroxime axetil is a 2nd generation oral cephalosporin, and it is widely available. The recommended dose is 1 gram twice daily. Cefuroxime can be used during pregnancy and breastfeeding, and can be given to children.

In general, while 3rd generation cephalosporins are considered more effective than 1st and 2nd, cefuroxime has great benefit as it also has activity against Staph, so it is good for treating atypical EM rashes that may contain bacteria other than Borrelia.

Cell-wall Deficient Forms of Borrelia
Macrolides
Erythromycin:
This is not an effective medication for Borrelia and is not recommended.

Azithromycin:
Azithromycin is a gentle medication that is typically well tolerated. While it is not among the most effective for Borrelia itself nor used as a first-line therapy, it has its place in Lyme treatment protocols. I choose it as a starting medication in patients who have high sensitivity levels to prescription medications, sometimes dosing it just three days per week. It

is more effective for musculoskeletal symptoms such as joint and muscle pain than neurological symptoms. Some individuals who would not be able to tolerate doxycycline can handle azithromycin. Typical doses are 500-600mg daily given in a single dose. Azithromycin has a very long half-life so once daily dosing is possible.

Clarithromycin:

Somewhat more potent and more effective than azithromycin, clarithromycin also has greater tolerability issues. Many people experience some gastrointestinal side effects such as nausea, as well as a metallic taste in the mouth. Clarithromycin may cause more significant Candida overgrowth problems when compared with azithromycin, in part because it must be dosed more frequently due to its shorter half-life.

Azithromycin and clarithromycin are not considered first line drugs for Lyme due to their limited effectiveness. This may relate to the fluid pocket created around the Borrelia bacteria in the cell. The fluid is quite acidic, meaning it has a low pH, and that acidity may inactivate azithromycin and clarithromycin. A way to overcome this is to give hydroxychloroquine (Plaquenil) or amantadine, which can raise the pH of the fluid and allow the two medications to work better. (This does not apply to telithromycin, which is not affected by the pH levels).

In spite of their limitations, azithromycin and clarithromycin still have a significant place in Lyme disease therapy especially when combined with other antibiotics. They are just not stand-alone medications. Mepron, a medication for Babesia, requires either azithromycin or clarithromycin for it to work effectively, so sometimes that dictates the inclusion of such medications in an individual's protocol. Also, azithromycin and clarithromycin, having the same purpose as the tetracyclines such as doxycycline and minocycline (which is to target cell-wall deficient forms), tend to work well along with them. They act slightly differently as they work on slightly different ribosomes, but they fulfil the same goal and are often used concurrently for that reason.

Clindamycin:

Clindamycin is sometimes used for Borrelia and also Bartonella. It can be effective as it penetrates the central nervous system and gets deep into other tissues to address deep-seated infection in the body. The biggest caution with clindamycin is its propensity to cause pseudomembranous colitis, which will cause unrelenting diarrhoea. Prevention is the key with high doses of mixed strain probiotics including Saccharomyces boulardii. The dose of clindamycin is 300mg two to three times daily.

Telithromycin:

Telithromycin, although not widely used, may be the most effective of the macrolide antibiotics. It has more serious side effects such as cardiac irregularities and liver enzyme elevation, so it requires close monitoring (EKG and liver enzymes every two weeks). It also has numerous interactions with other medications due to its effect on liver enzyme systems that regulate the metabolism of certain drugs. Telithromycin can provoke strong and prolonged Herxheimer reactions. It is dosed at 800mg once daily, and does not need amantadine or hydroxychloroquine to boost its efficacy. Given its toxicity and side effect profile, many Lyme-literate medical doctors in the United States will not prescribe telithromycin.

Tetracyclines

Doxycycline:

Doxycycline is perhaps the most widely used medication in Lyme disease treatment. It is used in acute Lyme but is equally effective in more chronic cases. Doxycycline has broad-spectrum activity against Borrelia along with co-infections such as Bartonella, Ehrlichia and Mycoplasma.

Doses of doxycycline are typically 200mg twice daily and as high as 600mg daily. 200mg twice daily has been shown to be more effective than 100mg four times daily. It should not to be used during pregnancy or breastfeeding, or in children younger than eight years of age (it can cause irreversible tooth staining in kids). Side effects of doxycycline include headaches, gastrointestinal disturbance and increased sun sensitivity. It is best taken two hours away from metronidazole and tinidazole due to its ability to bind with them and impede absorption, and also two hours away from dairy products and minerals such as calcium and magnesium.

It has a broader spectrum of activity than minocycline when addressing Lyme with co-infections.

Minocycline:

Minocycline is not used as widely as doxycycline in Lyme disease treatment. It is more lipid soluble than doxycycline so it may have greater benefit in neuroborreliosis, but for this same reason it tends to have more vestibular side effects such as headache and dizziness. The dosing of minocycline is 100mg three times daily. It creates slightly less sun sensitivity and GI side effects as compared with doxycycline, but despite this, doxycycline remains the preferred choice. Minocycline is sometimes used for its profound anti-inflammatory effects which can be particularly helpful in reducing neurological symptoms.

Tetracycline:

Tetracycline dosed at 500mg 3-4 times daily may be used if well tolerated. It is not used as frequently as minocycline or doxycycline, perhaps due to its lower central nervous system penetration or tolerability issues.

Cyst Forms of Borrelia

Metronidazole (Flagyl):

Metronidazole can be used for cyst forms of Borrelia but has gastrointestinal side effects and tolerability issues. For this reason it is not my first choice. It is dosed 500mg twice daily and can be pulsed 2 weeks on/ 2 weeks off. Optimally it is dosed separately from doxycycline or minocycline by two hours.

Metronidazole is not safe in pregnancy as it can cause birth defects, but it can be used in children. Metronidazole will heighten one's sensitivity to alcohol and cause severe reactions, so patients on metronidazole are warned to avoid all alcohol. Since herbal tinctures are often preserved with alcohol, more sensitive patients put their herbs in hot water to evaporate off the alcohol before drinking them. For most patients the amount of alcohol in drop doses of herbs will not be enough to cause them problems.

Tinidazole:

Tinidazole comes with many of the same cautions as metronidazole, as it is in the same family of drugs. It cannot be used in pregnancy and does not combine well with alcohol, yet tinidazole seems to be much better tolerated and causes less GI upset. The dosing schedule is the same— 500mg twice daily, pulsed two weeks on/ two weeks off. Tinidazole is my first choice in cyst-form medications for Borrelia. As with metronidazole, it can provoke quite significant Herxes, however most notice that after the first two or three cycles, the Herx reaction is lessened. Professor Eva Sapi studied metronidazole and tinidazole and found that the latter was much more effective in destroying colonies of Borrelia.

Plaquenil:

Plaquenil is essentially an anti-malaria drug, although it has multiple uses in medicine. In Lyme treatment we primarily use it to address cyst forms of Borrelia.

Plaquenil is widely used by rheumatologists for Rheumatoid Arthritis. It has anti-inflammatory effects, and appears to have immune modulating effects. I have found that Plaquenil can lessen pain and inflammation in Lyme patients with severe musculoskeletal symptoms. Unlike prednisone, which is immune suppressive (*and should never be used in patients with Lyme*), Plaquenil is more immune modulating and balancing, thus reducing the autoimmune process without wiping out the beneficial and necessary parts of immune function.

Another benefit of Plaquenil as mentioned above is the way it can shift the pH of the cell to make azithromycin and clarithromycin work better.

One of the major cautions with Plaquenil is that long-term use can cause retinal artery problems. Patients are advised to get an eye exam before starting treatment and every three months thereafter.

Alinia:

Alinia has less of a track record in chronic Lyme disease treatment but in recent years has been used as a cyst-form medication. It may also be effective for Babesia, thus having double benefit. The dosage is 500mg twice daily. Alinia's on-label use is intestinal parasitic infections such as Giardia and Cryptosporidium, and some patients do find that they have some diarrhoea when starting Alinia. It is unclear whether that is medication sensitivity or a response to the die-off of existing intestinal parasites, although new research indicates that Lyme disease may in fact involve various parasitic infestations of not just the intestinal tract, but also other areas throughout the body.

REFERENCES

1. Horowitz RI. Lyme Disease & Babesiosis: updates on diagnosis and treatment 2011 [Video]. ILADS, producers. Toronto (CA): ILADS Conference; 2011. 10:58 min., sound, color. Available from: http://www.ilads.org/media/videos/videos_horowitz.php.

2. Sapi E, Kaur N, Anyanwu S, et al. Evaluation of in-vitro antibiotic susceptibility of different morphological forms of Borrelia burgdorferi. Infection and Drug Resistance [Internet]. 2011 [cited 2012 May];4:97-113. Available from: http://www.dovepress.com/evaluation-of-in-vitro-antibiotic-susceptibility-of-different-morpholo-peer-reviewed-article-IDR-MVP DOI: http://dx.doi.org/10.2147/IDR.S19201

17. MEDICATION PROTOCOLS FOR CO-INFECTIONS AND RELATED TOPICS

Babesia

Of all the co-infections, Babesia has the most distinct regimen of medications because it is a protozoal parasitic infection, not a bacterial infection as are Borrelia, Bartonella and Ehrlichia. Until recent years, the usual treatment regimen was clindamycin plus quinine; however, this regimen has been abandoned due to an unacceptable incidence of severe side effects.

Atovaquone:

One of the primary medications of choice for Babesia, atovaquone goes under the brand name of Mepron in the United States and Wellvone in Australia. Nicknamed "liquid gold", mostly because of its price, it has a good track record in Babesia treatment. Standard dosage is 750mg twice daily, which equates to 1 teaspoon twice daily, however some patients need higher doses, up to 2 teaspoons twice daily. Atovaquone can cause a mild yellowish discoloration of the vision and mild gastrointestinal side effects but is generally quite well tolerated.

An important point about atovaquone is that it must be taken with significant amounts of fatty food to facilitate its absorption. Research shows that 22 grams of fat is the ideal amount. There are healthy ways to get this amount of fat without justifying a large helping of chips or a burger. See Appendix C for a list of healthy fats and fatty foods.

Atovaquone in the form of Wellvone must be combined with a macrolide such as azithromycin, clarithromycin or telithromycin, in the standard dosages listed previously. Patients on Wellvone should not take supplements containing CoQ10 or milk thistle, as those two supplements can reduce the efficacy of the Wellvone.

When Babesia is chronic, at least four to six months of treatment is required. Multiple medications are often needed, as it can be a difficult infection to eradicate. Babesia duncani may be more aggressive and treatment resistant than Babesia microti.

Malarone:

Malarone is a combination of atovaquone and proguanil. Although the standard dose of malarone contains only 1000mg of actual atovaquone compared with 1500mg in 10 mL of Wellvone, the proguanil helps to boost its effectiveness. Malarone is dosed at 2 tablets twice daily of the 250/100mg strength. It does not need a macrolide antibiotic along with it, so may be a better starting point in more sensitive patients. When cost is a major issue, Malarone is marginally less expensive than Wellvone. Both need high amounts of fatty foods taken at the same time to help with absorption. Overall, I consider Wellvone to be a more potent medication than Malarone; concurrent use of Bactrim DS or Septra may boost its efficacy. CoQ10 and milk thistle should also be avoided when taking Malarone.

Lariam (Mefloquine):

Mefloquine is another medication that is used in malaria treatment and prophylaxis. It is a tablet dosed at 250mg once every five to seven days. It can be taken along with atovaquone. I typically use atovaquone for six to eight weeks to reduce the overall parasitic load before introducing mefloquine, however I have seen mefloquine be very effective on the neurological aspects of Babesia such as anxiety and depression.

Mefloquine carries with it some possible neuropsychiatric side effects. On the milder end, vivid dreams or an exacerbation of depression or

Medication Protocols for Co-infections and Related Topics

anxiety may occur; on the more serious end, hallucinations, suicidal ideation and even psychosis have been reported.

My experience with mefloquine in my patients is that it can definitely cause a temporary worsening of psycho-emotional symptoms; however I have observed that to be consistent with a Herxheimer-type pattern where a patient's existing symptoms flare up at the beginning of treatment. I have not seen any cases of the more severe psychiatric side effects. Individuals with a history of bipolar disorder, schizophrenia or other serious mental illness would be poor candidates for mefloquine, but I consider it a very effective medication in Babesia treatment, particularly where Babesia is affecting the brain and causing psycho-emotional symptoms.

Coartem/ Riamet:

Under brand names of either Coartem or Riamet, these medications are a combination of artemether and lumefantrine. Again, they are used in malaria treatment, as well as Babesiosis. The advantage of Coartem is that it is only dosed twice a day for three days each month. The down side is that other Babesia medications and macrolide or quinolone antibiotics must be stopped for those three days plus two to three days on each side, so that can create quite a disruption in the treatment protocol.

Alinia:

Alinia has already been discussed as a possible cyst-form medication for Borrelia, but it also used in the treatment of Babesia. Dosing is 500mg twice daily. Alinia does not have as much of an established track record for Babesia as atovaquone, however I often use it in combination therapy, when either atovaquone ceases to have beneficial effect or the cost becomes prohibitive.

Septra/ Bactrim:

These two medications are a combination of trimethoprim and sulfamethoxazole. They are referred to as sulfa drugs, so anyone with an allergy to sulfa drugs cannot take either of these two medications.

Septra and Bactrim are good choices in combination therapy where Borrelia and co-infections are present. Subsequently I will choose these especially for treatment protocols for Borrelia along with the co-infections of Babesia or Bartonella. Significant Herxheimer reactions can be expected, sometimes lasting several weeks.

Bartonella

Rifampicin:

Rifampicin is one of the primary medications used in the treatment of Bartonella. It is not particularly effective for Borrelia but is a good medication to be used in combination therapy.

Rifampicin may cause a harmless orange discoloration of urine, and even sweat and tears. This is due to the inherent colour of the medication and not liver problems, as some people assume. Having said that, rifampicin can be liver toxic, so liver enzymes must be monitored regularly (at least monthly).

Rifampicin combines well with doxycycline for Bartonella treatment. Azithromycin and clarithromycin may increase its action and are commonly used along with it. In some cases, through influence on liver enzyme systems, it can impact the rate of metabolism of other drugs, so interactions should be monitored closely. Theoretically rifampicin can be given with Wellvone or Malarone, but it may reduce their efficacy. Dosing is 300mg twice daily, but is often commenced at 150mg twice daily to monitor sensitivity and Herx reactions.

Rifampicin can cause hormone dysregulation including an increase in Sex Hormone Binding Globulin (SHBG), so people with hormone irregularities should be monitored closely or should not use Rifampicin.

Septra/ Bactrim:

As in Babesia treatment, Septra or Bactrim DS can add a powerful boost to co-infection treatment protocols and both have been used in the treatment of Bartonella. See the section above on Babesia treatment for more information about these drugs.

Ciprofloxacin:

Ciprofloxacin is in the quinolone category of antibiotics. In the United States, a related medication called Levaquin is primarily used from this category; however Levaquin is not available in Australia. Dosing of Ciprofloxacin is 500-750mg daily.

Ciprofloxacin can be effective for Bartonella, but it is not my first choice due to its significant potential side effect of causing tendonitis, and even tendon rupture. Tendons are the connective tissues that connect bones to muscles, and tendonitis is the inflammation of these structures. Pain and swelling at the site are the primary signs, although in some cases rupture has occurred spontaneously, requiring surgical repair. Typically the larger tendons are affected first, such as the Achilles tendon behind the ankle, and tendons in the elbows and knees. Ciprofloxacin must be stopped at the first sign of tendon pain, although the risk of inflammation and even rupture may continue for several weeks or months. Preloading with magnesium may prevent issues, and high dose magnesium and vitamin C may be used to relieve pain and inflammation should it occur.

Other medications in this family are gemifloxacin (Factive) and moxifloxacin (Avalox).

Because of the tendon issue, the preferred choice of medications for Bartonella is a combination of doxycycline, rifampicin and azithromycin. Septra/ Bactrim DS may be added in patients who are not allergic to sulfa drugs.

Ehrlichia/ Anaplasma and Rickettsia

Doxycycline:

Given in similar doses to Borrelia, doxycycline is effective against both Ehrlichia and Anaplasma. Higher doses over several months are typically required for chronic cases – 400-600mg per day.

Rifampicin:

In treatment failures with doxycycline, or in combination therapy, rifampicin is the next medication of choice. 300mg twice daily is the dose, similar to Bartonella.

Mycoplasma

The role of mycoplasma in tick-borne illness is not fully understood, but many Lyme patients are also infected with mycoplasma.

Treatment regimens for mycoplasma involve combination therapy using doxycycline or minocycline, hydroxychloroquine, and azithromycin. Rifampin or Septra can also be helpful. In cases that do not respond to these medications, a quinolone such as Ciprofloxacin may be used; however the cautions given above regarding tendon damage apply.

Candida

While by definition more of a side effect than a co-infection, Candida overgrowth seems to be a common feature in tick-borne illness. Candida albicans is yeast that is naturally and normally found in the intestinal tract. In antibiotic therapy where both the "bad" flora and the "good" flora are indiscriminately killed, overgrowth of yeast can occur. This will be discussed in more detail in the next section on naturopathic treatments for tick-borne illness, but there are two primary medications that warrant discussion here.

Nystatin:

Nystatin is an anti-fungal medicine that targets intestinal yeast but is not absorbed through the gut into the blood stream. For this reason, it is a very safe and non-toxic medication as it does not put any stress on the liver. It is taken orally, goes on to kill yeast in the intestinal tract and is excreted through the bowels.

Nystatin is a valuable preventive medication and can be taken along with any antibiotic regimen. It needs to be dosed continuously, with a common dosage of 500,000 units given three times daily, since it does not build up in the system. Especially for women with a tendency towards vaginal yeast infections, Nystatin is recommended concurrently with antibiotic treatment protocols. Nystatin can be used to treat intestinal yeast overgrowth once it has arisen, although it is of limited benefit in more systemic manifestations.

Fluconazole:

Fluconazole (brand name Diflucan) is the heavier hitter of the anti-fungal medications. It does absorb systemically, which makes it more effective for systemic symptoms such as brain fog, vaginal yeast infections, and itchy skin rashes related to yeast overgrowth. On the other hand, the systemic absorption does make it more toxic, and it can add to liver stress when given alongside other medications. Whether used alone or with other drugs, liver tests should be administered periodically while using fluconazole.

If systemic yeast is suspected, one option is to take a 30-day course of fluconazole before long-term antibiotics are commenced, switching then to Nystatin along with antibiotics. Other patients take fluconazole just two to three days per week.

■ ■ ■ ■

Intravenous Versus Oral Administration of Antibiotics

Intravenous (IV) administration of antibiotics is another route that can be used in Lyme treatment. At the time of writing, access to IV antibiotics for Lyme in Australia is very limited, but hopefully, with increased education of the medical community, this situation will change and IV antibiotics will be accessible to a larger cohort.

IV therapy may be indicated in the following conditions –

- ▸ Illness duration longer than one year
- ▸ Major neurological involvement
- ▸ Lack of response to oral and/ or intramuscular medications

- Gastrointestinal function compromise to the point where oral medications are either not getting properly absorbed or are causing excessive GI side effects.

Some of the benefits of IV therapy include:

- Medications can be given in higher doses than oral to achieve higher blood levels.
- Medications given via IV bypass the gastrointestinal tract therefore have fewer GI side effects.
- Most of the medications given orally can be given via IV including doxycycline, azithromycin and metronidazole.

IV antibiotics are not necessarily the easy road or the magic bullet, however. Here are some of the potential issues:

- Having a PICC line or a central line can be very disruptive to activities of daily living. It requires daily maintenance, and risks of infection are always present.
- IV therapy may continue over several months, not just a few weeks. The minimum duration recommended for chronic Lyme is 14 weeks, however if the patient is showing improvement but is still symptomatic, even longer times may be required.
- IV ceftriaxone does not cover all phases of Borrelia nor does it address co-infections, so oral/ IM medications must still be administered for those. Very few patients do all of their three or four mediations via IV.
- IV ceftriaxone can cause biliary sludging and put the individual at risk of having to have their gall bladder surgically removed. (Interestingly, Dr. Burrascano believes that the gall bladder might be a reservoir of infection and has observed that his patients who do not have a gall bladder fare slightly better overall). Any surgery can be stressful for a Lyme patient, as it involves chemicals, anaesthesia, heightened risk of infection, adrenal and immune stress, and should be avoided where possible.
- IV ceftriaxone still clears through the liver and may still cause imbalances in the intestinal flora. Preventive measures to keep gut flora balanced must be undertaken.

Medication Protocols for Co-infections and Related Topics

Given that IV antibiotic therapy for chronic Lyme disease is not readily available in Australia at the current time, a good alternative is intramuscular administration of Bicillin LA. This is a very effective medication, has good central nervous system penetration, and relieves some of the burden on the gastrointestinal system. While still only addressing the spirochete form of Borrelia, and is therefore not a stand-alone therapy, Bicillin LA is one of the most effective antibiotics available for use in patients who do not have penicillin allergies.

Cautions With All Antibiotic Therapy

Long-term antibiotic therapy does have some potential side effects. Many possible issues can be easily detected with simple blood work done on a regular basis and sensible prophylactic measures.

Liver and kidney function must be checked every month. Multiple antibiotics for long durations can elevate liver enzymes and put stress on the kidneys. Labs include a complete blood count and a comprehensive metabolic panel that includes BUN, creatinine, AST, ALT and GGTP. If liver enzymes become elevated or kidney function is affected, medications may have to be slowed down, doses lowered or ceased for a duration of time until levels normalize.

Some oral antibiotics cause gastrointestinal side effects and imbalances in gut flora. If diarrhoea occurs, it may be a sign of yeast (Candida) overgrowth. Severe, ongoing diarrhoea should be evaluated for C. difficile (both toxins A and B) as a cause of colitis. Any antibiotics can predispose a person to C. difficile, but ceftriaxone and clindamycin may create a higher risk.

Medications such as telithromycin can prolong the QT interval and interfere with heart rhythm, so patients on this medication should have cardiac monitoring.

Women (and men!) also need to know that antibiotic therapy, especially the tetracycline family, may reduce the effectiveness of the oral contraceptive pill. Alternative birth control should be used while on antibiotic therapy.

While there are some risks to long-term antibiotic use, many of them can be prevented with naturopathic support such as herbs and adequate probiotics. This will be discussed in the next section. In general terms the benefits of long-term therapy usually outweigh the possible risks, and with careful monitoring, there can be minimal impact on the body from long-term treatment.

Antibiotic Therapy During Pregnancy and Breastfeeding

According to Dr. Joseph Burrascano and Dr. Charles Ray Jones, the optimal medications in pregnancy are –

Amoxicillin – 1 gram four times daily.
Bicillin LA – 1 injection three times weekly.
Cefuroxime – 1 gram every 12 hours.
Azithromycin – 500mg daily.

Starting in the early 80's, the Lyme Disease Foundation in Hartford, Connecticut kept a pregnancy registry over an eleven-year period. They found that women who took adequate amounts of antibiotics during pregnancy showed a very low, in fact almost zero, transmission rate to their baby. Doctors Burrascano and Jones have found similar statistics in their private practices.

At the ILADS annual conference in 2011, paediatric Lyme specialist Charles Ray Jones cited the following figures:

- Women with active Lyme disease who do not take antibiotics have a 50% chance of passing the infection to their child.
- Women who take one antibiotic during pregnancy have a 25% chance of passing Lyme disease to their child.
- Women who take two antibiotics during pregnancy have less than a 5% chance of passing Lyme disease on to their child.

Obviously, many women are reluctant to take antibiotics during pregnancy for fear of harming their baby. Certainly, there are specific medications that are not appropriate, such as the tetracycline class of antibiotics, and metronidazole and tinidazole. The medications cited in the prior paragraph are deemed safe in pregnancy. Still, it is a very personal and difficult decision to make. In my opinion, although taking antibiotics during pregnancy is not ideal, it is a far better choice than risking the transmission of Lyme disease to a baby, which could then impact his or her entire life. Since Borrelia spirochetes have been detected in breast milk by PCR testing, the antibiotic regimens above should be continued during this time also, or breast-feeding avoided.

Antibiotic Therapy for Children

Children can be treated with antibiotic therapy, but the medication choices and dosages will be adjusted for them. Tetracyclines are not used in children eight years and younger because of their ability to cause a permanent discolouration of the teeth.

Antibiotics considered safe and effective for children include:

Amoxicillin – 50mg/ kg/ day divided into doses every 8 hours
Cefuroxime axetil – 125mg-500mg every 12 hours based on weight.
Azithromycin – 250-500mg daily depending on their weight.
Tinidazole -125-250mg daily depending on their weight. May be pulsed two days per week.
Grapefruit seed extract—may be a better option for covering cyst-forms in children.

Practical Application

To summarize, the general principles of antibiotic prescribing in chronic Lyme disease are:

- ▶ Start with one medication at a time and assess reactions, side effects, Herx reactions and benefits. More resilient patients may add a new medication after two weeks; more sensitive ones may need 4-6 weeks.
- ▶ Layer in medications for all three forms of Borrelia.
- ▶ Prioritise co-infection treatment based on symptom picture as well as lab results—decipher which co-infection is dominant. If

LYME DISEASE in Australia

evidence or suspicion of Babesia consider treating that early along with Borrelia.
- Base the aggressiveness of a person's treatment on Herx levels and patient sensitivity.
- Recognize that Lyme disease requires higher doses of medications and for longer durations than typically used. Two years of treatment is not unusual.
- Treat for two months beyond resolution of symptoms.

Following is a summary of medications to consider along with dosing information and some sample protocols. For convenience this information is reprinted in Appendix D.

Medication Summary

Form of Borrelia	Medication class	Commonly used examples
Spirochetes	Penicillins	Amoxicillin, Bicillin LA
	Cephalosporins	Cefuroxime, Ceftriaxone
Cell-wall deficient	Macrolides	Azithromycin, Clarithrocin
	Tetracyclines	Doxycycline, Minocycline
Cyst forms		Tinidazole, Metronidazole Hydroxychloroquine (Plaquenil), Alinia

The ultimate goal of therapy for Borrelia –

- 1 cell-wall active medication (for spirochetes)
- 2 intracellular medications (for cell-wall deficient forms)
- 1 cyst form medication (for cysts)

Plus medications added for relevant co-infections.

Medication Protocols for Co-infections and Related Topics

Common Dosages

Penicillins:
Amoxicillin	1000mg	3-6 daily
Augmentin XR	2000mg	2x daily
Bicillin LA	0.9 mill	2 vials injected IM 3x weekly

Cephalosporins:
Cefuroxime	500mg	3x daily
Ceftriaxone	2 gram	2 grams twice daily IV 4 days/week

Macrolides:
Azithromycin	500mg	1x daily
Clarithromycin	500mg	2x daily
Telithromycin	800mg	1x daily

Tetracyclines:
Minocycline	100mg	3-4x daily
Doxycycline	100mg	2 twice daily
Tetracycline	500mg	3-4x daily

Cyst-form medications:
Metronidazole	500mg	2x daily; 2 weeks on/ 2 weeks off
Tinidazole	500mg	2x daily; 2 weeks on/ 2 weeks off
Plaquenil	200mg	2x daily

Babesia medications:
Wellvone	750mg/ 5mL	1-2 teaspoons twice daily
Malarone	250/ 100mg	2 twice daily
Lariam	250mg	1 every five days
Alinia	500mg	2x daily

Bartonella, Ehrlichia, Anaplasma, Rickettsia medications:
Rifampicin	300mg	2x daily
Ciprofloxacin	500mg	1x daily
Bactrim DS	800/160mg	2x daily

Sample Medication Protocols

Borrelia:

Doxycycline 200mg twice daily

After two weeks add Tinidazole 500mg twice daily 2 weeks on/ 2 weeks off

One month later add Bicillin LA 0.9 million units 3x weekly

One month later add Clarithromycin 500mg twice daily

Borrelia in a highly sensitive patient:

Azithromycin 250mg given Monday-Wednesday-Friday

Add Plaquenil 200mg twice daily

Build up azithromycin dose until tolerating 500mg daily

Add oral amoxicillin 1 gram three times daily

Add minocycline 100mg twice daily

Borrelia in a patient with a penicillin allergy:

Doxycycline 200mg twice daily

Cefuroxime 500mg three times daily

Tinidazole 500mg twice daily, 2 weeks on/ 2 weeks off

Babesia as the dominant infection:

Plaquenil 200mg twice daily

Clarithromycin 500mg twice daily

Mepron 750mg/ 5mL – 1 teaspoon twice daily

After 6-8 weeks – add Mefloquine 250mg every five days

After 12-14 weeks – add Bactrim DS twice daily

Borrelia + Babesia:

Doxycycline 400mg daily

Plaquenil 200mg twice daily

Azithromycin 500mg daily

Mepron 5mL twice daily

Bicillin LA 0.9 mill units 3 times weekly

Medication Protocols for Co-infections and Related Topics

Borrelia + Bartonella:

Doxycycline 200mg twice daily

Tinidazole 500mg twice daily, 2 weeks on/ 2 weeks off

Rifampicin 300mg twice daily

Bicillin LA 0.9 mill units 3 times weekly, or Cefuroxime 500mg three times daily

Can add Bactrim DS twice daily

18. FUNDAMENTALS OF NATURAL MEDICINE IN LYME DISEASE

NATURAL MEDICINE PLAYS SUCH A SIGNIFICANT ROLE IN THE treatment of Lyme disease. In fact, I do not believe in using antibiotic protocols without also using supportive natural therapies alongside them – that is where side effects and unwanted effects on the body occur. Some people decide not to do antibiotic therapy at all and rely solely on natural treatments, while others turn to natural treatments as they either cannot tolerate antibiotics or have seen limited benefit from them. As a practitioner I will only treat Lyme disease with antibiotics in conjunction with the profound benefit and protection of naturopathic support. In my opinion, a combination of both is the preferred approach.

Natural medicines and therapeutics do everything from supporting detoxification and offsetting Herx reactions to actually killing bugs, balancing hormones and supporting immune function.

Different kinds of naturopathic modalities include nutrition, herbal medicine, homeopathy, manual therapies such as the Bowen technique, detoxification therapies, chelation agents (for heavy metal detox), frequency-based therapies such as Rife therapy, salt/ C protocol, enzyme therapies and the list goes on. There are literally hundreds of modalities that can be implemented.

In my practice, I rely heavily on herbal medicines, the use of specific nutrient combinations, and dietary modifications to support and enhance Lyme disease treatment.

The Role of Natural Therapies with Antibiotic Protocols

Naturopathic therapies are primarily used with antibiotics to prevent or offset any possible side effects. The three main aspects to be addressed are -

1. Supporting detoxification to minimize Herxheimer reactions

2. Preventing liver and kidney stress during antibiotic therapy

3. Keeping gut flora balanced and preventing yeast overgrowth

1. Supporting detoxification to minimize Herxheimer reactions

We have already discussed how Herxheimer reactions can occur when antimicrobial therapy is undertaken, whether natural or pharmaceutical. Herx reactions involve a worsening of a person's current or typical symptoms, caused by the release of endotoxins when bacteria, yeast or parasites are killed off, and caused by inflammatory processes as the immune system is engaged to target the exposed infections.

If a Herx gets too severe, antibiotics may need to be reduced or even stopped while the body catches up and clears the toxins. Many people with Lyme have somewhat limited detoxification capacity anyway, and so Herx reactions can become a major issue. Herxes can also be dangerous to the patient, especially when vital functions such as heart function and breathing or swallowing are affected. And of course, Herxes simply make people feel terrible – they can intensify symptoms of pain, inflammation, joint swelling or stiffness, cognitive problems, sleep disturbance, debilitating fatigue and so on. Lyme disease never feels great, so the concept of it getting worse with treatment can be daunting for many, especially when it can last for days to weeks.

In many ways, one's success in recovering from Lyme disease is closely related to one's ability to detoxify, and Herxheimer reactions can be the limiting factor in the progression of treatment if these mechanisms are compromised. Thankfully, naturopathic treatments can greatly improve this by facilitating detoxification in the body. *I prefer detoxification support to be given in advance of any antibiotic therapy to prepare the body.* The body's detox systems should be upregulated before the neurotoxins are kicked up – trying to get control of it mid-way through will be a more difficult task.

There are a couple of remedies that I use to minimize Herxheimer reactions, and they work well together.

The first is a herb called Smilax, or Chinese Sarsaparilla. It works by neutralizing neurotoxins so it is a first-line choice in Herx reactions. In a very few patients, it can cause a slight detox reaction itself, but only in the most sensitive few. For most, it provides relief from Herxing, and is considered a gentle herb that is neuro-protective.

It also has anti-inflammatory properties so it can help joint and muscle pain. I have had patients who were able to reduce or eliminate pain medications with the introduction of Smilax due to both its detox and anti-inflammatory properties.

It is important to use Smilax glabrae (as opposed to other kinds of smilax) as it crosses the blood-brain barrier. This gives it an edge in neurological Lyme, where it can help with cognitive symptoms such as brain fog and memory issues, numbness/ tingling, nerve pain and other neurological deficits.

Glutathione is my next favourite remedy for supporting detoxification and minimizing the impact of Herx reactions. Glutathione, which protects every cell against oxidative stress and damage, is one of the key antioxidants in the body. It helps other antioxidants in cells remain in their active form and also plays a role in DNA synthesis and repair, enhancement of the immune system, and prevention of fat oxidation. Glutathione is a key element in liver detoxification and is liver protective.

I find that glutathione tends to improve cognitive issues in patients, which is usually most welcome. Interestingly, studies have shown glutathione levels to be lower in patients with Parkinson's disease. While we do not have copious research data to demonstrate this, it is a logical prediction that many Lyme patients have reduced glutathione levels also.

Glutathione must be taken in a specific form. If simply taken as a generic glutathione capsule, it will not be highly usable and absorbable by the body. More sophisticated delivery systems have been developed, my favourite being the liposomal reduced L-glutathione. The reduced glutathione is superior over the oxidized; do not worry about the biochemistry – one is useful, the other is not. You want the useful one. The liposomal delivery system means that even though it is taken orally, it is absorbed through the mucous membranes of the mouth and digestive tract, rather than being "digested" in the gut (which is where the loss of absorption occurs as it literally is converted into an oxidized form).

Glutathione can also be very effective when given intravenously – higher doses can be administered, and it goes directly into the blood stream. Availability and cost of this route are usually limiting factors. Transdermal (on the skin) glutathione creams and gels are other options and absorb well. I still prefer the oral liposomal form for convenience and effectiveness. As anyone who takes glutathione can attest, it is a sulphur-based compound and that is evident in the taste. Most people do not want to rub that smell into their skin and carry it around on them all day! Researched Nutritionals, the brand I prefer for glutathione, has released an orange-flavoured version, which most people prefer.

The other aspect of minimizing Herx reactions is to bind the toxins to facilitate their removal. Smilax and glutathione are great at neutralizing toxins, but we also have to get them out of the body.

Chlorella can be a good binding agent and works well for drawing out heavy metals also. Some people find it upsetting to the gastrointestinal tract. Other good binders include apple pectin, bentonite clay and activated charcoal. Generally speaking, a diet high in fibre will help elimination through the bowels by its sweeping effect. Ground flax seed or psyllium husk integrated into a daily protein smoothie work well. Binders are generally considered to be substances which stay in the digestive tract and absorb toxins which are dumped there via the bile, as most fat soluble toxins are.

A summary of ideas to manage Herxes is given in Appendix E.

2. Preventing liver and kidney stress during antibiotic therapy

When taking long-term antibiotics and multiple antibiotics, one of the risks is the extra work the liver and kidneys must do to detoxify and eliminate the medications. As a caution, we check liver and kidney function through lab testing at least once a month.

More common than kidney problems is an elevation in liver enzymes, which can be mild or severe. In some cases, medications must be reduced or ceased to allow enzyme levels to come down, which interrupts treatment.

As always, prevention is better than cure. Natural remedies that support liver function should be in place even before any medications are commenced.

Glutathione is definitely one of the key nutrients for the liver as it helps the liver remove chemicals that are foreign to the body. It is no coincidence that in the body, glutathione levels are highest in the liver and kidneys, two of the major organs of elimination. Glutathione also helps with the detoxification of heavy metals, which are often a problem for Lyme patients (more on that later). Its upregulation of liver enzyme systems and its ability to bind toxins in the body including chemical residues of antibiotics and other medications make it a valuable remedy for assisting the liver and kidneys.

There are several herbs that have great liver protective and liver cleansing properties. Dandelion root is one of my favourites because it is safe, gentle, effective and will not interfere with medications. Dandelion leaf can be used too, although it has a greater affinity for the kidneys, restoring mineral balance as it flushes out toxins.

Dandelion root's benefit comes from oils and bitter resins that stimulate digestive function and bile flow, combined with a viscous fibre which binds and transports toxins out of the body. It can be taken as a herbal tincture or as a tea. A product such as Bonvit's Dandelion Root makes a great coffee substitute and is actually better for the liver than coffee, which just adds to the toxic burden!

Milk thistle is perhaps the best-known liver herb. It has been used extensively to protect liver cells against toxins and the toxic effects of medications. It contains flavonoids, which prevent liver cells from damage and also aid in their regeneration. The only drawback of milk thistle is that is does not combine well with Wellvone and Malarone. It can interfere with their absorption, so people taking these two Babesia medications should not take milk thistle.

RestorMedicine Detox Support Formula #1 is a liver formula that contains milk thistle and is used in patients not on Wellvone or Malarone; Detox Support Formula #2 has the milk thistle removed so that is a good choice for those on Wellvone or Malarone.

Liquorice root is another herb that has great benefit for the liver. Studies have shown that liquorice can increase the body's production of interferon, which supports both liver function and immune function. Its anti-inflammatory effects reduce medication-related liver inflammation and at the same time provide antioxidants to protect liver cells.

3. Keeping gut flora balanced and preventing yeast overgrowth

Antibiotics can disrupt the gut flora. In the intestinal tract there are billions of naturally occurring yeast and bacteria. The gut contains an entire ecosystem, which maintains a delicate balance. This ecosystem functions to maximize assimilation of nutrients and provides a complex immune system of its own. The gut has a complex system of defence in place given that the gut is one of the first-line points of entry into the body and consequently is exposed to so many outside influences.

Antibiotics may be good for eradicating bacteria in the body, which we want in bacterial illnesses such as Lyme disease. However they are not discriminating. They will also have an effect against the healthy bacteria in the gut. If the healthy bacteria in the gut are reduced, opportunistic yeast such as Candida can gain a foothold and grow beyond their normal and healthy levels. Candida albicans and other strains of yeast are completely natural and normal in the gut; it is when they overgrow that problems arise.

Yeast overgrowth may appear as intestinal gas and bloating, a white coating on the tongue, vaginal irritation or infections for women, itchy skin rashes, increased brain fog and fatigue, among other things.

You will not be surprised to hear me say that here, prevention is the key. High potency, high quality probiotic supplements must be used along with antibiotics to help keep the gut flora in balance and prevent yeast overgrowth. Optimally, a variety of different strains of acidophilus and bifido bacteria will be used, and many good probiotics provide that. There is a type of yeast called Saccharomyces boulardii that is actually supplemented to prevent yeast also. It is counterintuitive to give a yeast to prevent yeast, but the goal is simply to supply enough of the "good yeast" that the "bad yeast" cannot get a foothold.

Most probiotics contain living organisms and therefore must be refrigerated to maintain their potency. The exception to this is soil-based probiotics (such as Prescript-Assist by Researched Nutritionals). Soil-based probiotics work slightly differently and are less susceptible to heat. They can be a good option while travelling or when refrigerated probiotics are not practical.

Probiotics must be taken at least two hours apart from antibiotics, otherwise the antibiotics can kill them off, too. This is true of prescription antibiotics, but it also applies to any natural remedy that has antimicrobial properties (such as teasel root, samento, olive leaf and grapefruit seed extract), as well as anti-fungal medications and herbs. I suggest taking probiotics at night before bed so that they have several hours to colonize in the gut before an assault by another dose of antibiotics. At least 100 billion live organisms per day must be taken as a prevention/maintenance dose; for people with yeast issues 200 billion live organisms per day are needed.

Natural medicine can be very helpful in anti-fungal therapy if yeast overgrowth does arise and we will cover than in the next section. For now, the important thing is to recognize the importance of probiotics in the prevention of gut flora imbalances during antibiotic therapy.

General Naturopathic Principles

Everything discussed above, while being crucial when taking antibiotics, is just as applicable for those not on antibiotics. Supporting detoxification is imperative for all chronic Lyme patients. Aside from the infection itself, most chronically ill patients have some component of toxicity contributing to their illness. This can worsen muscle and joint pain, brain fog, fatigue and neurological deficits.

More on Detoxification

Part of toxin build up may come from defects in the methylation pathway. The methylation pathway is responsible for a host of different metabolic functions, including detox, energy production and certain brain chemicals such as serotonin. If methylation pathways are not supported, then these functions will be compromised. Methylation, as the name suggests, requires "methyl groups" to feed it. Certain natural supplements can act as "methyl donors", feeding the raw materials to fuel the pathway, just like putting petrol in a car.

Supplements that support methylation include dimethylglycine (DMG), trimethylglycine (TMG) and methylcobalamin (a form of the vitamin B12). Methyl-B12 given by injection three times weekly can provide a great boost to energy and immune function, while supporting methylation pathways for detoxification. If injections are not available, sublingual forms of MB12 are the next best. Folic acid is also an important nutrient for methylation, and is best given in the form of 5-methyl-tetrahydrafolate.

MTHFR genetic markers can be tested to assess for defects in methylation and can help guide the appropriate supplementation.

Part of supporting detoxification is aiming for a more alkaline state. Nutritional principles for this will be covered in the next section. Supplementing with chlorophyll or chlorella can help. I encourage patients to drink a glass of warm water with the juice of one lemon squeezed in it on a daily basis. This can be especially helpful during Herxes as it seems to reduce the intensity of symptoms.

Other easy at-home remedies to support detox include taking baths with either Epsom salts or baking soda. Epsom salts are magnesium sulfate. The magnesium is very relaxing to the muscles, easing aches and pains, while also promoting relaxation and sleep; the sulfate part promotes detoxification. Baking soda is used more for its alkaline effects, not as much to help detox.

Castor oil packs are an age-old remedy but still have benefit. When placed over the liver, castor oil packs have been known to stimulate gall bladder function and bile flow, and clear stagnation and toxic build up in the liver. If liver enzymes become elevated during antibiotic therapy, castor oil packs are a good addition to the program to help reduce them. They can be done daily during these times, but generally 3-4 times weekly is sufficient. I have also found castor oil packs to be useful when used on specific areas of pain and inflammation. Instructions as to how to use castor oil packs are given in Appendix F.

As previously mentioned, while the liver is responsible for detoxifying chemicals, hormones and metabolites of our foods, it is not the only organ of elimination. Once the liver converts harmful toxins into non-harmful types, they are excreted through the skin, lungs, bowels and kidneys. Subsequently anything that can be done to support these organs can be helpful. An example is far-infrared (FIR) sauna. FIR sauna operates at lower temperatures than regular saunas, but being a different type of heat wave it actually penetrates the tissues more deeply assisting the cells in releasing toxins and clearing them through the skin. FIR sauna is especially good for heavy metal detox, which will be discussed later in this section, as it helps release toxins from fat cells.

Helping to flush the kidneys by drinking two litres of water a day is beneficial. For the lungs, either sauna therapy or some aerobic exercise stimulates their function. The bowels are a major channel of elimination. It is crucial to have at least one, preferably two, bowel movements per day. Ground flax or psyllium husk can be added to smoothies or food; extra magnesium or vitamin C promotes bowel motility (too much will give diarrhoea however); and some will need to supplement with soluble and insoluble fibres such as apple pectin, guar gum and aloe.

Binding agents are generally not absorbed from the intestinal tract and can help remove toxins by holding on to them and "escorting" them out of the body, after the toxins are dumped into the gut via bile (bile is one of the major routes of elimination for many toxins, but since 90% of bile is reabsorbed, it is important to take binding agents so that toxins do not get reabsorbed by the body). Activated charcoal is a good binder – it has a lattice structure that can trap toxins – and for this reason is often given in cases of accidental poisoning. Taken 2-3 hours after an antimicrobial that is creating die-off can ease Herx-type symptoms. Chlorella is often used in heavy metal toxicity as a binder especially in the gut. Chlorella alone will not be sufficient to mobilize heavy metals from the tissues, but can be taken alongside chelation protocols and also may be a good idea to take when eating a meal containing seafood which may possibly be contaminated with heavy metals such as mercury. In cases of severe neurotoxicity during Herx reactions, a medication called Wellchol is sometimes used. It is a prescription medication that it used to lower cholesterol (again, by binding the fatty acids in bile), but has been used in some cases of chronic infectious illness and particularly where mould toxicity may be a factor. Again, binding to the bile to prevent reabsorption is one of the keys to eliminating toxins from the body.

The other detoxification channel that is often forgotten is the lymphatic system. The lymphatic system is like the storm drains of your body – it filters the blood and removes toxic debris, bringing it back through a series of vessels towards the heart where it can be dumped into the larger blood vessels to be taken to the liver. Essentially, it keeps the toxic muck from clogging up the blood vessels, and can also function to deliver foreign invaders such as viruses and bacteria to the immune system. Lymphatic flow can be supported using herbs such as cleavers, burdock and poke root. Dry skin brushing can also be an easy way to gently enhance lymphatic drainage (see Appendix G for detailed information on how to do skin brushing). Lymphatic drainage massage is a specific massage technique that accelerates lymph flow; however it can also release a flood of toxins and make people feel temporarily worse afterwards. Exercise will also help keep the lymphatic system moving.

Inflammation

Inflammation is a major part of chronic infectious illness such as Lyme disease. Inflammation also arises from Herxheimer reactions, which increases immune chemicals called cytokines. Inflammation causes much of the pain and swelling in the joints, muscles and other connective tissue in Lyme disease. It can also cause swelling around the lining of the heart, and in the brain.

Managing inflammation is an important aspect of Lyme treatment, and natural remedies can certainly support this. The dietary influences on inflammation will be discussed in the next section on nutrition. I use herbs extensively to reduce inflammation. One of the main ones is white willow. It is used to make aspirin and is the plant from which salicylic acid is derived.

Another effective anti-inflammatory agent is turmeric. Often as effective as pharmaceutical anti-inflammatories but without the side effects, turmeric can be a potent pain reliever through its inhibition of Cox-2 pathways. It has the added benefit of being a great liver detoxifier.

Another approach to reducing inflammation is to use proteolytic enzymes. Whereas digestive enzymes are taken with food to help break the food down into easily absorbable molecules, proteolytic enzymes are taken away from food and are intended to be absorbed systemically and break down the by-products of the inflammatory process. They can help reduce the signs and symptoms of inflammation, which are heat, redness and pain. Used extensively in musculoskeletal inflammation, proteolytic enzymes can have a much broader impact by facilitating healthy immune response and preventing auto-immunity that may occur when the body is in a chronic inflammatory state.

Certain healthy fats can be taken to reduce inflammation. While the "good fats" are omega-3, omega-6 and omega-9's, the omega-3 fats have the most potent anti-inflammatory effects and they should be supplemented. We will discuss this more in the next section on nutritional strategies for Lyme disease. Fish and flax oil can both be supplemented at doses of two to six grams per day to provide omega-3 fatty acids and to help dampen inflammation.

Immune Function

Immune support is a crucial part of Lyme disease treatment. Our immune systems are our body's defence systems. They help to fight the infection, regulate inflammation and provide protection against other foreign invaders such as other viruses and bacteria.

In medicine we use the term "host defences", which refers to the immune system of the person with the disease (the host). Largely, one's immune system regulates one's ability to fight disease. Lyme patients need to support their immune function so that their body can contribute to the cause by killing off some of the infection through natural mechanisms. The stronger the immune system, the greater the ability to overcome and eradicate infection. While we do not want an overactive immune response, which can lead to auto-immunity, we do want a well-balanced and highly regulated immune system with sufficient power to fight infection.

Unfortunately, Lyme disease and related co-infections can dampen immune function. The co-infection Ehrlichia is particularly renowned for lowering the white blood cell count (white blood cells are immune cells); Borrelia can have the same effect. As previously discussed this is one of the reasons that lab testing for Lyme disease is so challenging – the immune reaction needed to register a positive result is lessened by the infection itself.

Fundamentals of Natural Medicine in Lyme Disease

To boost immune function, we have a variety of natural options. Since the immune system has different components – B cells (antibodies), T cells and natural killer (NK) cells - it is preferred to choose a variety of immune agents to support all aspects.

Transfer factors are small protein molecules that serve as messengers for the immune system, allowing for a faster and more efficient immune response. They train your immune system to function optimally and respond better to invaders. What is amazing about transfer factors is that they can be targeted for specific infections. A Lyme-specific transfer factor can actually help the immune system to identify Borrelia and go into attack mode on that specific infection. A combination of general transfer factors and targeted transfer factors is ideal for the highest level of immune support.

Transfer factors also support Natural Killer (NK) cell activity. NK cells are the Pac-Men of the immune system running around after the foreign invaders (bacteria, yeast, parasites etc). They are also designed to kill cancer cells. If you recall we discussed the CD-57 as being a marker on the NK cell – this can be quantitatively measured to assess how burdened the immune system is with Lyme disease. NK cells are a vital part of immune defence.

Beta glucans are also immune-fortifying molecules. They are sugars that are found in the cell walls of bacteria, fungi, yeasts, algae and some plants such as oats and barley. The beta glucans found in most supplements are extracted from the cell walls of the yeast Saccromyces cerevisaie (the final product is an extract only and does not contain yeast). Once extracted, they function to enhance recognition of invaders, and they bind with macrophages, a type of immune cell, to set off a cascade of heightened cellular response.

Colostrum is a high-protein substance that is found in the milk of mammals. Colostrum contains immune and growth factors including antibodies. Antibodies include IgG, IgE, IgA, IgM and IgD (we talked about IgM and IgG antibodies in relation to laboratory testing). Colostrum is considered a natural source of such immune cells. In fact, the purpose of colostrum in mammal's milk is to confer immunity to the offspring while their own immune system is still developing. Colostrum is extracted from the milk so only very scant traces of lactose and milk proteins are left behind. Those avoiding dairy can still safely take colostrum.

Medicinal mushrooms such as reishi, shitake and maitake have been used for centuries in traditional Chinese medicine, and evidence shows the ancient Egyptians also relied on their health benefits. Mushrooms benefit the immune system with their naturally occurring beta glucans, but they also contain other polysaccharides that upregulate the immune system and provide antimicrobial activity. Mushrooms may also have hormone-modulating properties. Some people with extreme Candida and yeast overgrowth, or with sensitivity to fungi, may not do well with medicinal mushrooms; however for many, they are a great addition to an immune protocol.

Herbs that support immune function are a helpful addition too. While some herbalists do not support its use in chronic health issues, astragalus is a herb that I use with good results. Along with its immune benefits, it also has mild antibacterial and anti-inflammatory activity.

While healthy levels of all vitamins and minerals are necessary for healthy immune function, vitamins C and D are particularly important.

Vitamin C boosts the immune system through its influence on the production and function of white blood cells and antibodies, and it enhances interferon which coats the cell surfaces to help ward off infection. It is also a powerful antioxidant, and in that role it protects immune cells from being damaged by toxins in the body.

Vitamin D has received much attention in recent years. It is associated with reducing inflammation and can have pain-modulating benefits. It also functions both as a fat-soluble vitamin within the body and also as a hormone, and has known benefit to the immune system. Adequate levels of vitamin D are necessary for the signalling and activation of T cells (one of the branches of the immune system) when a foreign invader is detected. When the immune cell is presented with a pathogen, it will put out a receptor for vitamin D, and once bound, that complex will signal T cells to mobilize, producing either NK cells to kill off the pathogen, or T-helper cells that train the immune system to remember that threat, allowing it to be more efficient next time it encounters it. Studies have found that a deficiency of vitamin D will hinder this process and reduce immune response.

Given that a strong immune system is a key component in being able to fight infection, moderate inflammation and recover from Lyme disease, it seems only sensible to utilize some of the powerful tools nature has given us.

Natural Antibiotics and Antimicrobials

Some people opt not to take pharmaceutical antibiotics, some are restricted by drug allergies or medication side effects, and some feel that they need extra antimicrobial help along with their antibiotics. I have seen natural antimicrobial agents work effectively against Lyme disease, its co-infections and some of the other commonly found pathogens in chronic illness such as yeast and viruses. When starting any antimicrobial therapy, I like to start out with herbs instead of antibiotics. It is easier to gauge sensitivity levels and a person's tendency to Herx with plant based medicines that have fewer side effects than antibiotics.

Please note that the below information is just a sampling of available non-pharmaceutical treatments for these infections. Literally dozens of other options exist, and the below information is intended as an introduction to the topic, not a comprehensive guide.

Borrelia

Samento – perhaps one of the best-known herbs for Borrelia, samento (also known as Cats Claw and Prima Una de Gato) has been used widely as a stand-alone therapy and in conjunction with antibiotics. The plant contains constituents known as quinovic acid glycosides, which are natural precursors to quinolones, a class of pharmaceutical antibiotics (of which ciprofloxacin is one).

Teasel root – possibly my favourite herb for Borrelia, teasel root is highly effective while still being gentle on the body. It is a potent antimicrobial and also has some anti-inflammatory properties. Drop doses (up to 10-15 daily) are typically all that is required. Teasel can provoke significant Herx reactions at the start of treatment.

Guaicum – this herb gained popularity in the sixteenth century as a cure for syphilis. Although it is not widely used in the United States, it is still used in Europe for spirochetal illnesses, of which Lyme disease and syphilis are categorized. Guaiacum also has anti-inflammatory properties and as such is used for arthritic and rheumatological manifestations of Lyme.

Grapefruit seed extract (GSE) – not to be confused with grapeseed extract, which is an antioxidant, grapefruit seed extract can be given to address the cyst forms of Borrelia. While human studies are not available, GSE did appear to eradicate Borrelia cysts in vitro (in the test tube). While perhaps not as potent as the medications for cyst forms, GSE is definitely a good option when medications are not tolerated or not available. (Samento and Banderol are options for cyst forms and biofilm too).

Babesia

Artemisinin – this is the active ingredient from the plant Artemesia annua, an anti-malarial, anti-parasitic herb (also known as Sweet Wormwood). It is effective against the co-infection Babesia, which is an intracellular parasite that creates an illness similar to malaria. Some practitioners give high doses of artemisinin (up to 500mg three times daily) but the Herx reaction can be profound. Lower doses of 200-400mg per day are more manageable. Because of its potential to create liver stress, it is advised to take one week off per month from dosing.

Cryptolepis – with less of a track record, Cryptolepis has still been used more recently for Babesiosis with seemingly good results. Accessibility and supply can be an issue; it is made from plants grown in Africa and can be challenging to source.

Enula – this product is made by NutraMedix, and is a combination of three different herbs – Elecampane, Jalapa and Blood Wiss. It is used in the treatment of Babesia, as well as parasitic worms. Also as an antimicrobial it has been shown to be effective in the treatment of MRSA.

Byron White's A-BAB formula is another effective option and can be used in conjunction with artemisinin.

Bartonella

Houttuynia is an herb used by QingCai Zhang, author of *Lyme Disease and Modern Chinese Medicine*. His product is called HH2 and is highly effective against Bartonella. This is the primary natural remedy I use for Bartonella.

The Nutramedix herbs developed by Dr Cowden including Cumanda and Banderol, and the newer Byron White A-Bart formula, have also been used to treat Bartonella.

Stephen Buhner recommends the herb Sida acuta stating that it protects the red blood cells against invasion by the Bartonella organisms.

Candida/ Yeast

There are many effective anti-fungals found in nature. The following are just a sampling, but I have found them to be effective. Anti-fungals seem to produce the best results when rotated – some people switch them every week, others every month. I tend to use combinations of anti-fungals at the same time for maximum coverage.

Grapefruit seed extract – already mentioned for its cyst-busting properties for Borrelia, grapefruit seed extract is also an effective anti-fungal. For this dual benefit it is often used in Lyme treatment. A 1990 study published in the Journal of Orthomolecular Medicine also showed grapefruit seed extract to be effective against moulds such as Aspergillus and Penicillium species.[1]

Garlic – one of nature's best anti-fungals, garlic has many other health giving properties. It is antimicrobial against a wide variety of pathogens while concurrently supporting the immune system. It also has a beneficial influence on cholesterol and blood sugar levels. Garlic cloves added to food are an easy and inexpensive way to get garlic, but for more potency, it can also be supplemented in liquid or capsule forms.

Caprylic acid – found in coconut oil, caprylic acid not only kills yeast by interfering with the cell wall of Candida but also restores healthy stomach acidity, allowing for better digestion of foods, especially proteins. Caprylic acid is typically well tolerated.

Oregano oil – oil of oregano is a potent anti-fungal that has been used in Mediterranean regions for many years. The chemical compounds in oregano react with the water in the bloodstream to dehydrate and kill the Candida yeast. It produces less resistance than other anti-fungals so it can be used effectively long term. Gastrointestinal side effects can be an issue, especially with liquid forms, so gel caps are usually better tolerated. Oregano oil also has some activity against Bartonella.

Pau d'Arco – originating from the Amazon basin, Pau d'Arco contains a range of constituents that have yeast-fighting activity. The primary way this herb is taken is as a tea, although it can be taken in a tincture too.

Olive leaf - another herb that supports the immune system, while also having potent anti-fungal properties. Olive leaf is also very effective against parasites and viruses, making it a good supplement for chronic Lyme sufferers. High dose olive leaf should not be taken while taking antibiotic therapies, but moderate doses show considerable benefit.

Viruses

While not theoretically co-infections of Lyme, many chronic Lyme patients have chronic viral infections, notably Epstein Barr virus (EBV), Cytomegalovirus (CMV), Human Herpes Virus 6 (HHV-6), and Herpes Simplex 1 and 2 (HSV 1 & 2). Natural remedies can assist the body in managing these viruses and prevent them from adding to Lyme symptoms.

Olive leaf – already mentioned as an anti-fungal, olive leaf has excellent anti-viral properties. It works by interfering with critical amino acid production essential for viruses, by inactivating viruses or by preventing virus shedding, and by directly penetrating infected cells to stop viral replication in the case of retroviruses.

Lauricidin – this extract is derived from coconut oil. It works by binding to the lipid-protein envelope of the virus, preventing it from attaching to and entering host cells, and therefore preventing it from replicating. Lauricidin is also used as an anti-fungal and anti-bacterial, and has immune strengthening properties. One of the advantages of lauricidin is that it kills off unwanted pathogens without killing off the good flora in the gut.

Biofilm

Biofilm, as we discussed in section two, is the mucopolysaccharide matrix (aka "sticky goo") in which Borrelia hide to evade detection by the immune system and resist antimicrobial treatment. It is probable that biofilm needs to be addressed in every Lyme patient; however, it should definitely be considered in a person who is doing a lot of antimicrobial therapy with very limited improvement. A summary of biofilm protocols is given in Appendix H.

Most of the remedies used to help break down biofilm are enzyme based and blood-thinning agents. Their goal is to break through the sticky substance so that the bacteria can be exposed to antimicrobial agents.

Lumbrokinase is one of the blood-thinning agents used to address biofilm. Its cousin, nattokinase, is also used but has somewhat lesser efficacy (but also less expense). Proteolytic enzymes such as those used in anti-inflammatory supplements can be helpful too. Calcium EDTA, while often thought of as a heavy metal chelator, is given along with lumbrokinase to break down the bonds within the biofilm substance. It does this by forming complexes with the ions in the matrix, rendering it less able to hold together. Also, biofilm is known to contain various metals, which may also explain why Calcium EDTA is effective here.

Once biofilm is being dissolved, there may be a greater Herx reaction, as more bacteria and parasites are newly exposed and open to being killed off. This, of course, is the goal, but an acceleration of the process should be anticipated and extra detox support given.

Another aspect of the biofilm protocol is to increase fibre intake to ensure that the bowels are getting adequately swept, and that microbial debris and toxins are being eliminated. Finally, adequate probiotics are needed to replace and rebalance healthy microbial flora.

Digestive Health

We have already discussed the need for probiotics to maintain healthy digestion, and some of the natural remedies used to control yeast overgrowth in the gut. However, naturopathic remedies can also be used to address other problems in the digestive system.

Gastrointestinal Infections

Infections in the gut can be bacterial or parasitic in nature.

Helicobacter pylori (H. pylori) are bacteria that infect the stomach, causing reflux/ heartburn, burping, stomach pain, and compromised ability to digest food, particularly proteins. The bacteria interfere with the cells in the stomach that produce hydrochloric acid (HCL), which is necessary for the proper digestion of food. H. pylori is often treated with antibiotics. From a natural standpoint, mastic gum is one of the key agents that can eradicate H. pylori. Zinc carnosine is also helpful. Deglycyrrhizinated liquorice (DGL) assists by coating and healing the oesophageal and stomach tissue that may have become irritated by the infection.

I have observed that sometimes stomach issues are assumed to be a side effect of medications, when really they may be caused by H. pylori. Many people taking proton-pump inhibitors and other antacids could be spared from years of these medications by an accurate diagnosis of H. pylori.

Intestinal parasites are common in chronic Lyme patients, perhaps because of a general lowering of immune function and increased susceptibility to pathogens. Intestinal parasites such as Cryptosporidium parvum, Blastocystis hominis and Entamoeba histolytica can cause symptoms such as gas, bloating, constipation, diarrhoea (sometimes alternating between the two) and abdominal pain. Again, long-term antibiotic use can often be the assumed cause of gut issues such as these, but ongoing, evaluation for parasites can be useful.

Herbs that have strong anti-parasitic activity include black walnut, wormwood, gentian, clove and yellow dock. Garlic and olive leaf are used here too.

Side Effects of Antibiotics

Certainly, gastrointestinal side effects, predominantly nausea and diarrhoea are among the most common in Lyme treatment.

One of the best remedies for nausea is ginger. Whether it is taken as a tea, added to food, or ingested in dried forms, ginger has a long history of use for nausea, whether caused by medications, pregnancy or motion sickness. I prefer the ginger root cut into small pieces and boiled for 10 to 15 minutes. Stevia (a natural sweetener and sugar-alternative) can be added for sweetness.

Peppermint is also good for nausea as well as irritable bowel type symptoms and indigestion. It can be taken as a tea, which is preferred, or drunk with one or two drops of peppermint oil mixed in water.

Some people find that essential oils of peppermint and lavender can help relieve nausea when diffused into the air.

Mild diarrhoea caused by medications can often be offset by increased probiotic use, anti-fungal therapies such as those listed earlier in the section, and/or the gut healing nutrients listed below under "leaky gut". Peppermint tea is also useful here. Any ongoing or severe diarrhoea should be evaluated for Clostridia difficile, which is a possible result of antibiotic therapy.

I have also seen increased fibre intake help diarrhoea (probably due to its binding capabilities) – especially soluble fibres such as apple pectin and chia seeds. Insoluble fibres such as psyllium husk can be too irritating for some. As a binder, activated charcoal can mop up toxins, which reduces diarrhoea and also the severity of Herxheimer reactions.

For bowel regularity I suggest a tablespoon of ground flax seeds taken daily, either sprinkled on food or blended into a smoothie. If constipation is an issue, the safest approaches are fibres such as flax or rice bran, or high dose vitamin C or magnesium.

Leaky Gut

Leaky gut refers to the phenomena where the cells in the wall of the small intestine become spaced out beyond what they should be. Ordinarily, the junctions between the cells are only large enough to let single particles of digested food into the blood stream for transport to other parts of the body. When the junctions open up, larger food particles can get through. This causes an immune reaction, as the immune system is trained to see single particles as "good" and clusters of particles as "bad". Of course, whenever "bad" happens, the immune system rushes to attack, which inherently leads to inflammation that can affect the entire body.

Eating foods that are inflammatory (more about this in the next chapter) or that one has allergies or intolerances to, having yeast imbalances and having unresolved chronic infections in the gut are also precursors to leaky gut.

Of all the nutrients that can be used to repair leaky gut, perhaps the most effective is the amino acid L-glutamine. Glutamine is healing to the intestinal wall, and can calm symptoms fairly rapidly. Slippery elm used as a gruel (powder mixed with water and eaten) is also very effective, as is aloe vera juice. Deglycyrrhizinated liquorice can be used for intestinal healing (as well as oesophageal healing) in combination with the other nutrients. Marshmallow tea is of great benefit for soothing and healing the gut.

Energy

One of the primary symptoms of chronic Lyme disease is fatigue. To some extent, fatigue will improve as the infection is eradicated, however there are things that may help to improve it along the way.

Three of the major causes of fatigue in chronic illness are adrenal fatigue, mitochondrial insufficiency and methylation defects. Let us explore each in more detail.

Adrenal Fatigue

The adrenals are the stress management centres of the body. Cortisol, one of the hormones they produce, is nicknamed the "stress hormone". When there is a stress on the body – whether an emotional stress, or equally a physical stress such as chronic infection, pain and inflammation – the adrenals respond by increasing cortisol output. This is a healthy mechanism that helps the body to compensate for the stress by giving the body an extra boost to deal with whatever is happening.

The problem lies in the fact that so often the stress becomes chronic, it does not go away. Subsequently the adrenal glands work harder and harder to maintain their cortisol output. Their compensatory mechanisms break down and over time cortisol levels will start to fall. Eventually, adrenal exhaustion ensues, reflected by low cortisol readings on labs and feelings of total physical, mental and emotional exhaustion. Cortisol is a natural anti-inflammatory, so it follows that chronically low cortisol allows for more inflammation, and more pain, in the body.

The first step in evaluating adrenal health is accurate testing. While blood levels can be measured, they will only reflect levels at that one particular time of day and are lowest at night. Cortisol has a circadian rhythm, so its levels start high in the morning, and ordinarily fall gradually throughout the day. Low cortisol at night is essential for the immune system to kick in and do its housekeeping (which it does during the night); and to allow restful sleep.

A saliva test can be a convenient way to get that information and can be done at home. A tube of saliva is collected at 8am, 12 noon, 4pm and 8pm, and then cortisol levels can be charted reflecting their levels throughout the day. It is not uncommon to see cortisol levels slump in the afternoon, in line with the typical afternoon energy crash, or levels elevated at night in those with major sleep issues. Granted, blood levels could be measured too, however it would require four samples during the same day, so that is not as practical.

Adrenal support is an important part of the Lyme treatment protocol. Herbs and glandulars (extracts from animal adrenal glands) can both be used. Some herbs are called adaptogens, which means that they balance function. They will upregulate sluggish adrenals, or tone down overactive adrenals. Basically they normalize function whether it is high or low. This is a great option if levels are unbalanced during the day (high at some times and low at others) as there is minimal risk of creating further imbalance.

Some of the more popular adrenal adaptogens include:

- Panax Ginseng (Korean Ginseng)
- Eleuthrococcus (Siberian Ginseng)
- Ashwaghanda
- Rhodiola

Of these, I think of panax ginseng being more energizing and stimulating (too much for some people) while eleuthrococcus and ashwaghanda are more gentle and balancing. Rhodiola is great for the mental and emotional impact of chronic stress.

Liquorice root is another great adrenal herb. It can build cortisol levels and is used in adrenal insufficiency for this reason. Over time it can cause slight elevations in blood pressure, and it can be slightly oestrogenic, so either of those pre-existing issues may make long-term administration problematic in some individuals.

There is also a product called Isocort that contains plant-based cortisol in very small doses (approximately 2-2.5mg per pellet). In people with very low cortisol levels, supplementing this way can bring quick relief from debilitating fatigue and help the adrenals get back on track.

Balancing low cortisol using plant-derived cortisol is very different to giving immune-suppressive steroid drugs such as prednisone. Prednisone is an immune suppressant and *should never be given to a Lyme disease patient* as it further renders their immune system unable to fight the infection. Even if the prednisone reduces inflammation and reduces symptoms, the long-term effects totally negate the benefit. Low dose plant-derived cortisol gives the body the cortisol it needs for the various roles it plays until such a time that the adrenals can recover and take over healthy production. Cortisol is closely tied with the immune system, so chronically low cortisol output restricts immune response just as boosting cortisol levels too much with prednisone also restricts immune response. It is a delicate balancing act.

Another approach to balancing adrenal hormones is to supplement with the precursors DHEA and pregnenolone. Pregnenolone is nicknamed the "grandmother hormone" because it supplies the material needed to produce a host of other adrenal hormones, including progesterone, cortisol, oestrogen and testosterone. DHEA can be used as it is, or converted by the body to oestrogen or testosterone.

If cortisol levels are too high - as may be the case in less chronic cases where night time elevations interrupt sleep or the adrenals are still trying to compensate for the stressors - the adaptogenic herbs may also be used to regulate those elevations.

Phosphorylated serine is a nutrient (serine is an amino acid) that has been used to dampen elevated cortisol levels. It is taken several hours before bed for nighttime elevations, and in the morning and afternoon for overall high levels.

Finally, full recovery from adrenal fatigue typically requires a reduction in overall lifestyle stressors, as well as a healthy diet low in inflammatory foods and high in B vitamins, especially pantothenic acid (vitamin

B5). Additionally, vitamin C is one of the primary nutrients used by the adrenal glands; liposomal vitamin C can have profound healing effects on the adrenal glands.

Mitochondrial Dysfunction

Another cause of low energy in chronic illness is mitochondrial dysfunction. The mitochondria are the little engines within each of our cells that produce our energy. This energy is called adenosine triphosphate, or ATP. If the little engines are not well oiled and well fuelled, slow downs can occur in the production of the ATP, which reduces the energy available for the body to use.

Certain nutrients have been shown to support mitochondrial function. NADH and CoQ10 are two that feed and support the cycle. Alpha-ketoglutaric acid and L-carnitine are others. It is important to note that patients who are taking Wellvone or Malarone for Babesiosis should not supplement with CoQ10 while they are on those medications, as the CoQ10 will interfere with the medications and make them less effective.

The other consideration here is that the membrane of the mitochondria contains its own DNA. Therefore if the membrane integrity is compromised, function will be impaired. NT Factor is well researched to provide phospholipids that can be transported from cell to cell and integrated into the mitochondrial membrane, keeping both structure and function optimal.

Supplementary mitochondrial support can help energy production tremendously. Typically, higher doses of the above nutrients are taken for the first two months to facilitate repair of the membrane and accelerate the biochemical pathways, then more moderate doses can be taken after that.

Methylation Defects

We have already discussed methylation defects as a cause of toxin build-up in the body, but it can also be a contributor to fatigue. In part, it ties into adrenal dysfunction, as methylation pathways can be impaired secondary to adrenal exhaustion.

Supporting methylation with methyl-B12 therapy can provide a generous boost of energy and improved mental outlook. One might think that simply taking the vitamin B12 in any form could do this, as B12 is a vitamin that is associated with energy, and to some extent, that is true. Some patients respond well to the forms of B12 that are not methylation-boosters (eg cyanocobalamin and hydroxocobalamin). However, I have seen clinically that far more patients derive benefit from the methyl-B12 therapy, indicating the methyl groups are equally significant. While beyond the scope of this discussion, biochemical markers can be measured through laboratory testing of the blood (MTHFR genetic markers as well as levels of amino acids methionine and cysteine), that indicate whether a person is an under-methylator or over-methylator. This can guide appropriate supplementation.

Hormone Health

Along with adrenal dysfunction, chronic Lyme patients often develop thyroid issues. There are two factors behind this. First, Lyme and co-infections impact the hypothalamus and the pituitary gland, the master regulators in the brain of hormone function; this is why all the hormones can easily get out of whack. Second, the thyroid is quite susceptible to autoimmune issues, and given that Lyme can trigger autoimmune processes within the body, it follows that the thyroid might be in the path of that. Hashimoto's thyroiditis is an autoimmune thyroid condition that often starts with a phase of hyperthyroidism (high thyroid function) but then moves into a longer phase of hypothyroidism (low thyroid function). Antibodies such as anti-TPO and anti-thyroglobulin antibodies are helpful markers to evaluate this autoimmune component. General testing for TSH, free T3 and free T4 show actual levels of thyroid hormones. Reverse T3 can be helpful as some people convert T4 to reverse T3 instead of the more active form of T3 itself. Even patients in the lower end of the normal ranges may have clinical signs and symptoms of hypothyroidism and would benefit from thyroid support.

Some people need to take thyroid hormone supplements to boost their thyroid function. The optimal way to do this is with bio-identical thyroid, which is a combination of T3 and T4 (our bodies produce mostly T4 in the thyroid gland, send it out to the body where it is converted into T3, the active form). Bio-identical thyroid hormone is created to mimic the human hormone exactly, so the body can use it most efficiently. Many compounding pharmacies offer bio-identical thyroid.

Natural support for thyroid includes iodine, which is needed for the production of thyroid hormones (T3 has three molecules of iodine; T4 has four). Iodine is contraindicated in Hashimoto's thyroiditis, however, as it may trigger an autoimmune attack. Herbs such as bladderwrack and kelp boost thyroid, as does the amino acid tyrosine. The nutrients zinc and selenium are necessary for the healthy conversion of T4 to T3 in the body.

■ ■ ■ ■

Reproductive hormones are also impacted by hypothalamic-pituitary dysregulation. Many men experience a drop in testosterone levels with chronic illness, and this contributes to loss of libido, sexual dysfunction, muscle weakness, loss of stamina, depression and sleep interruption. While herbs such as tribulus, maca and yohimbe can be potent tonics for men and help the situation, quite frequently a bio-identical testosterone supplement is best to normalize levels and improve function.

Any time reproductive hormones are out of balance or low, it is important to look at the adrenals. In both men and women, the adrenal glands are responsible for producing approximately 35-50% of the reproductive hormones oestrogen, progesterone and testosterone. It follows then that exhausted adrenals are not producing adequate levels of those as well as cortisol. Supporting adrenal function can improve symptoms that are related to reproductive hormones, too.

Lyme typically follows a pattern of four-week flares, even in men. However, in women, the flares usually coincide with the menstrual cycle, creating a double whammy. PMS symptoms can be severe in combination with the flare of general Lyme symptoms. And chocolate is off the list as a coping mechanism!

Herbs to support progesterone function such as Vitex (chaste tree) can be helpful. Some women do well with bio-identical progesterone in the second half of their menstrual cycle to lessen the severity of PMS.

For menopausal women, black cohosh, red clover, liquorice root and other more oestrogenic herbs are indicated along with the chaste tree. Anecdotally, I have found black cohosh to be helpful for the bladder irritation associated with Lyme disease in any gender and age group.

The night sweats of Babesia can be confusing for a woman of menopausal age, as often doctors attribute that symptom to their hormones when it may in fact be infection related. Sometimes both factors play a role, and both need to be addressed. Bio-identical hormone support with oestrogen, progesterone and/ or testosterone can be hugely beneficial to women with chronic Lyme disease.

Pain Management

Pain management is a huge issue in Lyme disease as pain is present in some form for most people. There are different types of pain and causes of pain. Sometimes pharmaceutical pain management is necessary while a person is undergoing treatment to make pain levels manageable. Natural approaches may be enough for some while others may need complement medications.

Joint and Muscle Pain

Magnesium is one of the best natural remedies for muscle pain. Magnesium relaxes skeletal muscle so it can help take away some of the tightness of painful, aching muscles. Epsom salts baths contain magnesium sulfate, and this is why they too can cause easing of muscle pain (some people who are sensitive to sulfates or sulfur compounds may feel worse with Epsom salts baths). Magnesium's relaxing effect also works on smooth muscle. Since the intestinal wall contains smooth muscle, magnesium is an effective treatment for constipation.

Malic acid is good for muscle pain too, working through a slightly different mechanism. Research has shown that muscle pain with chronic illnesses such as Lyme and fibromyalgia is associated with low muscle tissue oxygen pressure in the affected muscles. This hypoxia results in a low output of ATP in the muscle cells. Essentially, this represents a block in the energy production cycle, which malic acid can overcome.

Some of the herbal anti-inflammatories, which include white willow and holy basil, work well for joint pain and muscle pain. Curcumin, which is found in turmeric, has well-researched anti-inflammatory activity.

Proteolytic enzymes can modulate inflammation by helping to break down some of the chemical mediators and tissue by-products. These are not digestive enzymes, which are taken with food to assist in digestion, but are systemic enzymes that are deliberately taken away from food to allow their uptake into the blood stream and through the tissues. Examples of these are bromelain, papain and protease.

Another pain modulating remedy, which requires a prescription from a compounding pharmacy, is Low Dose Naltrexone (LDN). LDN is an immune modulator, meaning it balances immune function. For this reason, it is used not only in conditions of low immunity but also in autoimmune issues such as rheumatoid arthritis and Hashimoto's thyroiditis. It has a mild blocking effect on opioid receptors in the brain, which stimulate the body to upregulate its production of both enkephalins (immune balancing chemicals) and endorphins (feel good chemicals). It has one negative side effect of a transient sleep disturbance, which occurs in one or two people out of ten (based on my clinical observations), but there is a subset of people for whom LDN gives great pain relief.

Nerve Pain

Lyme patients often suffer from nerve pain, which can be burning, shooting or stabbing, and can range from mild to debilitating.

Some people get relief from nerve pain from methyl-B12 injections. B12 has a long track record of being used to treat neuropathy; some find it helps with the neuropathic pain also.

Herbs that can offset nerve pain include St John's Wort, Jamaica dogwood, lemon balm and skullcap. Curcumin can be helpful here too, both internally and in topical preparations.

Sleep

Sleep disturbance is one of the more common symptoms in Lyme disease. It is a catch-22 situation, since sufficient duration and quality of sleep is critical for the body to heal, and yet sleep is often elusive for Lyme sufferers.

Natural aids for sleep can be helpful. Melatonin is a hormone that we produce naturally to regulate our day/ night, light/ dark cycles. Melatonin can safely be supplemented and can aid in falling asleep; however it has a short span of activity and is less effective for sleeping through the night. Sustained release melatonin is available and would be a better choice for that.

5-HTP is an amino acid precursor to serotonin, and in higher doses can assist sleep. Up to 200mg at night is needed. Herbs for sleep include valerian, passionflower, chamomile, skullcap and California poppy.

Epsom salts baths at night have proved helpful for relaxing both the muscles and the mind.

Mood

Lyme disease impacts moods, which can present as anything from mild depression, irritability or anxiety to paranoid thinking and obsessive-compulsive traits. Mood changes in Lyme can be looked at from two viewpoints. The first is that Lyme disease is a painful, life-changing, often debilitating illness; with very little information or acknowledgement from the medical community; limited understanding even from the most well meaning family and friends; and until recently very little support or hope. It is quite natural, in the light of all that, to feel depressed, anxious and even quite hopeless.

The second is that Borrelia and co-infections do infect the brain and do have a physiological impact on both neurotransmitters and brain wave patterns. Neurotransmitters are the chemicals created in our central nervous systems that regulate our thoughts, moods, behaviours and cognition. These infections directly impact the brain and subsequently impact moods as well.

So the problem is twofold – the infections themselves create mood and personality changes. Then there is the very valid issue of the mental and emotional struggle to cope with a crippling and highly misunderstood illness.

Modulating neurotransmitters can be helpful to balance moods, and can be done through use of specific amino acids that provide the building blocks for the neurotransmitters.

5-HTP is one of the key supplements used because it supports serotonin, which is a calming brain chemical (we call it an inhibitory neurotransmitter). This is the first choice in depression. GABA and theanine are indicated for states of anxiety. If obsessive-compulsive traits are presenting (as they often do in Bartonella cases), inositol in high doses (5-10 grams) may take the edge off. Where depression is more an exhaustive state, with no physical or mental energy, tyrosine can be helpful as it fuels dopamine, epinephrine and norepinephrine, which are more energizing and stimulating neurotransmitters. Tyrosine has an added benefit of supporting thyroid function (low thyroid function is a cause of depression, too).

Heavy Metal Toxicity

One thing I see more and more is Lyme disease patients with high levels of toxic metals such as lead and mercury.

Toxic metals can come from a variety of sources. Lead, while more strictly regulated today, used to be found in pencils, petrol, paint and pipes, to name a few. Even older houses can still be sources of lead. Mercury can be found in vaccines, amalgam fillings and seafood. Both metals are inherent in pollution – both air and water – and so we all take in a certain amount of toxic metals daily. Coal burning power plants are a major source of mercury and other air-borne toxins. Aluminium, cadmium and arsenic are other metals that can accumulate in the body and cause problems. In fact, research shows a link between aluminium levels in the brain and Alzheimer's disease.

High levels of toxic metals in the system can cause neurological problems such as numbness, tingling and palsy as well as muscle aches, joint pain, cognitive dysfunction including memory loss and difficulty concentrating. It is easy to see how closely these symptoms resemble typical Lyme disease symptoms - and so an evaluation of whether toxic metals might be contributing to the Lyme disease picture is useful.

Not every Lyme patient has toxic metals, and not every person with toxic metals has Lyme disease. However, there does seem to be a correlation between Lyme disease and heavy metal toxicity. Recent research has also revealed that heavy metal toxins are often concentrated in the same parts of the body where Borrelia and co-infections make their home.

The question stands as to why Lyme disease patients are more impacted by heavy metals than other people in the population. My opinion is that Lyme patients have compromised detoxification mechanisms, and they are not able to rid themselves of heavy metals as they come into the body; hence, an accumulation occurs.

Lyme patients are also more neurologically stressed because they already have chronic infection impacting that system. So when another neurological stressor such as a toxic metal enters the picture, the impact is doubled.

Testing for Heavy Metals

There are a number of ways to test for heavy metals, each with its own merits and limitations.

Blood Test

This is the easiest and most readily available test through commercial laboratories. The problem with blood testing is that when metals come into the body, they only circulate in the blood stream for a period of a few weeks. After that they are taken up into the tissues – whether that be into the brain and neurological system, the joints and muscles, or the cardiovascular system (lead is implicated in cardiovascular disease through its presence in blood vessels and contribution to atherosclerosis). Therefore, unless there is a recent exposure to toxic metals, blood tests may well come back normal, completely missing the impact of metals already in the tissues.

Unprovoked Urine Test

An unprovoked urine test is a urine collection done without any provoking agent given beforehand. Again, this is a simple test to do, but the problem is that the urine is simply a filtration of the blood. Therefore an unprovoked urine test is going to carry the same limitations as blood testing. As with the blood, this test can be helpful if there has been a known recent exposure to metals, such as amalgam fillings being removed without proper precautions being taken to protect the body from mercury vapour. In cases of long-standing metal toxicity, it will be of limited benefit.

Provoked Urine Test

In many cases this is my preferred test. In this case, the patient is "provoked" with a dose of a heavy metal chelator prior to collecting the urine. Typically DMSA, an agent that bonds to the metal and "escorts" it out of the body, is used. DMSA is an agent that is known to chelate (bind) mercury in particular, and to a lesser extent, lead and other toxic metals.

The provoking agent serves to push the metals out of the tissues and back into the blood stream where they can be filtered by the kidneys. After a six-hour urine collection, levels of many different metals can be measured in the urine.

Granted, while this test is measuring how much toxic metal is dumped after a dose of DMSA, it does not measure remaining body stores. However, we know that high levels of metals in the body correlate with high levels being dumped in the urine, because as we repeat the same test using the same provocation every two months, and as metals are chelated out of the body, we see the amount dumped with the provocation lessening over time. This indicates that the heavy metal detox protocol is working.

In some cases we do an unprovoked urine test first, then do a provoked one after the dose of DMSA and compare the results to determine how much of the heavy metal burden is from recent exposure versus body tissue stores. For the provoked test, all urine excreted over a six-hour period is collected, with a small sample of that sent back to the lab.

Caution must be taken with patients who are very chronically and severely ill because the provocation dose may cause a detoxification reaction that could set them back. Heavy metals when mobilized can cause headaches, joint and muscle pain, fatigue and neurological problems – the body's detoxification mechanisms must be functioning adequately to handle this. Furthermore, there is the possibility that the chelator used for provocation, such as DMSA, may actually cause metals to be redistributed throughout the body, sometimes to more sensitive locations (such as the brain and liver) than their original storage sites.

The majority of people can tolerate the provoked metals test. In more sensitive patients we can reduce the dose of DMSA, slightly reducing the benefit of the test but also protecting them from severe detox reactions. There is a subset of patients who are too sick and too sensitive to safely carry out this test. In such cases, I will either do an unprovoked urine test or a hair analysis.

Hair Analysis

I am not a strong advocate of hair testing for heavy metals, but this can be a valid starting point in patients who are too sensitive to do the provoked urine test. It is an easy and non-invasive test since it only requires a hair sample; however, there can be inherent challenges in the interpretation of the results.

If a person's hair showed a high level of metals, it could indicate that they are metal toxic. However, if a person is showing low levels of metals in the hair, one could argue that they are unable to adequately excrete them and still have them in their system,

Also, the hair test may be skewed by contaminants such as hair dyes and styling products.

I use the hair analysis in patients where we do not feel they could tolerate the urine test or in very small children, and in some cases it provides useful information. However, it is not my first choice for heavy metal assessment.

Addressing Heavy Metals

There are a number of ways to address heavy levels, and treatment choices should be made based on the severity of the problems, as well as how ill the patient is and how sensitive they are. A Lyme disease patient who has debilitating symptoms and shows extreme Herx reactions with any new modality should be treated very gently, while a more functional person with some symptoms but a generally good tolerance can be treated more aggressively. It should be noted that detoxifying heavy metals can be a high-risk proposition, as these metals are extremely damaging to all systems of the body and they can end up being redistributed throughout the body if chelation protocols are not carried out correctly.

A viable starting point for heavy metal detox is to dose with an agent that binds metals without actually stirring up tissue stores too much. Chlorella, a single-cell green algae, is probably the best known example of this and is sometimes used to bind up biotoxins in Lyme disease also.

Cilantro is a herb that has been used for heavy metal detox. It has the ability to mobilize tissue stores of toxic metals so it may cause more of a detox reaction than chlorella alone. Cilantro is known for its ability to mobilize metals from the brain.

DMSA has been mentioned as we often use it as the provoking agent for urine metals tests. It preferentially pulls mercury but will also chelate lead and other metals such as aluminium and cadmium.

EDTA is another well-known chelating agent that has a stronger affinity for lead. It is not typically given orally as is DMSA, but instead either intravenously or via rectal suppository.

Other natural agents used to heavy metal detox include alpha-lipoic acid, high dose vitamin C, garlic and zeolite.

My preferred regimen for heavy metal detox in Lyme disease patients is a slow and steady approach, one that will not overwhelm the system, add stress to the detoxification processes or cause any worsening of symptoms. I use a product called Chelex that has small amounts of DMSA and EDTA, combined with cilantro, chlorella, garlic and alpha-lipoic acid. It can be taken every day without risk of depleting minerals, or every second or third day for an even more gentle approach.

For those who want or need a more rigorous protocol, DMSA or EDTA is used depending on which toxic metal showed to be more problematic on the provoked urine test. Cyclic dosing schedules are created, balancing stronger chelating protocols with mineral repletion.

One thing that is true of any heavy metal detox program is that fibres and binders are crucial to make sure the metals that are being dumped into the bowels via the bile are being excreted, and not reabsorbed into the blood stream and redistributed to the brain. Chlorella is helpful here, but adding fibres such as psyllium husk, ground flax seed, bentonite clay or apple pectin can be helpful.

Heavy metal toxicity is something that all Lyme patients should evaluate at some stage of their recovery. For many, it is not the primary priority – getting adequate Lyme treatment should be the first priority, and often with the amount of medications and supplements required for that, and the energy required to handle the Herxing, there is not a lot left over to deal with anything else! Patients on more established regimens that have had some improvement and are managing their Lyme disease protocol better might be better positioned to examine the toxic metal issue. Heavy metal detox should be done under the supervision of a health practitioner with expertise in this area, as doing it the wrong way or too quickly can make things worse.

■ ■ ■ ■

As you can see, there are many natural ways to help support the immune system, manage pain and inflammation, support digestion, balance hormones and eradicate pathogens using naturopathic therapies. The ones presented are just the ones I have primarily used and seen in my practice. There are literally hundreds of other tools and techniques in the world of natural medicine, and a wide variety of practitioners with unique expertise.

Sample Naturopathic Protocols

This list represents a sample of some of my favourite products that I use extensively in my practice. It does not necessarily cover all the individual ingredients listed, however it provides consolidated protocols that can be easily followed. Protocols using other products listed and respective dosages should be formulated on an individual basis in conjunction with a qualified naturopath. This list is not representative of a complete protocol, where every supplement is recommended. Specific supplements are selected depending on individual need.

Many of the following products are not available in Australia but can be shipped in for personal use. I have worked with a master herbalist in the design of the RestorMedicine herbal formulas, and all come from either organic or wildcrafted herbs. Researched Nutritionals is a supplement company based in California that designs formulas tailored to Lyme disease and other chronic illnesses, and I use their products because of their impeccable standards, the way they combine various nutrients so that protocols can be streamlined, and the efficacy of their products.

I have marked RestorMedicine products with * and Researched Nutritionals products with **. Full descriptions of products and ordering information is available at www.restormedicine.com. This information is reprinted in Appendix I.

Detoxification Support

Smilax*	40 drops twice daily
Detox Support Formula *	40 drops twice daily
Tri-Fortify Glutathione **	1 teaspoon in the morning in water
Dr. Nicola's Detox Plus Powder*	2 scoops daily

Immune Support

Transfer Factor Multi-Immune **	2 capsules before bed
Transfer Factor LymPlus **	2 capsules before bed

Digestive Support

RestorProbiotic Powder *	½ - 1 scoop before bed
(or) Inner Health Plus	2 capsules at night before bed
Dr. Nicola's Fibre Plus*	4 capsules at night
Anti-Parasite Formula *	40 drops three times daily
Anti-Fungal Formula *	40 drops three times daily

Pain and Inflammation

Soothe and Relaxx **	3 capsules twice daily
InflaQuell **	3 capsules twice daily between meals
Nerve Pain Formula *	40 drops three or four times daily

Mood and Sleep

Soothe and Relaxx **	3 capsules twice daily
Sleep Support Formula *	2 to 4 capsules before bed
200mg of Zen (ARG)	2 capsules twice daily
5-HTP	50mg 1 twice daily for mood; up to 4 before bed for sleep

LYME DISEASE in Australia

Cognitive Function
Tri-Fortify Glutathione **	1 teaspoon in the morning in water
Cognicare **	2 twice daily

Adrenal Support (Energy)
Energy Multiplex **	3 capsules in the morning
Liquorice Plus (Metagenics)	2 tablets twice daily
Adreset (Metagenics)	1 capsule twice daily
DHEA Plus (Douglas Labs)	1 capsule daily in the morning

Mitochondrial Support (Energy)
ATP Fuel **	5 capsules twice daily
CoQ10 400mg **	1 capsule daily
Ribos-Cardio **	1 scoop daily

Antimicrobial
Teasel Root *	5 drops twice daily
Lyme Support Formula*	10 drops twice daily
Artemisinin SOD **	2 capsules twice daily
HH2 Formula (Zhang)	1 capsule three times daily

Biofilm
Boulouke Lumbrokinase **	1 capsule twice daily between meals
InflaQuell **	3 capsules twice daily between meals
Interfase Plus (Klaire Labs)	2 capsules twice daily between meals

Heavy Metal Chelation
Chelex (Xymogen)	4 capsules one or two times daily
DMSA 250mg (Thorne)	1 capsule three times daily, 3 days on/ 7 days off
EDTA 750mg (compounded)	1 suppository every other night
Multiple Mineral (Klaire Labs)	2 capsules on non-DMSA/ non-EDTA days

REFERENCES

1. Ionescu G, Kiehl R, Wichmann Kunz F, et al. Oral citrus seed extract in atopic eczema: in vitro and in vivo studies on intestinal microflor. J Orthomol Med. 1990;5(3):155-57.

19. NUTRITION AND LYME DISEASE

LYME DISEASE SUFFERERS WHO PAY ATTENTION TO THEIR NUTRITION and make dietary changes invariably do better than those who do not. The right diet can make such a huge contribution to recovery and levels of symptoms. If nothing else, dietary modification is necessary while on antibiotic protocols to help prevent the yeast issues that can arise along the way.

I feel so passionately about this topic, and my patients were so eager for information on it, that I wrote a book about it. For detailed information on The Lyme Diet, including practical applications, meal suggestions, acid/ alkaline food lists and gluten-free food lists, I would refer you to my book, *The Lyme Diet: Nutritional Strategies for Healing from Lyme Disease.*[1]

What you will find below is an overview of the principles of The Lyme Diet including enough information to get you started and help you along the right nutritional path. My goal here is for you to see clearly how diet plays into your Lyme disease, and the ways in which changing your diet can help Lyme disease.

Inflammation

One of the key things nutrition can do is help moderate inflammation in the body. Lyme disease creates a lot of inflammation, which can fuel pain and swelling. Inflammation involves a complex cascade of processes, but the immune system and the chemicals it produces modulate much of it.

Inflammation can be systemic, all over the body, or localized to a specific area, as would be the case with an injury to a certain body part. In Lyme patients, inflammation can relate to joints, muscle tissues, the brain, cranial nerves or the tissues surrounding the heart, to name just a few.

Fats can be inflammatory or anti-inflammatory through their conversion to certain chemicals called prostaglandins. There are different types of prostaglandins (PG's): PG1 inhibits inflammation and has beneficial effects; PG2 has the direct opposite effects and fuels inflammation; while PG3 is a mixture of the two (but is thought of as more anti-inflammatory).

To reduce inflammation in the body we must promote PG1 formation and inhibit PG2 formation. Therefore we must choose foods that boost PG1 and avoid foods that boost PG2.

Saturated fats and trans fatty acids definitely fuel inflammation by increasing PG2 production and should be avoided.

Saturated fats are found in nature but are labelled the "bad fats". These include red meat and dairy. Trans fatty acids are processed chemically altered fats such as margarine and shortening. They are found in "junk food" such as chips, pastries, candies and so on.

This means that eating a lot of red meat, and any processed foods and deep fried foods, is going to worsen inflammation.

To reduce inflammation we want to choose fats that fuel PG1 production. These are the unsaturated fats, also called essential fats, containing omega-3 fatty acids. These are found in nature and have great health benefits. They are the "healthy fats".

Omega-3 fatty acids are perhaps the most important to deliberately take in the diet. They have the strongest anti-inflammatory effects, as

Nutrition and Lyme Disease

well as being very important for neurological function. Omega-6's and omega-9's are important too, but come more easily through the regular daily diet.

Omega-3 fatty acids are contained in flax oil and fish oil. I recommend 2-4 grams of either one of these (or a mixture) every day. A good way to get this is to put 1 tablespoon of flax oil in a smoothie or on a salad; then take a supplement of 2 grams of fish oil. Fish oil has the added benefit of being high in DHA, another important and healthy fat.

The other key to reducing inflammation is to reduce other inflammatory foods. Gluten and dairy are both inflammatory in nature. It is thought that many people are gluten intolerant and are unaware of it, as it does not always show pronounced digestive symptoms.

Gluten is found in wheat, oats, rye and barley, and is a hidden ingredient in many foods. Many people have trouble digesting the proteins in gluten, and it often triggers an immune reaction, leading to more inflammation. Gluten intolerance can also be an autoimmune process and can actually trigger the body's immune system to attack its own tissues including the brain. With all the immune problems inherent in Lyme disease, it makes sense that we want to lessen what the immune system has to deal with. Taking gluten out of the diet can relieve the immune system and the digestive system and create a much better picture of health.

Since gluten is contained in grains, it is typically found in carbohydrate foods such as breads and pastas. Lyme disease sufferers do best by avoiding too many carbohydrates anyway because of their inflammatory properties and the potential yeast overgrowth, so there is a dual benefit to avoiding them, and consequently gluten.

Many of my patients noticed a pronounced difference in how they feel when they removed gluten from their diets, and I highly recommend it.

Another food group that can cause inflammation is dairy. Dairy proteins found in milk, cheese, yoghurt, cottage cheese etc. are not easy for humans to digest. They can trigger immune reactions, and create mucous in the body. Anyone with respiratory conditions such as chronic sinus issues or asthma should definitely avoid dairy – but there is good reason for Lyme patients to avoid it too, or at least minimize it. Since yoghurt is fermented, it is somewhat easier to digest than milk or cheese; and goat dairy is easier to digest than cow dairy (sheep dairy is somewhere in the middle but closer to cow dairy).

Finally, any food that a person is sensitive to can fuel inflammation. In a full-blown food allergy, the reaction to the offending food is usually immediate and obvious. Most people know what their allergens are and avoid those foods. However, there are different types of food reactions, called food sensitivities or intolerances. They are mediated by different immune cells that can cause more subtle or hidden reactions, sometimes taking up to 72 hours from ingesting the food to manifest. The food sensitivities are caused by IgG immune cell reactions, while food allergies are triggered by IgE immune reactions.

To evaluate food sensitivities it is possible to do an elimination and challenge test. To do this, all the most common allergens are removed from the diet for a period of 21 days (gluten, dairy, soy, eggs, corn, citrus, peanuts). During that period of time the immune system has the chance to rest, recover and reset (when the foods are being eaten every day, typically the immune system cannot even register a problem as it is being constantly bombarded). After 21 days, foods are reintroduced one by one and any reactions noted. Usually after the 21 days of rest, the reactions to any problematic foods will be much stronger and more obvious, and therefore easier to identify.

The elimination diet requires a fair bit of discipline and effort, and it still has the potential to miss foods that might not have been excluded for the 21 days but are still causing problems. I have had patients with IgG sensitivities to garlic, bananas and pineapple – not things that we would typically consider problematic. Therefore the best way to assess for IgG food sensitivities is through a blood test. This testing is available in Australia (via Douglass Hanly Moir, Australian Biologics, Health Scope Functional Pathology and others) but as a word of warning, many medical doctors and allergists do not regard it as valid, so ask either an integrative or more open-minded medical doctor to order the tests for you!

Immunity

Many discussions have focused on immune function. Remember, your ability to fight Lyme depends on (1) your immune function, and (2) your ability to detoxify.

Nutrition can give immune function a boost. Fresh vegetables should be a large part of the diet. Vegetables contain vitamins, minerals and antioxidants, all of which the body needs in plentiful amounts. These nutrients facilitate cell growth and repair, cell-to-cell communication and metabolic processes. Enzymes in the body function to catalyse, or speed up, all of our biochemical reactions. Nutrients such as B vitamins, zinc and magnesium are required for those pathways to operate efficiently.

Green leafy veggies may well be the healthiest, but I suggest a broad range of colours. Different coloured vegetables contain different proportions of vitamins and minerals. A variety will ensure the best possible range.

High quality proteins are also important for immune function. Amino acids, the final breakdown product of proteins, are the building blocks of the body. Every cell and every tissue uses amino acids, including the immune system. High quality proteins include fish, chicken, some red meat (grass-fed red meat is ideal as it has a healthier fat content), eggs, nuts and seeds. This is one of the reasons I suggest a protein smoothie in the morning, to provide good quality proteins for the immune system to use. High quality proteins also keep the blood sugar stable and support adrenal function, which will in turn help the immune system.

The other part of supporting immunity is to avoid foods that suppress it. The main culprit in immune suppression is sugar. Studies have shown that one teaspoon of sugar can suppress immune function for up to 16 hours.

The mechanism by which sugar suppresses immune function involves insulin, the hormone that functions to shuttle sugar out of the blood and into the cells. When we eat sugar, insulin is released. The more sugar we eat, the more insulin is released. Insulin can circulate in the bloodstream long after the sugar has been metabolised, and an unwanted side effect of that is that the release of growth hormone from the pituitary gland is suppressed. Growth hormone is necessary for repair and recovery to occur in the body, and it is also a regulator of immune function. Therefore when sugar is eaten constantly, there is a constant flood of insulin in the blood stream, which in turn affects pituitary output of growth hormones and can create an immune deficiency.

Between the immune dampening and yeast-promoting effects of sugar, it is clear that Lyme patients are better off avoiding it altogether.

Digestion

There are several ways that nutrition can help digestive function. We already discussed that it is important to have gut function working optimally when treating Lyme disease – it is crucial to have a bowel movement at least once every day. If the bowels are sluggish and constipation is an issue, a high fibre diet along with supplementation with magnesium and vitamin C if necessary should be adopted to override this.

Fibre can also be used to sweep the bowels and clear toxins out. This is essential during antimicrobial therapy for Lyme and also during heavy metal detoxification.

As already discussed, good fibres for this are ground flax seeds and psyllium husk. I suggest a tablespoon of ground flax seeds in a protein smoothie every morning. Some people add flax seeds to salads or yoghurt. They must be ground, however, as whole flax seeds will pass through the intestinal tract without having the same sweeping effect as the ground ones. Psyllium husk is a little "rougher" than flax and does not contain the same cancer-preventing lignans, however for constipation it might be more effective.

Vegetables provide a great source of insoluble fibre. This is yet another reason to eat lots of fresh vegetables. Fruits contain more soluble fibre and they are beneficial too, but most Lyme patients restrict fruits because of their sugar content.

Candida, the naturally occurring yeast in the gut that tends to get overgrown during antibiotic therapy, feeds on sugar. All yeasts feed on sugar. One of the most fundamental principles of The Lyme Diet is to reduce sugar and carbohydrates, so as not to give the yeast a fuel source.

Avoiding sugars means not eating any refined sugars such as chocolate, candies, cakes, ice cream, etc. But it also means being mindful of all carbohydrates, even the "healthy" ones, as ultimately all carbohydrates break down into sugars. This includes fruit and whole grains.

Most of us have been brought up with the belief that fruit is a "good for you" thing, and in many ways it is. It is packed with vitamins and minerals and soluble fibre, and it is all natural. However, fruit is also a source of sugar, mainly fructose, and this too can feed yeast. For my patients with existing yeast issues, typically it is necessary to remove fruit from the diet for a period of time; for those without yeast issues but who still need to be mindful of prevention, one to two pieces a day is the limit.

Bear in mind that Candida and Lyme disease tend to go hand in hand, regardless of whether one is on antibiotics or not. In other words, many people with Lyme still struggle with Candida issues even when not taking antibiotics. Subsequently these guidelines apply to all Lyme patients.

The other way to foster good digestion is to avoid those food allergens and intolerances that we discussed in the section on inflammation. Any food that causes an immune reaction in the gut will cause some problems, whether or not they manifest overtly as digestive symptoms. Gas, bloating, constipation and diarrhoea are all possible symptoms of food intolerances.

Foods that cause inflammation in the gut can also lead to leaky gut. This is where the cells in the small intestine spread out, allowing larger than normal food particles to enter the blood stream. We discussed this in the section on naturopathic treatments for Lyme disease and gave some suggestions for gut-healing nutrients. But fundamental to improvement is removing the offending foods that are causing the problem in the first place – gluten, dairy and any other foods that trigger an IgG food sensitivity reaction.

Detoxification

Have you gathered by now the importance of detoxification for a Lyme patient?! We can help our detoxification pathways by the foods that we eat and those we avoid.

The liver, the primary organ of detoxification, is responsible for trapping toxins, converting them to less harmful forms and preparing them for excretion from the body. One of the kindest things we can do for our liver is simply to minimize the intake of toxins to reduce the load with which it has to cope.

This means eating organic fruits and vegetables whenever possible. It also means eating free-range meats, poultry and eggs – where the birds and animals have been raised without hefty doses of hormones and antibiotics. Remember, if they were fed antibiotics and hormones, residues of those will be entering your body when you eat them.

I understand that eating all organic produce and free-range or grass-fed meats and poultry can be expensive, and potentially more difficult to find. However, the reward is that the liver has a lighter load to carry, which can help the way you feel.

Fish is a contentious issue. I believe wild-caught fish to have a healthier fatty acid composition, however there are concerns about heavy metal levels. Mercury is a known neurotoxin and is bad for Lyme patients. Farm raised fish are often fed a grain diet and given medications along the way, so they are not really an ideal choice. The best solution in my opinion is to eat wild-caught fish. Choose the types of fish that are lower on the mercury scale (such as salmon) and limit seafood intake to twice weekly.

Foods that promote liver detoxification include artichokes, onions, garlic, beets, broccoli, spinach, cabbage, Brazil nuts, asparagus, avocado, pawpaw and cayenne. Any processed foods drag the liver down and should be avoided.

The other crucial element for detoxification is water. Since water makes up such a large proportion of our bodies, we must be constantly taking in fresh clean water for its cleansing and hydrating effects. Municipal water is high in chlorine and can potentially contain toxic elements such as heavy metals. Having adequately filtered water is important to avoid these pollutants. Most people should drink two litres per day.

Adding lemon juice to water helps to alkalinize the body (counterintuitive perhaps since lemon juice seems so acidic, but the overall effect in the body is alkaline), and to detoxify. The juice of one lemon squeezed into warm water is a good way to start the day, and is especially indicated during Herxes. Herbal teas are a good way to take in more water in a more holistic way while also naturally aiding various systems in your body. Peppermint helps digestive function, chamomile calms the nervous system, marshmallow soothes an inflamed gut, liquorice helps adrenal function, dandelion root boosts liver detox and dandelion leaf is a natural diuretic and kidney tonic. That is only a small sample of the herbs with medicinal effects that can be taken as tea.

Summary of Nutritional Principles

For a Lyme sufferer, the emphasis should be on:

- ▶ Vegetables
- ▶ Lean proteins
- ▶ Healthy fats

While eating less:

- ▶ Fruits
- ▶ Carbohydrates
- ▶ Processed foods

As mentioned before, vegetables should contain a range of different colours! Baby spinach, capsicum (green, red and yellow), tomatoes, beans, cauliflower and broccoli are just a few examples.

Ideally, eat less of the root vegetables such as potatoes, carrots, turnips and beets as they are starchier and can have a greater impact on yeast.

Lean proteins include fish, chicken, turkey, lean red meat (no more than once or twice a week) and eggs. Again, I strongly advise meats from animals that have been raised without hormones and antibiotics. Meats from grass-fed animals (as opposed to grain fed) have been shown to have a much more beneficial fatty acid profile. That is, they have less saturated fat (which as you remember are the ones that fuel inflammation). Historically, even beef contained healthy omega-3 fats, but when the cattle were taken off the fields, placed into stalls and fed a man-made, processed diet, their fat content became much more saturated, which was detrimental to the health of those who ate their meat.

Vegetarians will rely on tofu and legumes for their protein, and are strongly advised to drink a protein smoothie every day. In fact, everyone is strongly advised to drink a protein smoothie every day!

Healthy fats include the flax and fish oils discussed as anti-inflammatory oils, but there are also healthy fats found in avocado, olives and olive oil, and raw nuts and seeds.

Flax and olive oil are my preferred oils when used at room temperature or refrigerated, such as in salad dressings. For cooking, however, these oils will go rancid at higher temperatures, which counteract their health benefits. I recommend coconut oil for cooking, as it is stable at high temperatures. Coconut oil has two other benefits: It contains lauric acid, which is immune boosting and antiviral; and it contains caprylic acid, which is antifungal. While coconut oil was traditionally classified a saturated fat, it has a slightly different molecular structure to other saturated fats (containing medium chain triglycerides) which gives it more health benefits.

Foods to Avoid

As we have seen, fruits should not be eaten in abundance in Lyme disease, mostly because of their sugar content and effect on Candida. One or two pieces a day are acceptable for a person with no known yeast issues; during antibiotic therapy I suggest a limit of one piece a day; and if known yeast problems exist, fruit may need to be completely excluded for a period of time.

Fruit does contain lots of good vitamins and minerals. However, a wide variety of vegetables will also provide that without promoting yeast.

For the same reason, carbohydrates such as pastas, breads, potatoes, and rice may need to be restricted, as ultimately they get digested to sugars and can impact yeast. The starchy carbohydrates I prefer include quinoa, sweet potato and brown rice, mostly because they have a lesser impact on blood sugar, but even these can feed yeast in a susceptible individual. Decisions about how much fruit and starchy carbohydrates to eat are an individual one based on Candida, blood sugar and energy levels. Generally speaking those on antibiotics need to be stricter than those who are not, however I have seen both groups benefit from a low-carb diet.

Processed foods also need to be avoided. Full of saturated fats, hidden sugars, high-fructose corn syrup and gluten, processed foods add little in nutritional value to the diet. They can be a source of toxins and chemicals, and are rarely high in vitamins and minerals.

Drinks

The best fluids to take are water and herbal tea, approximately two liters daily. Lemon juice in water is also a good drink.

My single favourite nutritional boost is the protein smoothie. I encourage everyone to do a protein smoothie in the morning. The proteins provide a steady source of energy and help keep blood sugar balanced, which in turn helps the adrenal glands. A smoothie can also be a vessel for mixing other nutrients such as flax oil, and even nutritional supplements.

My favourite recipe is:

1 cup almond or rice milk

1 scoop protein powder (such as brown rice protein, whey protein, egg white protein, pea protein) *

1 tablespoon flax oil or coconut oil

1 tablespoon ground flax seed

1 cup fresh or frozen fruit (optional)

* Which protein powder to choose depends largely on your individual sensitivities.

Whey, although a dairy product, can be acceptable for some people. In dairy, the two major proteins are casein and whey. Of the two, casein is the more problematic and harmful. Whey, once isolated and purified, can promote liver detoxification and provide a high quality protein. Food sensitivity tests should indicate whether one is sensitive to whey and eggs, and that will help guide choices. For our highly sensitive patients we use a blend of rice, pea and chlorella proteins.

This is possibly the healthiest way to start your day providing not only proteins, but omega-3 fatty acids, fibre and lignans.

The other highly beneficial drink is a green smoothie. I am not a proponent of juices that are high in sugars such as fruits, and vegetables such as beets and carrots. I am also more of an advocate of high-powered blenders that completely liquefy vegetables, rather than juicers that extract the juice and leave all the beneficial fibres out. Not only is the fibre which benefits the bowels lost, the juice alone will transport through the gut and bloodstream more quickly without the effect of the fibre to slow it down, and can potentially have a detrimental effect on blood sugar. Vegetables such as spinach, cucumber and celery are good bases. Ginger and garlic can be added for flavour and their medicinal properties. I even add avocados to my green smoothies, and for those without major yeast issues who can do 1-2 pieces of fruit per day, a cup of berries or frozen mango sweetens it up.

Drinks to avoid are alcohol and coffee. Sorry about that.

Most Lyme patients become highly intolerant to alcohol, getting massive hangovers after only one drink. This typically provides enough of a deterrent. The liver, once again, is responsible for processing alcohol, so avoiding alcohol will remove one stressor, and that is worthwhile.

Lyme patients who are taking antibiotics should definitely avoid alcohol, as it can react adversely with the medications. Metronidazole (Flagyl), tinidazole (Fasigyn) and rifampicin are particularly harsh so no alcohol should be consumed at all while on those medications.

The amount of alcohol in drop doses of herbal tinctures is minimal and should not trigger a reaction. However for more sensitive patients or those wanting to be really thorough, herbs can be put into hot water, which will evaporate off the alcohol, then cooled before drinking.

Coffee not only provides one more thing for the liver to process but also acts as a stimulant on the adrenals. It is tempting to use coffee for a quick energy boost given the fatigue that is so common in Lyme disease, but the boost is short-lived, and ultimately it will add to exhaustion by taxing the adrenals. I am not categorically opposed to one coffee a day, but if several cups are needed just to get through the day, that is a sign of a bigger adrenal issue.

Lifestyle Factors

Exercise

Whether or not to exercise is one of the common questions that arise for Lyme patients. For some, it is not even a possibility – walking to the bathroom and back seems too far and a momentous task. Fatigue, pain, dizziness, and neurological issues can be prohibitive, even to activities of daily living.

For others, especially for those who had a regular exercise plan prior to their illness, it may be beneficial to do some light exercise.

I believe that as long as the exercise does not exhaust you, and so long as it does not set you back for the next couple of days, it is acceptable. My rule of thumb is that if the activity feels good at the time and you feel good the following day, then it is okay.

I am also not opposed to aerobic activity, which raises the heart rate and pumps oxygen around the body. In some cases, this can be revitalizing, and healthy for the body. Again, the rules of thumb are to *listen to your body* and *if in doubt, go slow*.

Good forms of exercise for Lyme patients are walking, swimming, yoga, Pilates and light strength training (weights, dyna bands, Kettlebells etc.). Running, tennis and other team sports are likely to be too intensive.

People with low cortisol need to be more careful as they have less fuel in the tank. Cortisol and the adrenals, among other things, are involved in the regulation of blood sugar. We think of insulin as the hormone responsible for this, and while that is especially true in the short term after we eat, cortisol also plays a significant role in the longer-term regulation of blood sugar. So people with erratic or insignificant cortisol production may be unable to adequately regulate their blood sugar post-exertion. The adrenals, through the hormone aldosterone, also play a role in salt and water balance in the body, and subsequently hydration. Poorly functioning adrenals may impact a person's ability to stay hydrated and maintain a healthy salt and water balance.

Those with low thyroid function, which is common in chronic Lyme disease may struggle with exercise due to the fatigue and lethargy associated with it.

Hypoxia, or low oxygen in the muscle tissues, is often seen in both fibromyalgia and Lyme disease patients. This will make exercise all the more painful as there is not sufficient oxygenation in the muscle cells, the mitochondrial energy-production pathways are not able to create as much ATP (which requires oxygen), and muscles will feel fatigued and achy, even with the lightest exercise. My patients have told me that the day after taking a slow walk around the block, they felt like they had run a half marathon instead because of their muscle aches and pains. This is due to the lack of oxygen and ATP, coupled with a rapid accumulation of lactic acid that was not cleared out of the muscles due to their slow metabolic processes.

This is where magnesium and malic acid can be very helpful, as the malic acid helps to support the oxygenation of the muscles while the magnesium aids muscle relaxation.

Many people find that supplementing with ribose before a workout helps their strength and overall energy levels. Ribose is a five-carbon sugar, but it is not a "bad" sugar since it does not impact blood sugar negatively (in fact, some people find it actually gives them a lowering effect, and need to take it with food to offset this), and it does not feed Candida. It is a sugar that feeds skeletal muscle and cardiac muscle directly. Taken prior to exercise it can provide a fuel source for the muscles and promote endurance. Even without exercising, many people with chronic fatigue, muscle weakness and lack of stamina benefit from supplementing with ribose and malic acid.

Any of the mitochondrial support nutrients – NADH, CoQ10, L-carnitine, alpha keto-glutaric acid – can be helpful for supporting energy production and thus helpful for sustaining exercise.

As a disclaimer, supplements should not be used to "prop you up" in order to exercise. They can be aids but should not be crutches. If you require two shots of espresso to get out and walk around the block, but you could not walk that far yourself without the two shots, then you probably should not be doing it. Anything with a stimulant effect can be harmful, especially when taken over time. Stimulants, while they might help at the time, wear down your adrenals even faster and contribute to more profound exhaustion down the road.

For those who are very sick and bedridden, you may set a goal to do some arm lifts and leg lifts a couple of times a day, or to walk to the end of the driveway and back. Even if this is your limit, still try to do it a couple of times a day. If you are in a wheelchair perhaps you could use one or two-pound weights for some arm exercises.

Remember that the bugs do not like oxygen so increasing oxygen throughout the body is putting them at a disadvantage. Maintaining some mild gentle activity can be strengthening and rejuvenating for the body. It can also be a game-changer for mental outlook. Exercise has been shown to be among the most helpful interventions for depression, and understandably, many Lyme patients struggle with depression. Activity, at whatever level is comfortable for you, increases oxygen flow to the brain and boosts the happy chemicals such as endorphins, growth hormone and serotonin.

Sleep

Before I say anything about sleep, I want to acknowledge that many Lyme sufferers have tremendous sleep disturbance. I understand that my advice to get eight hours of sleep may frustrate you, because you would happily sleep for four hours if you could, but sleep is elusive. People with chronic Lyme disease tend to either sleep many hours at a time out of sheer and perpetual exhaustion, or the complete opposite occurs and they have trouble falling asleep, staying asleep, or both. Insomnia affects most Lyme sufferers at some stage of their illness.

In the section on naturopathic interventions we looked at some of the natural sleep aids that can be helpful. While I am not a fan of prescription sleep aids, there are times when they can be necessary in the short term to promote healthy sleep patterns.

The body does a lot of healing while we sleep. Cortisol levels fall at night (hopefully), and the immune system kicks up to do its housekeeping. This is why symptoms sometimes feel worse at night, because the immune system is more active. This does not always hold true for all Lyme patients, partially because their immune system is operating on low levels to begin with, but it holds true for many.

Nutrition and Lyme Disease

The hours between 10pm and 2am are the most valuable hours in terms of physical regeneration. Therefore the more sleep you can get before midnight, the better off you are. Some people only need six hours sleep a night while others need eight or nine. Respect your body's need for sleep knowing it is using that time for healing. If in doubt, sleep more rather than less.

There are several things you can do to improve your sleep. Toxicity can be a major contributor to insomnia, so make sure your detoxification is sufficiently supported with smilax, glutathione, liver herbs, activated charcoal and so on. Magnesium sulfate (Epsom salts) baths at night are not only relaxing (the magnesium part) but they can give an extra boost to detox (the sulfate part).

Hormone imbalance also impacts sleep—low thyroid, while causing fatigue, can cause insomnia. Adrenal fatigue definitely impacts it, and many people find their sleep improves once their adrenals are better supported.

Electromagnetic fields can interfere with sleep patterns especially in highly sensitive people so remove as many electronic devices as possible from the bedroom, especially those with wireless or Bluetooth capabilities. Even getting rid of digital clock radios, cell phones by the bed, and cordless landlines makes a difference. A magnetic or earthing pad or sheet can offset the effects of electromagnetic fields.

Finally, create a cave for yourself. Get blackout curtains or blinds, have comfy bedding, make your bed a place you want to be. Have a protein snack before bed to keep your blood sugar stable through the night. And if sleep is elusive, make the decision that you will use that time to have productive, hopeful thoughts, not troublesome anxious ones. That might take some discipline at first, but the more you strengthen the neural pathways around positive thoughts, the easier it will be to draw on them.

REFERENCES

1. McFadzean N. The Lyme diet: nutritional strategies for healing from Lyme disease. Legacy Line Publishing; 2010. 216 p.

20. CAN NATURAL THERAPIES ALONE TREAT LYME DISEASE?

I AM FREQUENTLY ASKED WHETHER IT IS POSSIBLE TO RECOVER from Lyme disease without the use of antibiotics. It's a great question, but unfortunately not one for which I have a definitive answer. Rather, my answer is "sometimes". I wish I could tell people that they can treat their Lyme disease 100% naturally and have great outcomes every time, but that is just not realistic.

I definitely have patients that I work with without the use of antibiotics, where herbal antimicrobials and immune support, coupled with dietary changes and other supportive nutritional supplements have recovered them to the point where they are living their lives, either completely symptom free or at 90-95% of their normal (pre-Lyme) level of functioning. I love these cases as they really reinforce the power of natural medicine.

More often than not, when patients opt for all-natural treatment, it is necessary to select a variety of modalities to cover as many bases as possible. An example is to combine the immune-supportive properties of transfer factors (both general and Lyme-specific) with herbal antimicrobials (teasel, cats claw, olive leaf, etc) and Lyme-specific homeopathic remedies, and as I said, base all of that on a solid foundation of good nutrition. We want to address the infection from several directions at once to maximize the impact and our success. Of course supporting detoxification and digestive support are important, too.

In many cases herbs, nutrition and homeopathics will not be enough, and we need to step it up another notch. This is when I consider other therapies such as hyperbaric oxygen (HBOT). HBOT is a great way to improve oxygen flow to the cells, accelerating the cellular healing and regeneration. It also has antimicrobial action, as the bugs do not survive well in that high saturation of oxygen. It helps regenerate neurological function and sweeps the body of other microbes such as viruses and mycoplasma. HBOT can be time and money intensive, and accessibility can be an issue, but it is a very valuable treatment option.

If HBOT is not an option, another approach is to engage some kind of Rife or frequency-based therapy. This is based on the premise that if the frequency of a certain pathogen is introduced to the body, that pathogen will be killed by the energy/ frequency that matches it. Rife machines can be purchased for home use, and some practitioners offer Rife therapy in their office. For more information on Rife therapy, see Bryan Rosner's book, *When Antibiotics Fail: Lyme Disease and Rife Machines*.

Alas, there are cases where antibiotics are necessary. I wish it wasn't so, but it is. Some people just can't recover sufficiently without these medications, and antibiotics offer relief that other more natural therapies cannot give. I honestly think that the majority of Lyme patients require antibiotic treatment at some time during their treatment. Of course, I always vote for naturopathic support in conjunction with the meds, and nutrition is equally if not even more important here. But the bottom line is that in many cases, the medications are a necessary part of treatment.

There are a number of factors that determine whether a patient will respond well only to natural treatments. Duration of illness is one as well as severity of symptoms. Obviously a more recent case that hasn't gone as "deep" into the body will likely respond better. Also, I have had better success treating more naturally in cases where there is less neurological involvement. Arthritic-type Lyme seems to respond better to herbs and nutrient therapy, in part I believe because there are several great natural remedies for calming inflammation, which causes a lot of the pain. Minerals such as magnesium can offset a lot of the muscle aching, cramping and twitching.

So can Lyme disease be treated naturally? My answer is "sometimes". My general philosophy is to start with natural agents and build up to medications if the patient is not responding adequately. At least then we have laid a solid foundation of support and started doing some bug-killing before the medications are introduced, and have set up detox pathways to function better and handle medications and die-off better. In medicine this is called the "therapeutic order" – start with the least invasive therapy and work up in strength and invasiveness as needed.

Another important part of this puzzle is to ensure other issues such as hormone imbalance, heavy metal toxicity, thyroid issues and food intolerances are being adequately addressed. Sometimes if Lyme symptoms are not resolving there is a tendency to get more and more aggressive with medications, adding new ones and increasing doses, when the problem may not be originating from the Lyme disease at all, and may be helped with something completely different such as gluten avoidance or chelation therapy.

Of course, Lyme disease is complicated. There is no answer that is right for everyone, and the thing that might be right for an individual today may not be right for them six months from now. A lot of the answers come from listening carefully to what the body is saying, and not being afraid to make adjustments as needed. Whether natural treatments or antibiotics are used, a multi-system, multi-factorial approach is the key to recovery from Lyme disease. We need to treat the person, not the disease.

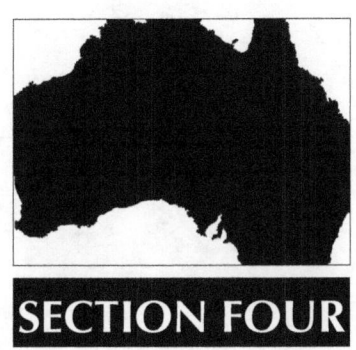

PUTTING IT ALL TOGETHER

21. WHAT DOCTORS SHOULD KNOW ABOUT LYME DISEASE

IF YOU ARE A PHYSICIAN OR OTHER HEALTH PRACTITIONER READing this book, the first thing I want to say is "Thank You". Thank you for your openness, your willingness to learn, and your courage in stepping outside the status quo and recognising that chronic Lyme disease is a real disease, a disease that exists in Australia, and one that affects some, maybe many, of your patients.

There are a few key take-homes that I would like to emphasize for healthcare providers.

1. The International Lyme and Associated Disease Society (ILADS) is a non-profit, multi-disciplinary, international medical society dedicated to disseminating accurate and practical information on Lyme and related illnesses. They hold annual conferences in the United States and in Europe, they have physician-training programs and they publish treatment guidelines. Their website is www.ilads.org. They are a great resource for new doctors; in fact, they may be the most important resource in existence at the time of this book's writing.

2. There is mounting evidence for the existence of Lyme disease in Australia. Case numbers are growing rapidly and will continue to do so as awareness grows. Please consider Lyme disease when you have a patient with a multi-system illness, where traditional medical testing and imaging does not show a valid explanation for the symptoms. A trial of antibiotic therapy can provide useful diagnostic information (either through improvement or flare of symptoms).

3. Patients often have no recollection of a tick bite or the typical EM rash. Lyme disease cannot be ruled out in the absence of these two things.

4. Lyme disease is a clinical diagnosis that can be made based on symptom picture and the patient's history. Lab work should be done to confirm the diagnosis and shed light on co-infections, but negative test results for Lyme do not rule out infection.

5. ELISA testing is not sufficiently sensitive to be considered reliable. Lab testing should be done through a specialist Lyme lab. IGeneX is the lab used by most Lyme-literate medical doctors in the United States and is considered the leader in the field of Lyme disease. Multiple test types should be run, including Western Blots, PCR and IFA for Borrelia; and antibodies and FISH tests for co-infections. The cost and extra work involved for the patient to send their blood to the United States is worth it for the information it can provide.

6. Lyme disease treatment protocols are complex and can be considerably different from standard antibiotic regimens. They are –

    ▶ Long duration – several months up to two years and even beyond.
    ▶ High dose – often these pathogens require higher than normal doses to be effective.
    ▶ Multiple medications – medications must be combined to cover the three different life cycles of Borrelia – spirochete form, cell-wall deficient form and cyst form, as well as addressing co-infections along the way. The medications needed will vary throughout the recovery process, depending on which infection or infections are most active at any given point in time.

These factors can make prescribing antibiotics for Lyme disease patients a challenging and intimidating task. Please continue to use this book, Dr. Burrascano's Advanced Topics in Lyme Disease and the ILADS Treatment Guidelines as resources (see Appendix A for Burrascano's 2008 Treatment Guidelines).

7. The Lyme Disease Association of Australia and the Karl McManus Foundation are good sources of information and are working to cre-

ate more physician training programs within Australia for the further education of doctors and other health practitioners.

8. Recognize that the best approach to chronic Lyme disease is multi-disciplinary. A team approach works well since no one practitioner can offer everything. A captain at the helm is always a good idea —one central doctor coordinating and overseeing the treatment—but recognising when counsellors, massage therapists, Bowen therapists, naturopaths and other allied health practitioners can be useful is a great bonus.

9. Please, please remain compassionate to the plight of Lyme disease patients. Please do not tell them they are crazy! Lyme patients need love and understanding and a kind, non-judgmental, listening ear. They have had way too many experiences of being cut off, dismissed, judged, ridiculed and shut down by other doctors. Please be the one that provides a different experience for them. None of us have all the answers, and Lyme disease is certainly a complex and challenging illness to treat. Sometimes, just being willing to listen and show compassion makes all the difference.

22. THE EMOTIONAL CHALLENGES OF LYME DISEASE

LYME DISEASE NOT ONLY TAKES A HEFTY PHYSICAL TOLL ON THE body but exacts a great emotional toll as well. Here is just a sampling of some of the challenges inherent in the world of chronic Lyme disease:

Lack of diagnosis/ answers – "there's nothing wrong with you"

Most patients have seen many doctors in their quest for answers as to why they are so sick. This is mostly because doctors are not trained to recognise the symptoms of Lyme disease, nor run adequate tests for it. Oftentimes many tests are run and studies undertaken, none of which return positive results, giving the appearance that there is nothing physically wrong with the person.

Further contributing to this problem is that in Western medicine today, the body has become so segregated. The nervous system is the domain of the neurologist, the bones are the domain of the rheumatologist, the stomach is the domain of the gastroenterologist. The General Practitioner is the physician designed to know a bit about everything, but realistically their training has conditioned them to refer out to the specialists when their knowledge and experience bank is tapped. So many Lyme patients are sent to various specialists who are unable to diagnose the problems they are having in any given organ or system in isolation; they do not see the global picture. Even when the patient's symptoms *do* match the symptoms of disease patterns they are trained to look for, they might discharge the patient telling them that there is nothing physically wrong with them.

The diagnosis of psychosomatic symptoms—"it's all in your head" or worse "you're crazy"

It is very common for Lyme patients to be told that their illness is all in their head, that it is stress related or related to depression or anxiety. This is because in the slew of medical tests and studies performed in the evaluation of their illness, nothing really shows up to explain the symptoms. Coupled with this, Lyme patients are often depressed or anxious by the time they have been sick for years, seen multiple doctors, not gotten any real answers as to what might be happening to their bodies, and to top it off, have bacteria and parasites messing with their brain.

Most Lyme patients at some point in their illness have been offered or given anti-anxiety medications or anti-depressants from their doctor. I am not saying that there is not a place for these therapies in the treatment of chronic Lyme disease – sometimes they can be highly beneficial to stabilise the psycho-emotional aspects of the illness while treatment is undertaken. However, Lyme disease is a physical disease with psycho-emotional manifestations. It is *not* a psychiatric illness. Telling a Lyme patient they are crazy and need psychiatric help is cruel, misguided and unproductive. I am sure 100% of Lyme patients would opt for a healthy life and a healthy body if given the chance. They did not "choose" their illness or bring it on themselves. Granted, as is the case with any chronic illness, suffering can be a great teacher and many people learn a lot about themselves, which they would not have gained otherwise. I would also say that in some, there can be psycho-emotional barriers to healing, and when these elements are addressed, the body recovers faster. However, that is a very different position from the claim that Lyme patients are making up symptoms or that the illness is purely a manifestation of stress or anxiety.

Symptoms that are not always visible to the world—"but you look fine to me"

Many Lyme patients feel like death warmed up, but on the outside they look quite healthy. Joint pain, headaches, buzzing in the limbs, rapid heart rate, aching muscles, and shooting pains may not be visible to friends, colleagues and neighbours, even though to the person experiencing them, they seem to be taking over their entire being. Drenching sweats in the privacy of one's bedroom at night are not recognized by others in the light of day.

Lyme disease patients do not look like cancer patients who may have lost their hair or a lot of weight during chemotherapy. They do not appear as rheumatoid arthritis patients whose joints are so red and swollen that they are clearly visible to the outside world.

The agony of Lyme disease can be very isolating. Lyme patients often feel very misunderstood, and very alone in their illness. Lyme is especially hard on spouses and families. When Mum might not be well enough to take the kids to school or to play or help with homework, it puts strain on the household. It is not uncommon for spouses to question the validity of their mate's symptoms and illness, as often they do not present outwardly with the things we associate with illness such as weight loss, looking pale, deformities of the body, or other visible signs.

Lyme patients often have to "soldier on", maintaining jobs outside the home, keeping house and coordinating kids' schedules. At the same time, while they might appear to be holding it together, there is often incredible pain and suffering on the inside.

The unknown – "how long is this going to last?" and "will I ever really be well again?"

We do know that chronic Lyme disease requires long-term treatment. Rarely is it less than one year, often two years, and many times even longer than that. It makes it particularly hard to plan for, given the potential loss of income, and the expense of treatments, medications, supplements, doctor visits and so on. This long-term nature of treatment places tremendous strain on families – in ways that are both financial and non-financial.

The million-dollar question of "do we ever really cure Lyme disease?" is one that I am asked all the time. The current belief is that acute Lyme, if caught early (in the first few weeks) and treated aggressively enough, can be cured. Chronic Lyme, however, is believed to remain in the body on some level even with treatment. BUT – there is always the possibility of full recovery, and that is always the goal. Once levels of infection are lowered, the immune system should be able to handle the load on an ongoing basis. If you have had glandular fever, the virus that causes it (Epstein-Barr virus) is always going to be in your system. That does not necessarily mean that it will ever cause you problems again. Similarly, there are Lyme patients who have made a full recovery, and who may never again experience any Lyme symptoms. Granted, once the infection is treated, care still needs to be taken to maintain a healthy immune system through nutrition and lifestyle factors such as adequate sleep, stress management and so on; but recovery *is* possible and should always be the goal. Also, many patients are able to live a very normal life even if they have a few small remaining symptoms. Sometimes, recovery to 90% well, along with some ongoing maintenance treatments, is a large victory and will allow patients to resume their normal lifestyle and activities.

If Lyme patients maintain hope that they can and will recover, then they actually stand a greater chance of recovering (the profound power of the mind). One of the real barriers to this is trying to stay optimistic that recovery is possible in the light of information that the infection will never fully be cleared from the body. I believe that working on emotional blocks and negative thought patterns around this through therapies such as Emotional Freedom Technique (EFT) can help people overcome this emotional hurdle.

The multiple costs of the illness—"am I going to lose everything over this?"

The costs of Lyme disease are painfully high. I have known many to lose their homes, exhaust their savings, have to borrow from friends and family, and live on social security income because Lyme disease has ravaged their financial wellbeing. But the costs go way beyond finances. Many people have lost jobs that they loved; careers that they worked so hard for; hobbies and interests that gave them joy. Many marriages have crumbled as they simply could not withstand the stressors that come with such a misunderstood chronic illness. A few have even lost the ability to care for their children, and had to entrust them to friends, relatives or the state to provide what they could not.

The loss that can come with chronic Lyme disease is profound and can be devastating – years of lost income, friends lost through confusion and lack of understanding, loved ones lost through the challenges of trying to maintain a relationship. Many times there is a significant grief aspect to this illness that needs to be compassionately understood and addressed.

The guilt factor—"did I give this to my children?"

I believe that congenital Lyme exists. I have treated children of mothers who have Lyme disease, some of whom were exhibiting symptoms from a very young age; some of whom had a concurrent autism diagnosis; and some of whom have never left Australia or who have no record of a tick bite. The guilt a mother feels if there is any chance that she passed Lyme disease on to her child can be tremendous. Of course, many women did not know that they had Lyme disease when they were pregnant and breastfeeding, and how could they have? But now, they have sick children and they wish that they had had more information back then as well as an accurate diagnosis of their own, so that they could have made more informed decisions (such as taking antibiotics during pregnancy, not breastfeeding, etc). This provokes a lot of guilt, and also a lot of anger at the medical system for not providing answers when those answers could have made all the difference.

LYME DISEASE in Australia

The Australian experience—"am I all alone?"

One of the most difficult challenges for Lyme disease sufferers in Australia is the brick wall they face as soon as the words "Lyme disease" are mentioned. Doctors shut down, friends look blank, insurance companies close their cheque books. Everyone denies that Lyme exists and goes on their merry way. Thankfully, some of the recent media coverage is extending knowledge of Lyme disease throughout the community, and people are recognising themselves and their experiences in the stories they hear. Through the Internet, email groups are forming, information is being shared, and people are finding some solidarity in their newly formed "pack". Support groups are sprouting up in various parts of the country, educational seminars are being planned, training programs are in development and Australian GP's are starting to make the trip to the U.S. or Europe for training with ILADS.

Australians are not alone any more, but understandably many still have that experience and have felt that way for many years. If this is you, I encourage you to take heart that you are no longer alone. The Lyme situation in Australia is changing and will continue to change because there are now enough motivated and passionate individuals and groups who will ensure it.

■ ■ ■ ■

23. COPING STRATEGIES

CONNIE STRASHEIM, AUTHOR OF SEVERAL BOOKS ON LYME DISease including *Insights Into Lyme Disease Treatment: 13 Lyme-literate Practitioners Share Their Healing Strategies*,[1] also wrote a great book entitled *The Lyme Disease Survival Guide: Physical, Lifestyle and Emotional Strategies for Healing*.[2] I recommend this book to provide thoughts and ideas that will support you.

There are a collection of tools and habits that my patients have used that seem to make a difference and keep them moving forward. These are also things that I believe in as being able to make a contribution towards healing.

Create a network of support and positivity

From an emotional standpoint, a positive attitude and a strong support system is central to "surviving" the Lyme experience. Positive thoughts, positive actions and positive surroundings can make the difference between giving in to illness, and being able to face it head on each day, striving for a better future.

It is impossible to stay positive and hopeful when surrounded by negative and pessimistic people. Surrounding yourself with the right people who prop you up, encourage you, celebrate your victories, and empathize with your struggles without letting you get into a big pity party about them will boost your outlook and your healing. Create that environment deliberately. Sometimes it helps to be direct: Tell people what you need from them; tell them exactly what support looks like to you; tell them if you just want them to listen to you or if you want them to offer ideas or opinions; tell them what it provides for you when they give you encouragement and understanding. People often want to help but they do not know how. It is your job to let them know. They cannot read your mind.

Do not be afraid to let go of people who pull you down and who are constantly negative about you or your illness as they will hinder your recovery.

Where possible, and especially if you do not have a good support system at home or in your close surroundings, get a counsellor or therapist whom you trust. They will always be there to support you and will provide you with compassion and understanding, which can be very healing. Just because a person has not experienced all you have experienced in your illness, does not mean they cannot be empathetic to what you are going through.

I have found Emotional Freedom Technique (EFT) to be a significant tool for patients. It is a technique that can be used to help release painful emotions. Once learned it can be done anywhere, anytime, and takes only a few minutes. It might be one of the best "coping tools" you can have in your arsenal. Another technique that is easy to do at home is binaural beat therapy (www.centerpointe.com). Listening to this CD daily helps the brain to reorganise itself into healthier patterns, leading to less anxiety and fear, better stress tolerance and a more positive outlook.

Also, do not be afraid to ask for help when the psychological and emotional aspects of the illness overwhelm you. Some people benefit from anti-depressant or anti-anxiety medications to get them through the hardest parts. You do not have to be a hero and suffer along needlessly. These medications, while I do not believe are the healthiest choice long term, can be life saving, or at least sanity saving, when used as a bridge to recovery.

Coping Strategies

Create an environment of positivity

Just as people can bring you up or down, so too can your environment make a big difference. Make sure to have things around you that represent freedom, health and wholeness. Do not pack your fishing gear or sporting equipment away in the back shed, assuming you will never be able to use them again. Keep them out. In fact, keep them handy (you may need them sooner than you think). The visual reminder keeps them in your present and future, not in your past.

I recommend people identify a few things that they enjoy doing and can manage, and do at least one every day. Examples are reading great books, talking to friends on the phone, listening to soulful music, sewing or writing – whatever are the things that you can do, do them. Even if it is just a few minutes each day, deliberately take time for something that brings you enjoyment.

Harness the power of the mind

Neuroscience is giving us amazing information about the brain that shatters all our pre-conceived notions. While once thought of as quite rigid and unchangeable, we now know that the brain is malleable. The term "neuroplasticity" has been coined to describe that phenomenon. What this means is that the brain is adaptable. If one part of the brain is damaged, a different part of the brain can take over its functions. That has been shown in conditions such as stroke, visual and auditory defects. It also means that the neural pathways can be shaped and strengthened, if we train them.

When we have a certain thought or thought pattern, that thought pattern travels along a neural pathway in the brain. There is both electrical activity and chemical activity associated with that. When we repeat that thought over and over again, the neural pathways representing it are strengthened. What started out as a "single lane dirt road" neural pathway can be grown and expanded into a "multi-lane superhighway" neural pathway. How? By repeated strengthening of that pathway, through repetition (the training effect). Given this information, it is easy to see that while positive thoughts may not seem like the easier ones to have in the midst of pain and illness, they are the ones you must have in order to strengthen those positive neural pathways. Giving in to chronic negative thinking will be self-perpetuating, self-fulfilling prophecy – you will literally train your brain to think negatively, and that will manifest in your body.

This is incredibly powerful information that can be used to significantly influence your health. I would highly recommend two books on this subject - *Molecules of Emotion*[3] by Candace Pert and *The Brain That Changes Itself*[4] by Norman Doidge.

Dare to dream

It is ok to dream of the days when you will be well again. Imagine what they will be like, think about what you will do – where you will travel, who you will spend time with, what you will eat and drink, what you always wanted to do before but never had the time/ money/ motivation. There is nothing like a painful, debilitating illness to make you realize what is truly important to you and what really matters in life. Make wish lists, gather information on exotic destinations you would like to see, research saxophone lessons or read up on the breed of puppy that might work well for you. Whatever it is, dream it, with the plan of living it.

We know now that our reality follows our thoughts. What we think, we will create; it becomes our reality. We already see that we can choose our thoughts, but thoughts are also sourced from our imagination. I used the term "daydream on purpose" because that resonates for me – if we "daydream on purpose" we create those visions - we make them real in our minds - then our minds set to work on making them real in our lives. I used to think this was airy-fairy nonsense, but having studied the neuroscience behind it, I now see that this is very real, and that our dreams and imaginings are distinct predictors of our future.

Develop your spiritual connection

Everyone has different religious and spiritual beliefs, and none are necessarily right or wrong. What I have observed in my years in practice and in my own life, is that feeling connected spiritually profoundly impacts the way we see the world, including the way we view suffering. I have noticed that the people who are more spiritually connected are more able to feel grateful for their life, even in the face of their illness, and feel less hopeless about their disease. They feel less alone and take solace in their spiritual connection. Spiritual practices such as prayer and meditation are also very grounding and calming for the mind, which can lead to a reduction in pain and suffering.

People with strong faith also tend to adopt an outlook of serving others. I realize that this may sound paradoxical as many Lyme patients struggle even to get themselves the help they need, but I have noticed that those who reach out and help and support others, even if it is just a two-minute phone call to see how an elderly or another sick person is feeling, tend to be less hopeless about their own situation. Lyme patients are now uniquely positioned to have compassion and understanding for those who are still struggling.

REFERENCES

1. Strasheim C. 13 Lyme-literate practitioners share their healing strategies. 1st ed. Lake Tahoe: BioMed Publishing Group; 2009. 444 p.
2. Strasheim C. The Lyme disease survival guide: physical, lifestyle and emotional strategies for healing. 1st ed. Lake Tahoe: BioMed Publishing Group; 2008. 296 p.
3. Pert C. Molecules of emotion. 1st ed. Simon & Schuster; 1999. 368 p.
4. Doidge N. The brain that changes itself. 2nd ed. Penguin Books; 2008. 427 p.

24. STORIES OF HOPE AND RECOVERY

THERE ARE PEOPLE WITH LYME DISEASE IN AUSTRALIA WHO ARE recovering, patients who have been through antibiotic treatment and are now off their medications and feeling well. There are many who have experienced significant improvement, and while not 100%, are back at work, living their lives, and functioning as they used to before they got sick.

Everyone's journey is different and everyone's concept of "better" or "recovered" is different. Some people will have to watch their nutrition more closely. Others may still feel a flare up of fatigue when they are under stress, or will one day have to do medications again. No one is claiming that they'll never deal with Lyme and its symptoms again. However, compared to what they suffered in the past, they are doing remarkably well. With a healthy diet, healthy lifestyle and healthy outlook, there is nothing to say that their recovery cannot be permanent.

I wanted to share some stories with you to show you this and encourage you along your recovery path. These are the stories of several of my patients.

■ ■ ■ ■

Aimee S., Sydney, NSW

I grew up in a tick endemic area on the east coast of the United States. I had deer living in my yard, our cats have brought mice into the house, I trained for half marathons in the woods and I have even pulled ticks off of my husband after his mountain bike rides. I thought that I knew about Lyme disease as my immediate family members and friends had contracted it after being bitten by a tick and getting the hallmark EM rash. So you would think that when I came down with every single symptom on the symptom checklist for Lyme, Babesia and Bartonella, I would have said to myself, 'Hey. I think I have Lyme.' Well, I wish it were that simple. You see, I never recall being bitten by a tick or having a bull's eye rash, so the diagnosis of Lyme never crossed my mind. And so I began my journey of discovery and more importantly, healing.

After years of symptoms, I had finally talked my GP into signing the paperwork and sending my blood off to IGeneX Labs. It is ironic because at this stage I was getting the tests done to rule out Lyme disease even though I thought it was a long shot. Although I did not have IGeneX test for Babesia or Bartonella, my tests came back IgM negative, but IgG positive, for Lyme. I had many positive bands and IND present on both of these Lyme tests. From conducting my own research on how to read and understand IGeneX lab results, I realized that the numerous positive bands I did have meant that I most likely had Lyme. I decided to make an appointment with a LLMD who gave me a clinical diagnosis of Lyme, Babesia and Bartonella.

My Lyme treatment lasted a little over three years, and I was treated by two different doctors. My first LLMD was located in the States as I was living in America at the time. He prescribed antibiotics to target Lyme first and then the co-infections. He used high doses of one antibiotic at a time, once I improved then plateau'd, I would move on to the next antibiotic on his schedule. I started with Doxycycline, then moved onto Zithromax, Ceftin, Flagyl and finally clindamycin & quinine. He also prescribed B-12 shots every other day, high doses of probiotics, magnesium, Diflucan for systematic yeast, Boulouke for biofilms and twice daily injections of heparin for thinning out my blood so the bacteria couldn't hide in the thick blood.

About a year into my treatment, my husband was transferred to Sydney, Australia for work. I tried coordinating overseas phone calls with my

LLMD in order to continue my treatments, but it never worked. I was living in Australia with no doctor to treat me. About this time, I felt ready to change doctors because all of my research indicated that it is best to treat with multiple antibiotics concurrently rather than consecutively. I was also looking for a more holistic and integrated approach. That is when I found Dr. N. through one of the Australian Lyme Support Groups. By the time I had my first appointment with her, some of my symptoms had improved, but I was still struggling with crushing fatigue, severe brain fog, air hunger, insomnia, some anxiety and depression, and pain on the bottom of my feet. Since my first doctor and I hadn't really addressed co-infections yet, Dr. N and I felt strongly that they were causing most of my symptoms. Dr. N and I focused on treating Babesia and Bartonella as well as Lyme. While under Dr. N's care I was on a multiple-antibiotics approach and taking Flagyl, Zithromax, Biaxin, Mepron, and Lariam. It was with her antibiotic combination that I saw my symptoms disappear.

While my main form of treatment was antibiotics, I did rely heavily on other adjunct treatment modalities. About three months after being diagnosed I bought a Rife machine and used that to not only target Lyme and co-infections but viruses as well. I do feel that my Rife machine was just as important as my antibiotics in terms of lowering my viral and bacterial load. Dr. N introduced me to colloidal silver, which I still use to this day. While killing the bugs is very important, detox was a top priority in my treatment protocol as well. Daily coffee enemas, Dr. N's herbal protocol, Dr. N's detox protocol, FIR sauna, Epsom salt baths, drinking three litres of lemon water a day, and lymphatic drainage massages were all used as part of my detox regime. After starting treatment with Dr. N., I began to see a chiropractor that knew about Lyme and we worked together to get my body realigned and functioning again. I believe this helped strengthen my immune system, provided relief from back & neck pain and gave me more flexibility and range of motion.

As part of my detox protocol I had to change my diet. I stopped eating gluten, wheat, soy, corn, starches, sugars and artificial sweeteners (I only use Stevia now). I have added more healthy fats such as coconut oil when cooking my meals. My new eating style is more aligned with a Paleo or Primal way of eating. Since making this change in my diet, I feel even better now than I did before I got sick with Lyme. I feel that cutting out these allergy and inflammatory type foods has allowed my immune system to get stronger, and I have been healthier to fight Lyme and its co-infections.

The three years that I battled with Lyme were some of the toughest and darkest days I had ever experienced. Just getting out of bed in the morning seemed like a small victory at times. I knew that having Lyme was going to be the ultimate test of my own self-determination and resilience. I had decided early on to take the approach of healing not only from a physical aspect but from an emotional & spiritual one as well. So while I was using antibiotics, Rife, colloidal silver, herbals and detox protocols for the medical aspect, I was also treating the emotional and psychological aspects. I made the decision not to get 'stuck' in anger, resentment or sadness at how my life had changed rather to look at my situation as a wake-up call or life lesson to be learned. I asked myself, 'How did I wind up in this predicament? Why did I get sick?' I don't believe that people just get Lyme for no reason. I believe that something in your body or in your lifestyle isn't healthy or working correctly and this allows you to get sick.

I am also a big believer that our thoughts and emotions are directly correlated to our state of health and wellbeing. I started seeing a therapist who specializes in Emotional Freedom Technique (EFT). This was a tremendous help and I was able to work through some of my mental blocks and negative self talk that I had been carrying around for years. I consider EFT instrumental in helping me get to where I am now. It also helped me realize that when I was in remission from Lyme, I didn't want to go back to my old life, because that old lifestyle is what got me sick in the first place - high stress, poor eating habits, no sleep, always putting other people's needs before my own, and basically not taking care of myself. I had to put me first.

It is still a struggle to change, but I know if I want to stay in remission, it is what I have to do. I never thought I would say this, but I am glad I got

Stories of Hope and Recovery

sick with Lyme. It was my wakeup call that I had to change in order to keep myself healthy. I realized that Lyme was my body's way of telling me, 'Hey, we can't go on like this anymore. Something has to give.' I listened and responded to that wakeup call. I consider myself an even better, healthier person today than before I got sick.

I consider myself in remission as I have been off antibiotics for 1-½ years. I continue to use my colloidal silver and sometimes my Rife machine. In addition, I have added the Salt and C protocol to my relapse prevention plan and it has kept me symptom free and living a full and active life for the past 1-½ years. I only think about Lyme disease when I take my daily dose of Salt and C. I do believe that remission is possible, but it has to be a multifaceted and holistic approach to healing. Now, when I make any life decisions, I ask, 'Is this in the best interest of my health?' I would have never thought this way three years ago.

■ ■ ■ ■

Greg W, Narooma, NSW

Up until a few months ago state and federal governments in Australia did not officially acknowledge the existence of Lyme disease in Australia. My story starts 40 years ago in 1972 when I first started work in the forestry industry in Australia. For as long as I can remember I've had tick bites every spring/summer - some years only a few, other years 20 or 30. In 1977 I traveled through Europe and West Africa and may have been exposed to ticks there, too. None of the tick bites stand out in my memory as exceptional in their symptoms. Bite site swelling, short-term headache and fever were common with every round of bites, but then in 1981 I started getting swollen, painful and 'hot' joints in my feet, ankles, wrists, neck and hands. This was diagnosed as arthritis, and I've been treated with anti-inflammatories ever since.

By the early 1990s I was finding it hard to get out of bed in the mornings. I'd wake up feeling more tired than when I went to bed, and my brain felt like it was in a fog all the time. I was treated for sleep apnoea. I'd get bouts of migraine-sized headaches. MRIs didn't show anything abnormal. I was working long hours and there was tragedy in my immediate family. The doctors put it down to fatigue and depression and put me on a course of anti-depressants as well as the anti-inflammatory medication. By this stage I was getting bone erosion in my joints and developing Baker's cysts in my knees, and I was being treated for high cholesterol. I had once done triathlons, but now it was painful just to walk a few hundred metres.

By 2010 I was convinced I had early-onset Alzheimer's - I couldn't remember nouns and place names and often became disoriented in familiar locations. I would get confused, uncoordinated and find it hard to string sentences together without concentrating. I suffered extreme bouts of paranoia. I was getting muscle twitches and pins-and-needles in the fingers, ringing in the ears, and sensitivity to loud noise and bright sunlight. My sense of smell disappeared.

In those 30 years none of the doctors had picked up that there might be a common cause for all these ailments. They had just been treating each symptom as it was presented. My own internet research in the late 90s had shown that a search for Alzheimer's + cholesterol brought up all these web pages showing bacteria as a common link, but my doctor said this was 'nonsense'; and further, the connection from bacteria to tick bites had not been explored.

Then in 2011 I read a newspaper story that changed my life. It dealt with the plight of an Australian, Karl McManus, and his fight with Motor Neurone Disease (MND), which was attributed to undiagnosed Lyme disease only after his death. I recognized his symptoms were the same as mine, and the prospect of MND horrified me. There was a link in the article to the Lyme Disease Association of Australia and they put me in touch with Aussie expat Nicola McFadzean, a Lyme specialist in North America. Nicola gave a clinical diagnosis and said, "If you were in North America you would have a positive diagnosis for chronic Lyme disease."

The symptoms indicated I probably had co-infections of Bartonella and Babesiosis and would need treatment for those as well.

After 30 years of dealing with undiagnosed symptoms, those words were a revelation. Nicola will always hold a warm place in my heart for her diagnosis.

Nicola initially started me on a regime of natural therapies – teasel root, smilax and therapies to support removal of toxins through my liver and kidneys. These natural therapies were insightful. I had an immediate reaction and for the first time in 30 years woke up feeling refreshed, and remembering dreams. The arthritis symptoms went away, and the brain fog began to lift. Unfortunately the initial benefits of the natural therapy were not sustained and we decided to move onto a regime of antibiotics. This was daunting. I took 200mg of Doxycycline twice a day, 500 mg of Tinidazole twice a day and 300mg of Rifampicin once a day over a four-month period, with fortnightly reviews of progress. I had a really strong Herxheimer reaction to the antibiotic regime as a result of the dead bacterial toxins in my system, and that made me very sick for a few days. In a way this was good because it confirmed that I did have a bacterial infection and that the antibiotic treatment was working.

Towards the end of the first four-month treatment schedule, I got caught out by not keeping up probiotics to my good gut bacteria and I developed colitis - my digestive system shut down with severe gastric reflux. I ended up in hospital for three days while it was sorted out.

Over the first four months of treatment, the Lyme symptoms slowly disappeared. All the arthritis symptoms that had plagued my daily activities for 30 years vanished. The joint problems and joint swelling disappeared. The constant back and neck pain were gone. The hot, painful feet were a thing of the past. The rosacea rashes disappeared. However the four-month review showed that the neurological symptoms, though diminished, were still present and needed further treatment.

The antibiotic treatment changed and it was even more daunting. I took 500 mg of Clarithromycin twice daily, 500 mg of Tinidazole twice a day and 300mg of Rifampicin once a day over a 4 - month period with fortnightly reviews of progress. In addition there were twice weekly injections of 0.9 million units of Bicillin to treat the stubborn neurological symptoms. This treatment regime was slowly working. I was feeling a little better every day, and the neurological symptoms were slowly disappearing.

Unfortunately seven months into what could be 24 months of treatment, I came up against the Australian medical bureaucracy, which is no longer supporting this treatment regime 'prescribed by a practitioner that is not registered in Australia'. My treatment has stopped while my doctor and pharmacist try to find a Lyme specialist in Australia prepared to sponsor the treatment schedule. It's a catch-22. At this time there are no true Lyme specialists in Australia. They have found a microbiologist who is interested in the case, but he wants to identify the specific bacteria before sponsoring treatment, and tests for Lyme in Australia often come back negative.

Nicola describes me as now 'mostly well'. I'm looking forward to the time when the Australian medical bureaucratic red tape that is strangling effective Lyme treatment in this country is sorted out, when Lyme is recognized in Australia and when I can start my treatment regime again. I'm looking forward to getting these bacteria totally out of my system and once again, waking up refreshed in the morning after a restful night's sleep.

■ ■ ■ ■

Jo M, Berwick, VIC

I consider the story of my illness odd as I was not sick until I started treatment for Lyme disease. I was always active and exercised, including running, bike riding and weights in the gym. I had a good diet and did not drink alcohol or smoke. I did suffer from asthma and was on a preventative for this. Other than that, I felt fit and healthy.

In 2009 I began to get headaches on a daily basis, which I would describe as a dull ache and throb at the back of my head. They did not seem to go

Stories of Hope and Recovery

away completely but just varied from day to day in their intensity. I put it down to stresses at work and thought nothing more of it.

Around the same time I also began to get lower back pain, most noticeable in the morning, as though I had been standing for hours. After I got up, showered and moved around for about an hour, the pain seemed to go.

During the year and predominantly at night, I started to notice that I was getting very minor heart palpitations while I was sitting and relaxing. I felt my heart racing for a few minutes and then it would stop. It was not a frequent occurrence and not enough to worry me. I had been to a cardiologist prior to this for a leaky mitral value and was told at the time that my heart was otherwise healthy.

The main symptom I noticed was extreme tiredness. I went for many months unable to physically stay awake after around 9.30 pm. I was getting about nine hours of sleep and would wake feeling really tired. There were times when I was being driven to work and would fall back asleep as soon as I got in the car. In time this seemed to pass so again, I thought nothing of it.

Apart from these odd symptoms, which I never linked to each other, I thought that I was in good health. I didn't get sick with the flu or colds during the year, and I was riding my bike through the hills five out of seven days a week for about 50 minutes a day.

In May 2010 my husband collapsed at work and was taken to the hospital. His health had been deteriorating over a year, and he had been undergoing numerous medical tests in an effort to work out what was wrong with him. At this stage I still had the daily headaches and lower back aches and assumed it was the stress of his ill health.

I spoke to a colleague at work about my husband's ill health and symptoms, and they told me of a friend of theirs with similar symptoms who had been diagnosed with Lyme disease. At this time I had never heard of Lyme.

LYME DISEASE in Australia

We flew from Melbourne to Sydney to see Dr. Peter Mayne, who clinically diagnosed my husband with Lyme disease and possible co-infections of Bartonella and Babesia. At the time I did not have what I thought were any similar symptoms, and so I did not have a clinical diagnosis made.

Shortly after my husband received his blood results from America, which indicated he had Lyme disease and the Bartonella co-infection, we were contacted by Dr. Mayne again. Dr. Mayne requested that I have blood taken to analyse my CD-57 count. A few days later and before the results were available, Dr. Mayne requested further blood tests from me as he suspected that my husband may also have the infection Mycoplasma fermentans, which we were advised, was highly contagious. If my tests revealed Mycoplasma fermentans, it would mean that my husband had it as well and would need additional antibiotics to treat it.

In April, 2011 I was contacted by Dr. Mayne who advised me that he had received my CD-57 results and that my count was 22, indicating Lyme disease. I was shattered by the results as I did not feel sick and I had no symptoms apart from the headaches and lower back pain.

At the start of June 2011 I was again contacted by Dr. Mayne who told me I had tested positive for Mycoplasma fermentans. Dr. Mayne started me on two tablets twice daily of 250 mg of Doxycycline and Clarithromycin to deal with the Mycoplasma fermentans only. About two weeks after starting this medication, I began to feel a little unwell but again put this down to stress, as it seemed to pass and I was still working 40 hours a week and exercising five days a week.

Towards the end of June I contacted the Australian Biologics laboratory as I still had not received my Borrelia results and was initially advised that I was negative. My husband and I then started to have monthly consultations with Dr. Nicola.

In August 2011 Dr. Mayne contacted me and told me that the initial test for the Borrelia species was incorrect. The laboratory had re-tested my blood and I showed a strong positive result for the Borrelia species.

He concluded that I also had Lyme disease, but my co-infections were unknown. Dr. Mayne initially prescribed me 400mg of Doxycycline daily, Clarithromycin 250 mg, two tablets twice daily, and Simplotan 500 mg, one tablet twice daily. I was to pulse the Simplotan in for two weeks, stop taking it for two weeks and then commence it again in the same cycle. When I started taking all this medication I felt nothing for about a week, and then I began to feel worse. My headaches worsened, my lower back pain increased, my joints seemed to ache and I felt like I had been hit by a truck, or was getting a flu which never came.

I also commenced two Bicillin injections a week. I would get my injections on Monday morning and by mid-afternoon the colour in my face had drained, I felt nauseous, and I ached all over. For the following two to three days I would also have shivering and sweating sensations. By the Thursday or Friday this feeling seemed to pass.

I stopped regular consultations with Dr. Mayne and made the decision to only consult with Dr. Nicola.

Towards the end of August my hands began to blister and were red and extremely painful. Dr. Nicola suggested I stop taking the Doxycycline and replace it with Ceftin (cefuroxime) 500mg three times daily. The blisters and redness went away in about two weeks.

From May 2011 until October 2011 my headaches appeared to worsen, and I had them day and night. I was still able to work but found it difficult to concentrate at times. My lower back pain increased slightly and my flu-like symptoms came and went intermittently. As time wore on, I felt like I was actually getting sicker.

In October 2011 Dr. Nicola was concerned that I showed no change in my headaches and suggested I commence taking two Artemisinin tablets twice daily. I pulsed in the Artemisinin daily for three weeks, stopped for a week and then resumed for three weeks. Within two days of commencing the Artemisinin tablets I began to feel sick. My body aches, headaches and back pain increased. At times I would have hot flashes and trouble sleeping. I also started to get extreme whole-body twitches whenever I laid down to rest. I would feel my whole body reacting and it was frightening. I had modified my diet after reading Dr. Nicola's *The Lyme Diet* book to give my body a chance to fight, but continued to exercise (bike riding) five days a week and always felt really healthy afterwards.

For the next three months I continued with this treatment and felt like I was getting worse as time progressed. I felt that I was getting very sick and this concerned me greatly. Generally when people feel unwell, they are prescribed medication, which makes them feel better. I was feeling well, and after I started the medication, I progressively got sicker. I suffered weight loss, loss of appetite and withdrew in myself. I did not suffer anxiety or depression but refused to talk about Lyme, I chose to take my medication and daily supplements, and continue to work and exercise as if I was well. I continued to work a 40-hour week and took up study for a promotion at work.

In January 2012 Dr. Nicola was still concerned about my continual headaches and felt that I was showing Babesia symptoms. She suggested I commence taking Mepron (Wellvone) 5 ml, twice daily. Within a few days of adding the Mepron to my treatment, I felt the sickest I had ever felt, and it was more noticeable when I was taking the Artemisinin tablets.

In February 2012 Dr. Nicola added Larium 250 mg, 1 every five days, to my treatment. Again within ten days I felt even worse, but after a month or two, I didn't seem to notice the Larium. Dr. Nicola changed the Larium dosage to 1 tablet every four days but I still find that on the day I take the Larium, I feel a little sick that night.

By March 2012 I had been on treatment for 11 months and felt that I was in worse health than before I took any medication or had the blood tests. I really struggled with the concept of taking the medication as it is meant to make you well but it felt like it did the opposite for me! Many friends and colleagues told me to stop taking the medication as I looked so sick compared to before I started treatment. I decided to continue with my treatment as I had seen how sick other people had become without treatment.

By April 2012 after a year of this treatment, I started to notice that I was having two or three days where I felt a bit better. Between April and May 2012 I begin to notice the several days in a row of feeling better rather than the odd day when I felt worse. I didn't feel back to normal, just better than I had.

I continued my treatment program until May 2012 when Dr. Nicola increased my Bicillin injections to twice weekly, on Monday and Thursday mornings. The evening of my injections I would ache and get very cold. The following morning I would feel better. I actually felt like I was getting healthier. I no longer had the lower back pain, and my headaches only seemed to appear twice a week. My twitches had ceased as well.

In late May 2012 Dr. Nicola increased my Mepron dosage to 10 ml, twice daily. Upon commencing this double dose I felt really sick for first few days. For the four weeks prior, I had felt healthy. With the new dosage, however, I felt like I had been hit by a truck, and my headaches appeared four out of seven days a week. The pain was still significantly less than it was at the end of 2011.

In hindsight, I don't think any of the medication was unhelpful, but at the time, I hated it all as it felt like it was making me sicker.

I have been on treatment for 14 months but I would say the most significant improvement began after 9 months of treatment when I commenced the Mepron. For the last six months, my health has been constantly improving.

When I reflect on my Lyme journey so far, I wouldn't do anything differently. I read Dr. Nicola's book and Dr. Singleton's book and researched the medications prescribed to me on the Internet. I refused to speak to people within the Lyme community or watch documentaries on how sick Lyme patients can become. I chose to follow the treatment plan of Dr.

Nicola only, as I felt her holistic approach was far better than antibiotics alone. I saw other Lyme patients suffer from depression and anxiety and the more they spoke about the illness the more it appeared to affect their mental health. I know that by not involving myself in these conversations and getting on with my life has greatly increased the time frame of my recovery.

I combined my antibiotics with natural supplements:

5 ml Fish Oil daily, Flaxseed Oil, Magmin, Vitamin D, Multi-vitamin, Vitamin B12, Vitamin C, Dr. Nicola's Detox Formula #2, Simlax, Lyme Support, Teasel root, probiotic powder and tri-fortify liposomal glutathione.

I did not drink alcohol before being diagnosed and still do not. I rarely ate bread but continued to have a small bowl of cereal and skim milk daily. I have never drunk coffee. I continued having weak black tea daily (three cups). I began to drink more water, reduced my chocolate intake although my diet was basically good prior to getting sick. I don't eat seafood, cheese or eggs because I am a fussy eater.

I understand the importance of giving your body the best chance to fight while the immune system is depressed but it needs to be balanced with sustaining your mental health and treating yourself on occasions. I hate being sick, and having to be so rigid constantly reminded me of my disease. This is why it was important for me to continue my exercise, which I changed to 50-minute walks seven days a week instead of bike riding.

The holistic approach of combining antibiotics with natural supplements was of greater benefit to me. With respect to detox I would say I was not strict with this. I did not use the sauna, nor take baths or exercise daily. I listened to my body, when I exercised I actually improved my feeling of wellness. Dr. Nicola advised I take her probiotic powder which I do daily.

I think what helped me was to believe that I would get better and that there was no other option other than getting well. I am not spiritual but believe in nature and the strength of my body to fight this disease. I know that continuing to work (I have only had four days off sick in the 14 months) has been a struggle at times but it has strengthened me and allowed me to keep going with the treatments that made me so sick.

I was lucky that I did not suffer anxiety from the disease or prior to it. At times I became sad but never depressed which I knew was a very real and devastating effect of the disease. I believe that my mental strength has increased my recovery. I am a fighter and will not give in to this disease. I had the mentality that the disease had taken my health for the time being but it wouldn't take the other areas of my life - exercise and work. I passed my promotional exam and sat a panel for a promotion, which I attained. I am currently undergoing courses for this new position and won't be stopped by Lyme. It has not been easy to achieve this but I did not want to give in.

One of the hardest elements to my recovery was the lack of medical support in Australia. I was lucky to have found Dr. Nicola to support me through my recovery. My two local doctors have been so supportive of my treatment plans despite the lack of medical knowledge of this disease. At times I get upset that there is no support in Australia but I don't allow this to consume me; I get on with the treatment rather than looking for medical support from doctors. I put my faith in Dr. Nicola and I have been rewarded with improving health. I am now having more periods of wellness, and I begin to think about when I can stop treatment. This has been one of the hardest battles in my recovery as no one can tell you how long in terms of months or years it will take. It is frustrating but you need to move on from this, otherwise, you spend mental energy worrying about something you cannot change, instead of the things you can.

■ ■ ■ ■

Paul M, Berwick VIC

I have traveled the world extensively, Europe, Africa, Middle East, Canada and USA. In 2006 I traveled to Canada where I suspect I received a tick bite. I have a very vague recollection of a large pimple-like mark on my neck.

Leading up to my diagnosis I had many bouts of the flu, tiredness and fatigue. This did not stop me from living a normal work and social life. Up until my diagnosis I was keeping fit by running, bike riding and going to the gym regularly, but felt my fitness and health slowly deteriorated.

In May 2010 I collapsed at work with pain in my right loin area and my blood pressure dropped. An ambulance was called and I was taken to the Emergency Department. All tests indicated everything was normal, but they could not account for my blood pressure dropping every time I sat up. This subsided in time. The hospital doctors stated they could not find anything wrong with me, and they believed I was in good health, though I knew and felt differently.

After leaving the hospital I felt consistent pain to my right loin and kidney area, headaches, and dizziness; I felt like I had been hit by a truck. It took 14 days of rest to feel well again.

I continued to have bouts of feeling sick with pain in the kidney area off and on, and dizziness. I was referred to a cardiologist who conducted the following tests – 24-hour heart monitor, stress test and tilt table test. I failed the tilt table test, and because of this, was diagnosed with Neurally-Mediated Hypotension but my heart was otherwise healthy. Even after this diagnosis I still felt it was not the cause of my problems, as I continued to have off and on loin (kidney) pain and headaches. After visiting my GP several times because I still felt poorly, she referred me for an ultrasound for the kidney pain and an MRI for the headache, which all came back normal.

During this period I was feeling fatigued and tired but put it down to working excessive hours.

In early March my wife Jo was speaking to a work colleague about my ill health and the inability of the doctors to determine what was wrong with me. Her colleague had a friend with similar symptoms who had recently been diagnosed with Lyme disease, and subsequently supplied details of a Lyme doctor in Sydney.

On 12 March 2011, I saw Dr Peter Mayne in Sydney for a clinical assessment for Lyme disease. After the assessment Dr Mayne suspected I had Lyme disease as well as the co- infections Babesia and Bartonella.

At this time my symptoms consisted of pain in the loin (kidney) areas. I had trouble thinking, brain fog, poor concentration, tiredness and fatigue. I had neck and back stiffness, chest pains, palpitations of the heart at times (like my heart drops) and a tingling feeling in my lower legs, like a crawling feeling. I had headaches at the back of my head, and at times my head felt hot. I was sensitive to alcohol and caffeine, felt unbalanced and light-headed, and experienced periods of diarrhoea. I suffered from bouts of anxiety and had the occasional panic attack, which I had never experienced.

On 15 March 2011 I had a blood test conducted, which showed I had a CD-57 level of 30. This was followed up with the IGeneX Lyme IgG Western Blot test showing a positive result.

I commenced antibiotic treatment on 23 March 2011 in consultation with Dr Peter Mayne in Sydney. Dr Mayne is a true champion in the treatment of Lyme disease in Australia. He provided sound treatment, advice and support.

Since 17 May, 2011 I have consulted with Dr Nicola McFadzean in the USA who has gone out of her way to make herself accessible to Lyme patients in Australia. Dr. Nicola is truly a professional, supportive Lyme doctor who genuinely cares and wants patients to recover from Lyme disease. She provides regular and consistent treatment with a sound holistic approach to Lyme treatment, which includes the use of antibiotics, diet, natural medicine and other treatments.

My wife and I were supported by two local GP's who accepted the fact we had Lyme disease, and though the treatment was unknown or counter to their training and education, they provided amazing support during our treatment. They assisted by administering Bicillin injections, providing prescriptions, requesting and monitoring blood tests and monitoring our general health throughout our treatment. These doctors are truly great doctors who displayed professionalism, care, empathy and understanding. Since commencing treatment these GP doctors have seen me slowly improve and have often commented on this.

One of the hardest things I had to come to terms with was the lack of medical support here in Australia and scepticism from medical practitioners in relation to Lyme disease and the ILADS treatment protocols. As part of my return-to-work plan, I was required to see an infectious disease expert after I had already been diagnosed with Lyme disease. The infectious disease doctor stated my tests were inconclusive and that I did not have Lyme disease. I replied, "I am chronically ill so what do you say is wrong with me?" He said, "I don't know. Mediated hypotension is a possibility." With that, I knew I had to place my faith in Lyme-literate practitioners who offered treatment, support and most importantly hope. At this point I found a determined resolve and belief that to recover from Lyme disease, I would have to take responsibility for my own health and treatment.

I was lucky that I had a GP who did everything in an attempt to determine why I was so unwell. When I told my doctor that I had Lyme disease, she said, "That would make sense, and I don't know if we would have ever worked it out". My GP has supported me totally with my Lyme treatment.

The antibiotic treatment has changed at different times and has included:

1. Doxycycline tablets 100 mg - Dosage 2 tablets twice a day.
2. Clarithromycin tablets 250 mg - Dosage 2 tablets twice a day.
3. Tinidazole tablets 500 mg - Dosage 1 tablet twice a day.
4. Bicillin injections LA 0.9 mill units - Dosage 2 injections twice a week
5. Rifampin capsules 300 mg - Dosage 1 tablet twice a day (for Bartonella)

6. Bactrim - 960 mg twice a day
7. Larium 250 mg 1 tablet every five days.
8. Mepron - initially commenced on 5ml twice a day and increased 10 ml twice a day.

About four weeks after commencing treatment with doxycycline, clarithromycin and tinidazole, I became extremely sick and my symptoms became significant, especially the head symptoms - brain fog, concentration, vision and noise sensitivity and fatigue. I had sustained moderate Herxes, which were at times severe.

Soon after this I commenced two Bicillin injections a week, which caused significant Herxes within 24 hours. These subsided in time and then about six months later, I commenced double injections twice a week which immediately caused significant Herxes which were mainly mild to moderate intensity. I felt this treatment was significant to my improvement.

After three to four months on Rifampin I noticed that my anxiety and Bartonella symptoms subsided.

After ten months of treatment I started on Mepron. After a couple of months, I felt significant improvement and my symptoms (stomach/back cramps, headaches - top and back of head, and general feeling of sickness improved). However once my dosage was doubled from 5mL twice a day to 10mL twice a day my symptoms became significant. I am currently on double Mepron for one month, and though I still feel poorly, I feel I am improving as a result.

I consume a detox diet based on *The Lyme Diet* book by Dr. Nicola, and I consume filtered water and green tea with lemon.

I regularly saw an Exercise Physiologist who set an anaerobic exercise plan based on Dr. Burrascano's guidelines. I walked for 30 minutes and did a series of anaerobic exercises and stretches every second day. During the initial stages I was very fatigued and didn't feel well, but I consistently exercised and never skipped a session.

My energy levels have improved significantly and I am currently going to the gym every second day and weight training using light to moderate weights as well as doing the series of exercises and stretches. I continue to walk regularly and am now capable of bike riding and running but choose not to because of the impact aerobic exercise would have on my immune system.

I feel exercise was so important to improving my health and my mental well-being. After exercising I feel better and feel my body and health improve. It was difficult at times especially because of how I felt, but I was determined to complete my exercises.

I also purchased a portable far infrared sauna and started using it daily for 30 minutes. Now I use it every second day. For the first six months of treatment I would have a hot salts bath every second day. At first, I wouldn't feel well after the bath, but that subsided in time.

I take a range of supplements, including probiotics, aloe vera juice, alpha-lipoic acid, fish oil, flax oil, vitamin C, CoQ10, magnesium, vitamin D, vitamin B and spirulina. Dr. Nicola also put me on some of her formulas including glutathione, detox support, teasel, and her Lyme support formula.

I struggle to identify what was the most helpful part of my treatment. Although my symptoms improved significantly with antibiotics, it is hard to determine which one was the most effective because of the number, dosage and frequency of medicines I took. The Bicillin injections and Mepron are most effective in causing Herx reactions, which resulted in the biggest improvement for me. I found it difficult at times to determine why I wasn't feeling well, whether it was as a result of Herx, medication, symptoms, the disease itself, or a combination.

One of the things that made this journey so difficult has been the lack of acceptance of Lyme disease and its treatment in Australia. Though I had a positive attitude from the beginning, I found it difficult to comprehend that I was unable to get medical treatment and support for Lyme disease here. Further, I had to tolerate scepticism from doctors who questioned the treatment.

I am still on the road of recovery but have had stages of improvement after about five months. I feel I have improved significantly since commencing treatment. It's only now that I realize how sick I was at the beginning of treatment.

At about the six-month mark I noticed the beginning of improvement; my symptoms were still present but not as severe. Anxiety subsided and the Herxes were mild to moderate.

After seven months on treatment I returned to work. At the twelve-month mark, I felt significant improvement and returned to work full time, eight hours a day, five days a week. Returning to work was a massive achievement and truly signified that I was reclaiming my life and that all the hard work and positive attitude was paying off. I am not going to let the disease determine the outcome of my life.

I still have mild to moderate symptoms at times, but I also have windows of feeling normal. I currently try to live an active life while not running myself down. I exercise regularly, eat a healthy diet, try to sustain consistent sleep/rest periods and actively socialize with friends and family in cafes and restaurants, and at parties. In the first six months this was very difficult to do, as I didn't feel well and was extremely noise and vision sensitive. I struggled to concentrate during conversations because I would zone out. Thankfully this has subsided significantly.

Through self-education and reading books such as Dr Nicola's *The Lyme Diet* and Dr Singleton's *The Lyme Disease Solution*,[1] I quickly understood that diet is one of the most important aspects of Lyme treatment and truly believe it is a key component to your recovery. Like in life, you get out of it what you put in. The same is true with your health. If you put good healthy food into your body, you will eventually get good health. I strongly believe the body has the ability to heal itself but needs the support of a healthy diet along with other positive treatment methods.

I based my diet on Dr. Nicola's book *The Lyme Diet* and was extremely disciplined with my diet especially during the first 10 months. After that I continued to stick to the Lyme diet but allowed myself to have other foods within reason when socializing. Even with the additions, I am still very disciplined in eating good, healthy food to support my Lyme treatment.

Through self-education I discovered that treatment needs to be supported by naturopathic medicine, and I believe that a holistic approach is required to recover from Lyme disease. I have placed my trust in Dr. Nicola's naturopathic medicine knowing that detoxifying is so important to eliminate toxins from the body. This is further supported with filtered water and caffeine-free green/herbal teas.

I am a strong believer in finding the inner strength within no matter how hard things become. I have a 'never give up' and 'never surrender' philosophy. Tough times don't last; tough people do. I take one day at a time, and I try to do positive things every day, no matter how bad I feel.

Helping or giving to others is important to me, whether it is friends, family or others. It gives one so much satisfaction and a sense of feeling helpful and useful. My father was extremely ill over the last 12 months until he passed away in March 2012. This was a difficult time and I wasn't feeling well, but rather than give into self-pity, I decided to help my father and mother through this difficult time. It made me realize that I could have it so much worse.

This illness was difficult for me as the anxiety, which I had never experienced previously was extreme at times. Once I realized that the Lyme was causing it and that it would pass, I managed much better and it has subsided. It is very easy to become obsessed with Lyme disease. I choose not to let it control my day-to-day life.

I strongly believe exercise, interacting with family, friends, getting back to work and finding some happiness every day goes such a long way in dealing with Lyme disease.

I sought assistance from a psychologist, which was of great benefit. It assisted in dealing with the illness and reinforcing my self-belief that I would reclaim my health.

Prior to my diagnosis, I lived an active and healthy lifestyle, which I believe has contributed to my body's ability to deal with the Lyme disease. I will continue with this lifestyle.

I am currently 14 months into treatment and experiencing windows of normalcy, but I still have such a long way to go. I know I am still required to undergo treatment for some time if I wish to recover. I have a self-belief and determination that I will reclaim my full health and recover from Lyme disease.

■ ■ ■ ■

Rhonda M, Melbourne, VIC

I was finally diagnosed with Lyme disease in April 2008 after returning from Scotland and Bavaria and being sick for four years. During this time I was diagnosed with a range of illnesses from meningitis and Bell's palsy to severe ongoing headaches, muscle weakness, extreme fatigue, depression, skin and bowel disorders to name a few. Each of the diagnoses had been individually treated. At this time I was put on doxycycline for three weeks. As I was not improving I had a lumbar puncture done which confirmed the disease was in my central nervous system, and then received 30 days of 2g intravenous ceftriaxone, after which a second lumbar puncture was done and came back negative for the infection.

Once the IV treatment started my symptoms increased to include speech and reading difficulties, and problems performing normal activities to the extent at times it became dangerous (e.g. pouring water into the electrical component of the bread maker and not the bowl). I found these mental difficulties to be very unsettling as I had gone from running professional development in curriculum development for teachers; along with parent information sessions; and modelling and mentoring colleagues in best teaching practice, to being unable to put sentences together correctly at times, and unable to read, to the extent that I felt like a child learning to read. My specialist could not explain this and put it down to Chronic Fatigue and Fibromyalgia, but my symptoms were constantly changing. What I experienced one day might not be what happened the next! I was referred to a neurologist who couldn't find anything during a physical examination but was going to access my history next time he was in the hospital. I never heard from him again.

As Lyme disease is not found in Australia (or so I was told at the time), it was difficult to get answers. My infectious disease specialist had seen very few cases of Lyme and had not treated someone who had been infected for four years. He told me that I had been given the best treatment possible (he kept referring to a little book from Stanford University, obviously the IDSA treatment guidelines) and that hopefully by Christmas, I would have more good days than bad. I started to improve and then would go backwards. It was difficult because I was not sure what to expect, and there was no one to really discuss it with.

I consulted an integrative medicine physician who found I was deficient in a number of vitamins and minerals. I had seven weekly IV treatments with Vitamin B, eight with vitamin C and zinc, and two with magnesium. I also took supplements for all of these except Vitamin C. This doctor picked up that I had a thyroid problem, as I had high thyroid antibodies and started treating me with thyroid medication.

Fortunately one of the nurses who had been treating me while I was having intravenous treatment visited Germany for a holiday and spoke to a friend about Lyme disease treatment in Germany. She returned to Australia and contacted me with the website details for the Borreliose Centrum Augsburg (BCA) in Augsburg, suggesting it would be worth contacting them to see if they could offer any advice on this disease.

After waiting a few months I was at my wits end and so one night, I emailed BCA. My husband thought that they wouldn't reply or would tell me to go to Germany. To our surprise we received a response the next morning from one of the doctors at BCA, saying I had not had the best treatment with oral antibiotics, and that the IV treatment was insufficient in both dose and the amount of time given. I was also told that after four years I had chronic Lyme disease. He suggested that I needed to be tested for co-infections and, "The first step for you is looking for Lyme activity in your blood by Elispot-LTT and CD-57 count." He also told me what treatment I needed and was happy to speak to my specialist, and so began my long journey towards recovery.

My infectious disease specialist started the new regimen of IV ceftriaxone at the increased dose, which was pulsed at four days on/ three days off each week, with weekly blood tests done here. He didn't think it was necessary to have the blood tested by the clinic in Germany, however after discussions with the doctor at BCA, we decided to send the blood sample to Germany. This was the best decision we could have made since the results came back showing both Lyme disease and Chlamydia pneumonia. I had IV treatment for nine weeks, and initially my specialist was supportive. However, as the weeks passed and I was admitted to the hospital a couple of times, he began to change his attitude and say that it was "all in my head". The clinic in Germany had sent articles regarding Lyme and co-infections and the necessary treatment, which we passed on to the specialist. When asked at one of the weekly consultations whether he had read the articles, his response was, "No, I don't have time." I found these weekly consultations to be very distressing but was always supported by the fantastic nurses from "Hospital in The Home" who were caring for me and the doctor from BCA, with whom I had regular contact and who would respond quickly to any concerns.

At the beginning of week eight I again sent blood to Germany, and my specialist had decided he was going to stop IV treatment straight away. We managed to persuade him to continue until the results came back a few days later. These indicated that I still had both infections but the Chlamydia needed to be treated. I changed to Phase 2 of treatment as recommended by BCA, which involved oral antibiotics - clarithromycin and Plaquenil for 12 weeks, fortnightly blood tests for liver, kidney and blood count and sending blood to Germany every eight weeks. By this stage I had experienced enough of the negative attitude of the specialist impacting negatively on my health, and after discussion with my local doctor, decided that I would be better off having him supervise my care. He has been fantastic and even organized for my blood to be taken at the clinic and transported to BCA. He could see that I still required treatment but believed that I should not have to go overseas to be treated. BCA's protocol involved having a break for four weeks and then sending blood again. After this I began Phase 3 of treatment. The oral antibiotics changed to azithromycin which was again a pulsed therapy and Plaquenil for 12 weeks, and we continued to send blood for testing.

In October 2009 after 12 months of antibiotic treatment, BCA recommended I go off all antibiotics for another 12 weeks and build up my immune system (the latest results still indicated that I had a very high cellular active Chlamydia pneumonia infection and a high cellular Lyme infection. I also had symptoms for a Bartonella-like organism co-infection). While I was happy to be off the antibiotics, I was very concerned and distressed about the possibility of the infections getting worse again.

After further discussion with BCA, I pointed out that right from the start, I had been building up my immune system as they had advised with the help of an integrative doctor, I couldn't see how I would improve without some sort of additional support over the next 12 weeks. I was really concerned that I wouldn't be able to function and would end back where I started. After much discussion and review of my symptoms, it was recommended that I change to a herbal and naturopathic pathway.

This presented a problem for me as the medical system here in Australia does not promote naturopathic therapies as is the case in Europe. In general our medical system does not practice "holistic" medicine, which is what I needed. BCA offered to send me the name and contact number of someone who could do phone consultations with my practitioner in

Australia. At this stage and after having read Dr. Whitmont's article in the book, *Insights Into Lyme Disease Treatment* by Connie Strasheim, I found a medically trained classical homeopath who had some experience in treating Lyme started homeopathic treatment. This homeopath was very caring and after doing some research recommended that I try Rife treatment via an F-Scan compact machine, which he ordered so he could treat me. I was responding and showing signs of improvement. It was then Christmas, and he loaned me the machine to use every second day while the clinic was closed, and then he continued the treatment himself. It was at this stage that I deteriorated rapidly and ended up worse than I had ever been. The homeopath recommended that I needed to see my doctor to determine the next steps. My doctor was still more than happy to support me in my treatment but wanted to be guided by someone who had considerable experience in treating Lyme disease. It was agreed that I would contact Dr. Nicola.

I was too ill to do anything so my husband sent an email to Dr. Nicola at the end of January 2010 and within two days we had scheduled a phone consultation. This was the beginning of many long distance consultations via the phone and Skype. I was also fortunate enough to be able to see Dr. Nicola in Sydney and Canberra. Dr. Nicola gradually introduced antibiotic, herbal and naturopathic supplements, which continued until January 2011. This treatment focused on Lyme, Babesia and Bartonella and was quite difficult at times. Apart from the Herxing, which I experienced, I also had a severe reaction to Alinia, which took me a couple of weeks to get over with the help of my osteopath and massage therapist (all my muscles had been adversely affected and I struggled to move). It was very much a case of working out which antibiotics worked for me. Progress was slow and seemed to be one step forward two steps back, but Dr. Nicola kept reassuring me that I would come through this, and that there was light at the end of the tunnel. The doctor at BCA had also said it was a very long process and that "patients needed to be patient". I would often think that I wasn't making much progress only to suddenly realise that I was able to do something again that I hadn't been able to do several months before. BCA had encouraged me to keep a record of symptoms, which was very helpful in recognising the changes in both symptoms and severity; when you are feeling so ill, it is easy to forget so you may not notice subtle changes.

In January, 2011 I looked at the possibility of going off antibiotics and returning to the naturopathic pathway. My doctor was concerned that I would regress after coming so far. At this stage it felt right to me, and I could always go back on antibiotics. After discussion with Dr. Nicola, we decided I would start coming off antibiotics one at a time and very slowly so we could monitor what was happening. These antibiotics were replaced with olive leaf and colloidal silver but I continued to use all the other supplements from Dr. Nicola. I was feeling quite well but would still experience setbacks.

Through the BCA I learned about the importance of a holistic approach to treatment. I needed to support my recovery on many levels as I was about to experience a roller coaster ride. They encouraged me to download the Burrascano guidelines, which I was able to give to my doctors, and to purchase Dr Kenneth Singleton's book *The Lyme Disease Solution*. These became constant resources along with BCA's website and Connie Strasheim's book *Insights Into Lyme Disease Treatment*.

As part of the holistic approach to regaining my health, I built up a team of supporting professionals to work alongside me in my journey, some of whom I had worked with prior to my diagnosis. Alongside BCA, Dr Nicola and my local doctor, these people helped to play a crucial role in helping me through extremely difficult times to regain my health.

I was fortunate enough to have the support of a psychologist who I had worked with while teaching. Being told that I had nothing wrong with me and needed to have counselling was very draining and set me back emotionally. The psychologist gave me strategies to deal with this setback and support to deal with the chronic illness and resulting depression. He offered strategies to ensure that my husband and I always had the appropriate support.

My osteopath took the time to research Lyme disease after I was diagnosed. He utilized a number of treatments over the years and I responded very well to Biodynamic Cranial Osteopathy. The osteopath said, "as the infection gets into all parts of your body, the biggest benefit is that this treatment helps your whole body work together to heal all of its parts and as such, all parts benefit from the treatment. It especially helps your neuro-endocrine-immune system work as a whole to fight the infection." He also worked closely with my massage therapist and myotherapist. He discussed my personal needs with my personal trainer and Pilates instructor, both of whom had been given the ILADS information about physical activity and its role in healing. It didn't matter how bad I was feeling, they encouraged me to attend my sessions and would adapt them accordingly, many times just gently getting my muscles moving. They also believed that getting me out of the house, even for a short time, would assist my general wellbeing.

Despite using several sleep remedies, sleep remained a major issue in my recovery. I was lucky to have one hour of sleep a night, and everyone was concerned about the impact on my body healing. At times I had to resort to strong sleep medication. As a result I tried hypnotherapy and acupuncture without success. I eventually came across Ondamed therapy, which is a form of energy medicine, and while reluctant and sceptical about this I was eventually desperate enough to give it a go. This was to become a core part of my treatment program because it addressed both my sleep and other health issues. I also used other treatments such as far-infra red sauna and Epson salt baths to assist with detox, aromatherapy and meditation.

Diet played a major role in my treatment and helped to reduce toxins and inflammation throughout my body. Just prior to my Lyme diagnosis I was diagnosed with Fructose Malabsorption, gluten intolerance and lactose intolerance, and as a result, my diet changed to gluten free. The BCA clinic recommended a Mediterranean diet as it was anti-inflammatory. This required some adjustments due to the fructose malabsorption issues but was easily managed as long I watched the type and quantity of fruit

I was eating at one time. Adjusting my diet has made a big difference to my general well-being.

My personal faith through prayer and meditation has been vital in coping with the illness. It was comforting to know that others within the faith communities were also praying for me.

From the time of diagnosis it has taken about 3-1/2 years to start feeling well enough to be able to participate more fully in everyday activities. Improvement was gradual and I would often suddenly realize I was able to do things I hadn't been able to do in a long time. The day I was able to start reading again and not feel like a child learning to read was truly wonderful. Being able to walk up and down stairs at a relative's home was another great step forward, quickly followed by realising that I could go for walks again no matter how small to start with. It was important to remember not to overdo things because I was feeling good that day, and even now, I try to follow the advice of my psychologist to only do 70% of what I feel I can do comfortably, and then have a break and go back to it. Of course, sometimes, I forget these wise words, and when I do, I always feel worse after pushing myself.

Last year I was able to travel through outback Australia for 13 weeks and coped very well. We did as much planning as possible to ensure things went smoothly for me, including buying a caravan that had an en-suite for the days when it would be too much for me to walk to the amenity block at the caravan park. I worked with my local doctor to ensure that I had enough medication plus a back-up plan for an emergency (which wasn't needed but was great to have). We also worked out how far I could comfortably travel within a day without getting tired, and we had a healthy diet of fresh and home-cooked food. This was a great experience and really lifted my spirits, helping me to feel like my old self again. We now go away once a month for a weekend with the caravan club, something I look forward to. As a rule, when we go out of a night, we don't stay out late, which gives me the best possible chance of staying well. This also means that I can participate in more social activities.

I don't know if I will ever fully recover. I still experience setbacks but these generally only last a day or two. Today I would consider myself to be somewhere around 90% recovered. But I believe it is important to remember that I have also gotten older and there are some natural aging changes. I find it helpful to think of the Lyme bacteria in the following way (pointed out to me by my local naturopath/homeopath): "Once you have had chicken pox, the bacteria stay in your body but your body is able to live in harmony with it for most of the time. Lyme bacteria could be the same as it may not be possible to eradicate every single bacteria" I am now more vigilant about my health and have learned to listen to my body and respond to its needs rather than pushing myself to keep going and meet other's demands.

Today I try to improve my current state of health by building and supporting my immune, adrenal and nervous systems, through the advice and support of a local Naturopath/Homeopath, Osteopath, Myotherapist, Ondamed therapist, Pilates instructor, Personal Trainer, regular meditation and diet as well as detoxing.

For those suffering with Lyme, don't give up hope of ever regaining your health. Be aware that lab results may not match your diagnosis, especially here in Australia. Fortunately my initial lab results showed Lyme infection, otherwise I would have never been diagnosed. However they didn't show the extent of the infection or the co-infections. If doctors here tell you to stop treatment, check with and be guided by doctors experienced in treating Lyme who work with symptoms. Be gentle on yourself and take things slowly. Do not take medical advice in Australia as gospel, which I naively did in the early days. Be proactive in your treatment and listen to your body. You will know what is right for you.

■ ■ ■ ■

Fiona B., Alexandria, NSW

One of the first things people ask me when they discover that I have Lyme disease is, "How long have you had it?" My answer is simply that

I have no idea. I have been unwell for many years but had plenty of justifications for all the symptoms individually, and I guess I also suffered from martyrdom and I just got on with it. It wasn't until I really couldn't stay awake after lunchtime, was in unbearable physical pain, vomited daily, had distortions with my vision and a brain that seem to find basic functioning hard that I sought medical advice. I fortunately have a GP in Sydney that took it seriously. After months and months of testing and eliminating lots of different possibilities, I got a CD-57 test result that allowed my GP to confidently but unofficially diagnose Lyme disease and immediately start me on an antibiotic program. Not long after this I was introduced to Dr. Nicola and as luck would have it my GP was very willing to work with her. For the next 18 months I trusted my treatment program entirely to those two. For the most part I took between three and five different antibiotics daily, and numerous naturopathic remedies to support it. I did do some IGeneX testing which came back unable to deny or confirm the diagnosis. Fortunately my GP wasn't swayed by this at all and continued supporting this intensive treatment plan.

One of the hardest parts of this medical/naturopathic plan for me was trying to manage and understand it. My brain didn't work so well and there was a complex concoction of dosing combinations! I focused on just trying to get the right doses on the right dates and happily left the planning to my medical team. To this day I am not entirely sure which drugs and herbs I took and when. Some people find this odd, but for me it was all just too much information that I couldn't manage. My Lyme disease story actually highlights that I compartmentalized it into areas that I needed to take responsibility for, and areas I could trust to others. I was happy with my medical team taking the responsibility for the treatment plan.

I did some research into the disease early on, which was necessary for me to get a sense of how serious this was. I needed some perspective. The next natural step for me was to grieve. I felt a real anger at the world and a sense of sadness at the loss of my life. I made contact with the Lyme community in Australia and read everything I could. After a while, this became counter-productive. I felt overwhelmed and ultimately despairing. It seemed such a hopeless situation and I struggled to find any positives.

I guess this is when my recovery changed for me. I asked myself, "If this is as good as it is going to get, then what could I be grateful for today?" So I began to put into practice what I as a coach helped other people do. I started to work on the mind, body, spirit approach to my disease.

Body - I looked at my diet and while far from perfect, I tried to eliminate food and drinks that didn't work. I cut out gluten, dairy, sugar and yeast. I ensured my vitamin and mineral intake was sufficient. I aimed to do a little bit of exercise every week to keep my body moving. Ten minutes walking was sometime my limit, but I committed to doing it. I allowed myself to sleep when I needed to and began listening to my body as to when to push a bit and when to rest.

Mind - This was the area in which I had the most control and also the area that not only assisted in feeling better, but made my journey to recovery easier emotionally. I did not want to stay in the place of being angry, overwhelmed and despairing, so I stopped fighting and started to accept that I had Lyme. I chose to focus on how I could maintain a positive attitude even if I felt terrible. I looked at what was still good, I made gratitude lists, I stopped feeling sorry for myself and took interest in other people, and I focused on what was good in my life, even if it was hard to find. Some days this was so hard when I felt so ill, and so sometimes I allowed myself to have a poor mental attitude day, knowing that this day would pass, and tomorrow I could be positive again. I also stopped believing that my fate would be the same as all the people talking to each other in the online communities. I started to *know* that I would recover and planned for the things that I would do as evidence of it. I watched people run up a hill and planned to cycle up it when I was well again. Daily I gave myself a pat on the back for a job well done! The actions I took regarding my mind were numerous but the intention was simply to cleanse my mind of toxins.

Spiritual - Fortunately for me I had developed a faith in a higher power in the last decade, and I turned to that during this period. I trusted that all would be fine, that it would all work out OK, and that I was being looked after. My spirituality is a personal experience and impossible to describe, but it was important for me to have this connection throughout.

After about 16 months of antibiotic treatment, I finally took my last tablet. I still had symptoms and felt unwell but I had a strong sense of knowing that the symptoms that persisted were not Lyme. I knew it was different. Five months later I am still off antibiotics and getting stronger daily. I have had to deal with other issues and am not 100%, but the comparison between now and last year is strikingly different.

I do not know if I have recovered from Lyme, am in remission, or what. All I know is that for the last few months I have begun functioning again. I am beginning to re-engage with life, and my biggest fear is losing it all again and going back into that dark, deep hole of two years ago. My journey of recovery will be life long. I need to continue doing all things that are good for my mind, body and spirit. I choose to remain positive, to enjoy each day, to set goals for the future and to keep perspective. Not every headache is an indicator that I am relapsing! I am still working on the goal of cycling up a hill and yet I know I will do it.

Given the opportunity again, I am not sure I would do anything differently. In a strange way I am grateful for my experience. My hope for my future though is that experiencing this once is enough in this lifetime!

■ ■ ■ ■

REFERENCES

1. Singleton K. The Lyme disease solution. 1st. ed. Charleston: BookSurge Publishing; 2009. 550 p.

CONCLUSION

WE HAVE COVERED A LOT OF GROUND IN THIS BOOK, BUT THERE is a lot of ground to be covered. That is the nature of Lyme disease.

Chronic Lyme disease is a very real, very serious illness. It has unique complexities and multiple facets that must be understood. Governments and health authorities have restricted knowledge and information about it, making it one of the most politicized illnesses of all time, and at the same time making accurate testing and treatment difficult for patients to obtain.

But let us not harp on that. The focus now needs to be changing the situation and getting accurate and appropriate recognition of Lyme disease in Australia. That in turn will translate to accurate and appropriate care for people affected by it.

Success in that area is dependent on raising awareness, supporting research efforts, and generating funding. Education of health practitioners is necessary so that they know what to look out for, and so that they consider Lyme disease as a diagnosis.

Thankfully, the efforts of groups such as the Lyme Disease Association of Australia and the Karl McManus Foundation have done a lot to raise awareness and promote education. They have disseminated fliers, generated media campaigns, and coordinated seminars. They have compiled doctor information kits and built websites dedicated to giving people more information. They are constantly seeking out doctors who are open to treating Lyme disease, and the list of such doctors who are treating Lyme disease nationwide is growing.

Research groups such as those at Sydney University are conducting studies, travelling to Infectious Disease conferences to present their information, and analysing data from Australian patients.

Internationally, ILADS is at the forefront of the promotion and education of doctors worldwide. They have email groups, physician training programs, annual conferences and treatment guidelines, all of which are available to Australian doctors.

Change is coming. In fact, change is already here. It might be slower than we would hope, and it might not originate from the sources we have traditionally trusted to give us accurate information about our health and the threats to our health within Australia, but thanks to the courage of the many Lyme disease sufferers who have spoken out, the tenacity of those who have seen their loved ones suffer and who are determined to make a difference, the curiosity of the media, and the truth, which ultimately always wins out, Lyme disease is gaining recognition as a recognised disease in Australia. As time goes on, treatment options will expand, doctors will be trained, and many more people will have their own stories of hope and recovery to share.

APPENDICES

A. Burrascano's Treatment Guidelines 2008

B. Summary of IGeneX Australian Panels

C. Healthy Fats to Take With Mepron and Malarone

D. Summary of Medications and Common Dosages

E. Coping With Herx Reactions

F. Castor Oil Pack Instructions

G. Dry Skin Brushing Instructions

H. Summary of Biofilm Protocols

I. Sample Naturopathic Protocols

APPENDIX A

Burrascano's Treatment Guidelines 2008

ADVANCED TOPICS IN LYME DISEASE

DIAGNOSTIC HINTS AND TREATMENT GUIDELINES FOR LYME AND OTHER TICK BORNE ILLNESSES

Sixteenth Edition
Copyright October, 2008

JOSEPH J. BURRASCANO JR., M.D.

*Board Member,
International Lyme and Associated
Diseases Society*

DISCLAIMER: The information contained in this monograph is meant for informational purposes only. The management of tick-borne illnesses in any given patient must be approached on an individual basis using the practitioner's best judgment.

TABLE OF CONTENTS

BACKGROUND INFORMATION
    What is Lyme Disease 3
    General Principles 3
    Hypothalamic-Pituitary Axis 4
    Co-Infection 4
    Collateral Conditions 5
LYME BORRELIOSIS
    Diagnostic Hints 6
    Erythema Migrans 7
    Diagnosing Later Disease 7
    The CD-57 Test 8
SYMPTOM CHECKLIST 9-10
DIAGNOSTIC CHECKLIST 11
LYME DISEASE TREATMENT GUIDELINES
LYME BORRELIOSIS
    General Information 12
    Treatment Resistance 12
    Combination Therapy 12
    Borrelia Neurotoxin 13
TREATING LYME BORRELIOSIS
    Treatment Information 13
    Antibiotics 13
    Course During Therapy 16
ANTIBIOTIC CHOICES AND DOSES
    Oral Therapy 17
    Parenteral Therapy 18
TREATMENT CATEGORIES
    Prophylaxis 19
    Early Localized 19
    Disseminated 19
    Chronic Lyme Disease (persistent/recurrent infection) 20
    Indicators for Parenteral Therapy 20
ADVANCED TREATMENT OPTIONS
    Pulse Therapy 21
    Combination Therapy 21
LYME DISEASE AND PREGNANCY 21
MONITORING THERAPY AND SAFETY 21
CO-INFECTIONS IN LYME
    Piroplasmosis (Babesiosis) 22
    Bartonella-Like Organisms 23
    Ehrlichia/Anaplasma 24
    Sorting Out Co-Infections 24
SUPPORTIVE THERAPY
    Rules 26
    Nutritional Supplements 27
    Rehabilitation 30
    Rehab/Physical Therapy Prescription 32
    Managing Yeast Overgrowth 33
BITE PREVENTION AND TICK REMOVAL 35
SUGGESTED READING AND RESOURCES 36

WELCOME!

Welcome to the sixteenth edition of the "Guidelines".
Amazingly, this edition is not only the sixteenth in the series, but as the first edition appeared in 1984, this reflects *twenty four years of effort!*

New information is constantly being uncovered, and my goal is to keep this monograph as current as possible. Very recently, increased sharing of information among practitioners who care for people with chronic conditions such as Lyme, CFIDS, autism, Gulf War syndrome, chronic toxin exposure, autoimmune diseases of unknown origin, and others marks the dawning of a new age of medical enlightenment. Unfortunately, the huge quantity of information that embodies these separate but related conditions makes it ever more difficult for any one practitioner to 'do it all". This current edition, admittedly a work in progress as I try to assemble this new data, is the beginning of my effort to incorporate some relevant information learned from my work in these other fields, in an effort to better diagnose and treat those who have become ill, especially those who are chronically ill, as a result of exposure to tick-borne diseases.

I once again extend my best wishes to the many Lyme patients and their caregivers whose wisdom I deeply appreciate, and a sincere thank you to my colleagues whose endless contributions have helped me shape my approach to tick borne illnesses. I hope that this new edition proves to be useful. Happy reading!

BACKGROUND INFORMATION

WHAT IS LYME DISEASE?
I take a broad view of what Lyme Disease actually is. Traditionally, Lyme is defined an infectious illness caused by the spirochete, *Borrelia burgdorferi* (Bb). While this is certainly technically correct, clinically the illness often is much more than that, especially in the disseminated and chronic forms.

Instead, I think of Lyme as the illness that results from the bite of an infected tick. This includes infection not only with *B. burgdorferi*, but the many co-infections that may also result. Furthermore, in the chronic form of Lyme, other factors can take on an ever more significant role- immune dysfunction, opportunistic infections, co-infections, biological toxins, metabolic and hormonal imbalances, deconditioning, etc. I will refer to infection with *B. burgdorferi* as "Lyme Borreliosis" (LB), and use the designation "Lyme" and "Lyme Disease" to refer to the more broad definition I described above.

GENERAL PRINCIPLES
In general, you can think of LB as having three categories: acute, early disseminated, and chronic. The sooner treatment is begun after the start of the infection, the higher the success rate. However, since it is easiest to cure early disease, this category of LB must be taken VERY seriously. Undertreated infections will inevitably resurface, usually as chronic Lyme, with its tremendous problems of morbidity and difficulty with diagnosis and treatment and high cost in every sense of the word. So, while the bulk of this document focuses of the more problematic chronic patient, strong emphasis is also placed on earlier stages of this illness where closest attention and care must be made.

A very important issue is the definition of **"Chronic Lyme Disease"**. Based on my clinical data and the latest published information, I offer the following definition. To be said to have chronic LB, these three criteria must be present:
1. Illness present for at least one year (this is approximately when immune breakdown attains clinically significant levels).
2. Have persistent major neurologic involvement (such as encephalitis/encephalopathy, meningitis, etc.) or active arthritic manifestations (active synovitis).
3. Still have active infection with B. burgdorferi (Bb), regardless of prior antibiotic therapy (if any).

Chronic Lyme is an altogether different illness than earlier stages, mainly because of the inhibitory effect on the immune system (Bb has been demonstrated *in vitro* to both inhibit and kill B- and T-cells, and will decrease the count of the CD-57 subset of the natural killer cells). As a result, not only is the infection with Bb perpetuated and allowed to advance, but the entire issue of co-infections arises. Ticks may contain and transmit to the host a multitude of potential pathogens. The clinical presentation of Lyme therefore reflects which pathogens are present and in what proportion. Apparently, in early infections, before extensive damage to the immune system has occurred, if the germ load of the co-infectors is low, and the Lyme is treated, many of the other tick-transmitted microbes can be contained and eliminated by the immune system. However, in the chronic patient, because of the inhibited defenses, the individual components of the co-infection are now active enough so that they too add to features of the illness and must be treated. In addition, many latent infections which may have pre-dated the tick bite, for example herpes viruses, can reactivate, thus adding to the illness.

An unfortunate corollary is that serologic tests can become *less* sensitive as the infections progress, obviously because of the decreased immune response upon which these tests are based. In addition, immune complexes form, trapping Bb antibodies. These complexed antibodies are not detected by serologic testing. Not surprisingly the seronegative patient will convert to seropositive 36% of the time after antibiotic treatment has begun and a recovery is underway. Similarly, the antibody titer may rise, and the number of bands on the western blot may increase as treatment progresses and the patient recovers. Only years after a successfully treated infection will the serologic response begin to diminish.

The severity of the clinical illness is directly proportional to the spirochete load, the duration of infection, and the presence of co-infections. These factors also are proportional to the intensity and duration of treatment needed for recovery. More severe illness also results from other causes of weakened defenses, such as from severe stress, immunosuppressant medications, and severe intercurrent illnesses. **This is why steroids and other immunosuppressive medications are absolutely contraindicated in Lyme. This also includes intra-articular steroids.**

Many collateral conditions result in those who have been chronically ill so it is not surprising that damage to virtually all bodily systems can result. Therefore to fully recover not only do all of the active infections have to be treated, but all of these other issues must be addressed in a thorough and systematic manner. *No single treatment or medication will result in full recovery of the more ill patient. Only by addressing all of these issues and engineering treatments and solutions for all of them will we be able to restore full health to our patients.* Likewise, a patient will not recover unless they are completely compliant with every single aspect of the treatment plan. This must be emphasized to the patient, often on repeated occasions.

It is clear that in the great majority of patients, chronic Lyme is a disease affecting predominantly the nervous system. Thus, careful evaluation may include neuropsychiatric testing, SPECT and MRI brain scans, CSF analysis when appropriate, regular input from Lyme-aware neurologists and psychiatrists, pain clinics, and occasionally specialists in psychopharmacology.

HYPOTHALAMIC-PITUITARY AXIS
As an extension of the effect of chronic Lyme Disease on the central nervous system, there often is a deleterious effect on the hypothalamic-pituitary axis. Varying degrees of pituitary insufficiency are being seen in these patients, the correction of which has resulted in restoration of energy, stamina and libido, and resolution of persistent hypotension. Unfortunately, not all specialists recognize pituitary insufficiency, partly because of the difficulty in making the laboratory diagnosis. However, the potential benefits of diagnosing and treating this justify the effort needed for full evaluation. Interestingly, in a significant number of these patients, successful treatment of the infections can result in a reversal of the hormonal dysfunction, and hormone replacement therapies can be tapered off!

CO-INFECTION
A huge body of research and clinical experience has demonstrated the nearly universal phenomenon in chronic Lyme patients of co-infection with multiple tick-borne pathogens. These patients have been shown to potentially carry Babesia species, Bartonella-like organisms, Ehrlichia, Anaplasma, Mycoplasma, and viruses. Rarely, yeast forms have been detected in peripheral blood. At one point even nematodes were said to be a tick-borne pathogen. Studies have shown that co-infection results in a more severe clinical presentation, with more organ damage, and the pathogens become more difficult to eradicate. In addition, it is known that Babesia infections, like Lyme Borreliosis, are immunosuppressive.

There are changes in the clinical presentation of the co-infected patient as compared to when each infection is present individually. There may be different symptoms and atypical signs. There may be decreased reliability of standard diagnostic tests, and most importantly, there is recognition that chronic, persistent forms of each of these infections do indeed exist. As time goes by, I am convinced that even more pathogens will be found.

Therefore, real, clinical Lyme as we have come to know it, especially the later and more severe presentations, probably represents a mixed infection with many complicating factors. I will leave to the reader the implications of how this may explain the discrepancy between laboratory study of pure Borrelia infections, and what front line physicians have been seeing for years in real patients.

I must very strongly emphasize that all diagnoses of tick-borne infections remains a clinical one. Clinical clues will be presented later in this monograph, but testing information is briefly summarized below.

In **Lyme Borreliosis**, western blot is the preferred serologic test. Antigen detection tests (antigen capture and PCR), although insensitive, are very specific and are especially helpful in evaluating the seronegative patient and those still ill or relapsing after therapy. Often, these antigen detection tests are the only positive markers of Bb infection, as seronegativity has been reported to occur in as many as 30% to 50% of cases. Nevertheless, active LB can be present even if all of these tests are non-reactive! Clinical diagnosis is therefore required.

In **Babesiosis**, no single test is reliable enough to be used alone. Only in early infections (less than two weeks duration) can the standard blood smear be helpful. In later stages, one can use serology, PCR, and fluorescent in-situ hybridization ("FISH") assay. Unfortunately, many other protozoans can be found in ticks, most likely representing species other than B. microti, yet commercial tests for only B. microti and B duncani (Formerly known as WA-1) are available at this time! In other words, the patient may have an infection that cannot be tested for. Here, as in Borrelia, clinical assessment is the primary diagnostic tool.

In **Ehrlichiosis and Anaplasmosis**, by definition you must test for both the monocytic and granulocytic forms. This may be accomplished by blood smear, PCR and serology. Many presently uncharacterized Ehrlichia-like organisms can be found in ticks and may not be picked up by currently available assays, so in this illness too, these tests are only an adjunct in making the diagnosis. Rarely, Rocky Mountain Spotted Fever can coexist, and even be chronic. Fortunately, treatment regimens are similar for all agents in this group.

In **Bartonella**, use both serology and PCR. PCR can be performed not only on blood and CSF, but as in LB, can be performed on biopsy specimens. Unfortunately, in my experience, these tests, even when both types are done, will presently miss over half the cases diagnosed clinically.

Frequent exposures to **Mycoplasmas** are common, resulting in a high prevalence of seropositivity, so the best way to confirm active infection is by PCR.

Chronic viral infections may be active in the chronic patient, due to their weakened immune response. PCR testing, and not serologies, should be used for diagnosis. Commonly seen viruses include HHV-6, CMV, and EBV.

COLLATERAL CONDITIONS
Experience has shown that collateral conditions exist in those who have been ill a long time. The evaluation should include testing both for differential diagnosis and for uncovering other subtle abnormalities that may coexist.

Test **B12 levels**, and be prepared to aggressively treat with parenteral formulations. If neurologic involvement is severe, then consideration should be given to treatment with methylcobalamin (as outlined below in the section on nutritional support).

Magnesium deficiency is very often present and quite severe. Hyperreflexia, muscle twitches, myocardial irritability, poor stamina and recurrent tight muscle spasms are clues to this deficiency. Magnesium is predominantly an intracellular ion, so blood level testing is of little value. Oral preparations are acceptable for maintenance, but those with severe deficiencies need additional, parenteral dosing: 1 gram IV or IM <u>at least</u> once a week until neuromuscular irritability has cleared.

Pituitary and other endocrine abnormalities are far more common than generally realized. Evaluate fully, including growth hormone levels. Quite often, a full battery of provocative tests is in order to fully define the problem. When testing the thyroid, measure free T3 and free T4 levels and TSH, and nuclear scanning and testing for autoantibodies may be necessary.

Activation of the **inflammatory cascade** has been implicated in blockade of cellular hormone receptors. One example of this is insulin resistance; clinical hypothyroidism can result from receptor blockade and thus hypothyroidism can exist despite normal serum hormone levels. These may partly account for the dyslipidemia and weight gain that is noted in 80% of chronic Lyme patients. In addition to measuring free T3 and T4 levels, check basal A.M. body temperatures. If hypothyroidism is found, you may need to treat with both T3 and T4 preparations until blood levels of both are normalized. To ensure sustained levels, when T3 is prescribed, have it compounded in a time-release form.

Neurally mediated hypotension (NMH) is not uncommon. Symptoms can include palpitations, lightheadedness and shakiness especially after exertion and prolonged standing, heat intolerance, dizziness, fainting (or near fainting), *and an unavoidable need to sit or lie down*. It is often confused with hypoglycemia, which it mimics. NMH can result from autonomic neuropathy and endocrine dyscrasias. If NMH is present, treatment can dramatically lessen fatigue, palpitations and wooziness, and increase stamina. NMH is diagnosed by tilt table testing. This test should be done by a cardiologist and include Isuprel challenge. This will demonstrate not only if NMH is present, but also the relative contributions of hypovolemia and sympathetic dysfunction. Immediate supportive therapy is based on blood volume expansion (increased sodium and fluid intake and possibly Florinef plus potassium). If not sufficient, beta blockade may be added based on response to the Isuprel challenge. The long term solution involves restoring proper hormone levels and treating the Lyme to address this and the autonomic dysfunction.

SPECT scanning of the brain- Unlike MRI and CT scans, which show structure, SPECT scans show function. Therefore SPECT scans give us information unattainable through X-rays, CT scans, MRI's, or even spinal taps. In the majority of chronic Lyme Borreliosis patients, these scans are abnormal. Although not diagnostic of Lyme specifically, if the scan is abnormal, the scan can not only quantify the abnormalities, but the pattern can help to differentiate medical from psychiatric causes of these changes. Furthermore, repeat scans after a course of treatment can be used to assess treatment efficacy. Note that improvement in scans lag behind clinical improvement by many months.

If done by knowledgeable radiologists using high-resolution equipment, scanning will show characteristic abnormalities in Lyme encephalopathy- global hypoperfusion (may be homogenous or heterogeneous). What these scans demonstrate is neuronal dysfunction and/or varying degrees of cerebrolvascular insufficiency. If necessary, to assess the relative contributions of these two processes, the SPECT scan can be done before and after acetazolamide. If the post acetazolamide scan shows significant reversibility of the abnormalities, then vasoconstriction is present, and can be treated with vasodilators, which may clear some cognitive symptoms. Therapy can include acetazolamide, serotonin agonists and even Ginkgo biloba, provided it is of pharmaceutical quality. Therapeutic trials of these may be needed.

Acetazolamide should not be given if there is severe kidney/liver disease, electrolyte abnormalities, pregnancy, sulfa allergy, recent stroke, or if the patient is taking high dose aspirin treatment

LYME BORRELIOSIS

DIAGNOSTIC HINTS
Lyme Borreliosis (LB) is diagnosed clinically, as no currently available test, no matter the source or type, is definitive in ruling in or ruling out infection with these pathogens, or whether these infections are responsible

for the patient's symptoms. The entire clinical picture must be taken into account, including a search for concurrent conditions and alternate diagnoses, and other reasons for some of the presenting complaints. Often, much of the diagnostic process in late, disseminated Lyme involves ruling out other illnesses and defining the extent of damage that might require separate evaluation and treatment.

Consideration should be given to tick exposure, rashes (even atypical ones), evolution of typical symptoms in a previously asymptomatic individual, and results of tests for tick-borne pathogens. Another very important factor is response to treatment- presence or absence of Jarisch Herxheimer-like reactions, the classic four-week cycle of waxing and waning of symptoms, and improvement with therapy.

ERYTHEMA MIGRANS
Erythema migrans (EM) is diagnostic of Bb infection, but is present in *fewer than half*. Even if present, it may go unnoticed by the patient. It is an erythematous, centrifugally expanding lesion that is raised and may be warm. Rarely there is mild stinging or pruritus. The EM rash will begin four days to several weeks after the bite, and may be associated with constitutional symptoms. Multiple lesions are present less than 10% of the time, but do represent disseminated disease. Some lesions have an atypical appearance and skin biopsy specimens may be helpful. When an ulcerated or vesicular center is seen, this may represent a mixed infection, involving other organisms besides B. burgdorferi.

After a tick bite, serologic tests (ELISA. IFA, western blots, etc.) are not expected to become positive until several weeks have passed. Therefore, if EM is present, treatment must begin immediately, and one should not wait for results of Borrelia tests. You should not miss the chance to treat early disease, for this is when the success rate is the highest. Indeed, many knowledgeable clinicians will not even order a Borrelia test in this circumstance.

DIAGNOSING LATER DISEASE
When reactive, serologies indicate exposure only and do not directly indicate whether the spirochete is now currently present. Because Bb serologies often give inconsistent results, test at well-known reference laboratories. The suggestion that two-tiered testing, utilizing an ELISA as a screening tool, followed, if positive, by a confirmatory western blot, is illogical in this illness. The ELISA is not sensitive enough to serve as an adequate screen, and there are many patients with Lyme who test negative by ELISA yet have fully diagnostic western blots. I therefore recommend against using the ELISA. The newly available C6 ELISA appears to be no more sensitive than standard ELISAs, and in my experience there are even more false negative C6 assays in late disease than in earlier stages of the illness. I therefore do not recommend or use this type ELISA either. Instead, order IgM and IgG western blots- but be aware that in late disease there may be repeatedly peaking IgM's and therefore a reactive IgM may not differentiate early from late disease, but it does suggest an active infection. When late cases of LB are seronegative, 36% will transiently become seropositive at the completion of successful therapy. In chronic Lyme Borreliosis, the CD-57 count is both useful and important (see below).

Western blots are reported by showing which bands are reactive. 41KD bands appear the earliest but can cross react with other spirochetes. The 18KD, 23-25KD (Osp C), 31KD (Osp A), 34KD (Osp B), 37KD, 39KD, 83KD and the 93KD bands are the species-specific ones, but appear later or may not appear at all. You should see at least the 41KD and one of the specific bands. 55KD, 60KD, 66KD, and 73KD are nonspecific and nondiagnostic.

PCR tests are now available, and although they are very specific, sensitivity remains poor, possibly less than 30%. This is because Bb causes a deep tissue infection and is only transiently found in body humors. Therefore, just as in routine blood culturing, multiple specimens must be collected to increase yield; a negative result does not rule out infection, but a positive one is significant. You can test whole blood, buffy coat, serum, urine, spinal and other body fluids, and tissue biopsies. Several blood PCRs can be done, or you can run PCRs on whole blood, serum and urine simultaneously at a time of active symptoms. The patient should be antibiotic-free for at least six weeks before testing to obtain the highest yield.

Antigen capture is becoming more widely available, and can be done on urine, CSF, and synovial fluid. Sensitivity is still low (on the order of 30%), but specificity is high (greater than 90%).

Spinal taps are not routinely recommended, as a negative tap does not rule out Lyme. Antibodies to Bb are mostly found in Lyme meningitis, and are rarely seen in non-meningitic CNS infection, including advanced encephalopathy. Even in meningitis, antibodies are detected in the CSF in less than 13% of patients with late disease! Therefore, spinal taps are only performed on patients with pronounced neurological manifestations in whom the diagnosis is uncertain, if they are seronegative, or are still significantly symptomatic after completion of treatment. When done, the goal is to rule out other conditions, and to determine if Bb (and Bartonella) antigens or nucleic acids are present. It is especially important to look for elevated protein and white cells, which would dictate the need for more aggressive therapy, as well as the opening pressure, which can be elevated and add to headaches, especially in children.

I strongly urge you to **biopsy** all unexplained skin lesions/rashes and perform PCR and careful histology. You will need to alert the pathologist to look for spirochetes.

THE CD-57 TEST

Our ability to measure CD-57 counts represents a breakthrough in LB diagnosis and treatment.

Chronic LB infections are known to suppress the immune system and can decrease the quantity of the CD-57 subset of the natural killer cells. As in HIV infection, where abnormally low T-cell counts are routinely used as a marker of how active that infection is, in LB we can use the degree of decrease of the CD-57 count to indicate how active the Lyme infection is and whether, after treatment ends, a relapse is likely to occur. It can even be used as a simple, inexpensive screening test, because at this point we believe that only Borrelia will depress the CD-57. Thus, a sick patient with a high CD-57 is probably ill with something other than Lyme, such as a co-infection.

When this test is run by LabCorp (the currently preferred lab, as published studies were based on their assays), we want our Lyme patients to measure above 60; a normal count is above 200. There generally is some degree of fluctuation of this count over time, and the number does not progressively increase as treatment proceeds. Instead, it remains low until the LB infection is controlled, and then it will jump. If the CD-57 count is not in the normal range when a course of antibiotics is ended, then a relapse will almost certainly occur.

CHECK LIST OF **CURRENT** SYMPTOMS: This is not meant to be used as a diagnostic scheme, but is provided to streamline the office interview. Note the format- complaints referable to specific organ systems and specific co-infections are clustered to clarify diagnoses and to better display multisystem involvement.

Have you had any of the following in relation to this illness? (CIRCLE "NO" OR "YES")
Tick bite   N Y   *"EM" rash (discrete circle)*   N Y
Spotted rash over large area   N Y   *Linear, red streaks*   N Y

SYMPTOM OR SIGN	CURRENT SEVERITY				CURRENT FREQUENCY				
	NONE	MILD	MODERATE	SEVERE	NA	NEVER	OCCASIONAL	OFTEN	CONSTANT
Persistent swollen glands									
Sore throat									
Fevers									
Sore soles, esp. in the AM									
Joint pain									
Fingers, toes									
Ankles, wrists									
Knees, elbows									
Hips, shoulders									
Joint swelling									
Fingers, toes									
Ankles, wrists									
Knees, elbows									
Hips, shoulders									
Unexplained back pain									
Stiffness of the joints or back									
Muscle pain or cramps									
Obvious muscle weakness									
Twitching of the face or other muscles									
Confusion, difficulty thinking									
Difficulty with concentration, reading, problem absorbing new information									
Word search, name block									
Forgetfulness, poor short term memory, poor attention									
Disorientation: getting lost, going to wrong places									
Speech errors- wrong word, misspeaking									
Mood swings, irritability, depression									
Anxiety, panic attacks									
Psychosis (hallucinations, delusions, paranoia, bipolar)									
Tremor									
Seizures									
Headache									
Light sensitivity									
Sound sensitivity									
Vision: double, blurry, floaters									
Ear pain									

MANAGING LYME DISEASE, 16^h edition, October, 2008

SYMPTOM OR SIGN	CURRENT SEVERITY				CURRENT FREQUENCY				
	NONE	MILD	MODERATE	SEVERE	NA	NEVER	OCCASIONAL	OFTEN	CONSTANT
Hearing: buzzing, ringing, decreased hearing									
Increased motion sickness, vertigo, spinning									
Off balance, "tippy" feeling									
Lightheadedness, wooziness, unavoidable need to sit or lie									
Tingling, numbness, burning or stabbing sensations, shooting pains, skin hypersensitivity									
Facial paralysis-Bell's Palsy									
Dental pain									
Neck creaks and cracks, stiffness, neck pain									
Fatigue, tired, poor stamina									
Insomnia, fractionated sleep, early awakening									
Excessive night time sleep									
Napping during the day									
Unexplained weight gain									
Unexplained weight loss									
Unexplained hair loss									
Pain in genital area									
Unexplained menstrual irregularity									
Unexplained milk production; breast pain									
Irritable bladder or bladder dysfunction									
Erectile dysfunction									
Loss of libido									
Queasy stomach or nausea									
Heartburn, stomach pain									
Constipation									
Diarrhea									
Low abdominal pain, cramps									
Heart murmur or valve prolapse?									
Heart palpitations or skips									
"Heart block" on EKG									
Chest wall pain or ribs sore									
Head congestion									
Breathlessness, "air hunger", unexplained chronic cough									
Night sweats									
Exaggerated symptoms or worse hangover from alcohol									
Symptom flares every 4 wks.									
Degree of disability									

DIAGNOSTIC CHECKLIST

To aid the clinician, a workable set of diagnostic criteria were developed with the input of dozens of front line physicians. The resultant document, refined over the years, has proven to be extremely useful not only to the clinician, but it also can help clarify the diagnosis for third party payers and utilization review committees. **It is important to note that the CDC's published reporting criteria are for surveillance only, not for diagnosis. They should not be misused in an effort to diagnose Lyme or set guidelines for insurance company acceptance of the diagnosis, nor be used to determine eligibility for coverage.**

LYME BORRELIOSIS DIAGNOSTIC CRITERIA	RELATIVE VALUE
Tick exposure in an endemic region	1
Historical facts and evolution of symptoms over time consistent with Lyme	2
Systemic signs & symptoms consistent with Bb infection (other potential diagnoses excluded):	
Single system, e.g., monoarthritis	1
Two or more systems, e.g., monoarthritis and facial palsy	2
Erythema migrans, physician confirmed	7
Acrodermatitis Chronica Atrophicans, biopsy confirmed	7
Seropositivity	3
Seroconversion on paired sera	4
Tissue microscopy, silver stain	3
Tissue microscopy, monoclonal immunofluorescence	4
Culture positivity	4
B. burgdorferi antigen recovery	4
B. burgdorferi DNA/RNA recovery	4

DIAGNOSIS

Lyme Borreliosis Highly Likely	7 or above
Lyme Borreliosis Possible	5-6
Lyme Borreliosis Unlikely	4 or below

I suggest that when using these criteria, you state Lyme Borreliosis is "unlikely", "possible", or "highly likely" based upon the following criteria"- then list the criteria.

LYME DISEASE TREATMENT GUIDELINES

LYME BORRELIOSIS:

GENERAL INFORMATION
After a tick bite, Bb undergoes rapid hematogenous dissemination, and for example, can be found within the central nervous system as soon as *twelve hours* after entering the bloodstream. This is why even early infections require full dose antibiotic therapy with an agent able to penetrate all tissues in concentrations known to be bactericidal to the organism.

It has been shown that the longer a patient had been ill with LB prior to first definitive therapy, the longer the duration of treatment must be, and the need for more aggressive treatment increases.

More evidence has accumulated indicating the severe detrimental effects of the concurrent use of immunosuppressants including steroids in the patient with active B. burgdorferi infection. **Never give steroids or any other immunosuppressant to any patient who may even remotely be suffering from Lyme, or serious, permanent damage may result, especially if given for anything greater than a short course.** If immunosuppressive therapy is absolutely necessary, then potent antibiotic treatment should begin at least 48 hours prior to the immunosuppressants.

TREATMENT RESISTANCE
Bb contains beta lactamases and cephalosporinases, which, with some strains, may confer resistance to cephalosporins and penicillins. This is apparently a slowly acting enzyme system, and may be overcome by higher or more continuous drug levels especially when maintained by continuous infusions (cefotaxime) and by depot preparations (benzathine penicillin). Nevertheless, some penicillin and cephalosporin treatment failures do occur and have responded to sulbactam/ampicillin, imipenem, and vancomycin, which act through different cell wall mechanisms than the penicillins and the cephalosporins.

Vegetative endocarditis has been associated with Borrelia burgdorferi, but the vegetations may be too small to detect with echocardiography. Keep this in mind when evaluating patients with murmurs, as this may explain why some patients seem to continually relapse after even long courses of antibiotics.

COMBINATION THERAPY
Treatment of chronic Lyme usually requires combinations of antibiotics. There are four reasons for this:
1. TWO COMPARTMENTS- Bb can be found in both the fluid and the tissue compartments, yet no single antibiotic currently used to treat Bb infections will be effective in both compartments. This is one reason for the need to use combination therapy in the more ill patient. A logical combination might use, for example, azithromycin plus a penicillin.
2. INTRACELLULAR NICHE- Another reason, discussed below, is the fact that Bb can penetrate and remain viable within cells and evade the effects of extracellular agents. Typical combinations include an extracellular antibiotic, plus an intracellular agent such as an erythromycin derivative or metronidazole. Note that some experts discourage the co-administration of bactericidal plus bacteriostatic agents, thus the recommendation to avoid a cell wall drug combined with a tetracycline.
3. L-FORMS (SPHEROPLAST)- It has been recognized that B. burgdorferi can exist in at least two, and possibly three different morphologic forms: spirochete, spheroplast (or l-form), and the recently discovered cystic form (presently, there is controversy whether the cyst is different from the l-form). L-forms and cystic forms do not contain cell walls, and thus beta lactam antibiotics will not affect them. Spheroplasts seem to be susceptible to tetracyclines and the advanced erythromycin derivatives. Apparently, Bb can shift among the three forms during the course of the infection. Because of this, it may be necessary to cycle different classes of antibiotics and/or prescribe a combination of dissimilar agents.
4. CYSTIC FORM- When present in a hostile environment, such as growth medium lacking some nutrients, spinal fluid, or serum with certain antibiotics added, Bb can change from the spiral

form ("spirochete") into a cyst form. This cyst seems to be able to remain dormant, but when placed into an environment more favorable to its growth, Bb can revert into the spirochete form. The antibiotics commonly used for Lyme do not kill the cystic form of Bb. However, there is laboratory evidence that metronidazole and tinidazole will disrupt it. Therefore, the chronically infected patient who has resistant disease may need to have metronidazole (or tinidazole) added to the regimen. More details are provided in the section on treatment options.

BORRELIA NEUROTOXIN (With thanks to Dr. Shoemaker)
Two groups have reported evidence that Borrelia, like several other bacteria, produce neurotoxins. These compounds reportedly can cause many of the symptoms of encephalopathy, cause an ongoing inflammatory reaction manifested as some of the virus-like symptoms common in late Lyme, and also potentially interfere with hormone action by blocking hormone receptors. At this time, there is no assay available to detect whether this compound is present, nor can the amount of toxin be quantified. Indirect measures are currently employed, such as measures of cytokine activation and hormone resistance. A visual contrast sensitivity test (VCS test) reportedly is quite useful in documenting CNS effects of the neurotoxin, and to follow effects of treatment. This test is available at some centers and on the internet.

It has been said that the longer one is ill with Lyme, the more neurotoxin is present in the body. It probably is stored in fatty tissues, and once present, persists for a very long time. This may be because of enterohepatic circulation, where the toxin is excreted via the bile into the intestinal tract, but then is reabsorbed from the intestinal tract back into the blood stream. This forms the basis for treatment.

Two prescription medications that can bind these toxins include cholestyramine resin and Welchol pills. When take orally in generous amounts, the neurotoxin present in the intestinal tract binds to the resin, is trapped, and then excreted. Thus, over several weeks, the level of neurotoxin is depleted and clinical improvement can be seen. Current experience is that improvement is first seen in three weeks, and treatment can continue for a month or more. Retreatment is always possible.

These medications may bind not only toxins but also many drugs and vitamin supplements. Therefore no other oral medications or supplements should be taken from a half hour before, to two hours after a dose of one of these fiber agents.

Cholestyramine should be taken two to four times daily, and Welchol is prescribed at three pills twice daily. While the latter is obviously much simpler to use, it is less effective than cholestyramine. The main side effects are bloating and constipation, best handled with increased fluid intake and gentle laxatives.

TREATING LYME BORRELIOSIS

LYME DISEASE TREATMENT INFORMATION
There is no universally effective antibiotic for treating LB. The choice of medication used and the dosage prescribed will vary for different people based on multiple factors. These include duration and severity of illness, presence of co-infections, immune deficiencies, prior significant immunosuppressant use while infected, age, weight, gastrointestinal function, blood levels achieved, and patient tolerance. Doses found to be effective clinically are often higher than those recommended in older texts. This is due to deep tissue penetration by Bb, its presence in the CNS including the eye, within cells, within tendons, and because very few of the many strains of this organism now known to exist have been studied for antibiotic susceptibility. In addition, all animal studies of susceptibility to date have only addressed early disease in models that behave differently than human hosts. Therefore, begin with a regimen appropriate to the setting, and if necessary, modify it over time based upon antibiotic blood level measurements and clinical response.

ANTIBIOTICS
There are four types of antibiotics in general use for Bb treatment. The TETRACYCLINES (tetracycline, minocycline and doxycycline, but not tigecycline- see below), are bacteriostatic unless given in high doses. If high blood levels are not attained, treatment failures in early and late disease are common. However, these

high doses can be difficult to tolerate. For example, doxycycline can be very effective but only if adequate blood levels are achieved either by high oral doses (300 to 600 mg daily) or by parenteral administration. Kill kinetics indicate that a large spike in blood and tissue levels is more effective than sustained levels, which is why with doxycycline, oral doses of 200 mg bid is more effective than 100 mg qid. Likewise, this is why IV doses of 400 mg once a day is more effective than any oral regimen. However, the newly available, parenteral-only tetracycline, tigecycline, represents a true advance, in that it inhibits efflux of the antibiotic (basically a minocycline derivative) out of the host cells, thus achieving far better results than even parenteral doxycycline. As with all tetracyclines, nausea remains the primary and use-limiting side effect of this drug.

PENICILLINS are bactericidal. As would be expected in managing an infection with a gram negative organism such as Bb, amoxicillin has been shown to be more effective than oral penicillin V. With cell wall agents such as the penicillins, kill kinetics indicate that sustained bactericidal levels are needed for 72 hours to be effective. Thus the goal is to try to achieve sustained blood and tissue levels. However, since blood levels are extremely variable among patients, peak and trough levels should be measured (for details, refer to the antibiotic dosage table). Because of its short half-life and need for high levels, amoxicillin is usually administered along with probenecid. An extended release formulation of amoxicillin+clavulanate ("Augmentin XR") may also be considered if adequate trough levels are difficult to attain. An attractive alternative is benzathine penicillin ("Bicillin-LA"- see below). This is an intramuscular depot injection, and although doses are relatively small, the sustained blood and tissue levels are what make this preparation so effective.

CEPHALOSPORINS must be of advanced generation: first generation drugs are rarely effective and second generation drugs are comparable to amoxicillin and doxycycline both in-vitro and in-vivo. Third generation agents are currently the most effective of the cephalosporins because of their very low MBC's (0.06 for ceftriaxone), and relatively long half-life. Cephalosporins have been shown to be effective in penicillin and tetracycline failures. Cefuroxime axetil (Ceftin), a second generation agent, is also effective against staph and thus is useful in treating atypical erythema migrans that may represent a mixed infection that contains some of the more common skin pathogens in addition to Bb. Because this agent's G.I. side effects and high cost, it is not often used as first line drug. As with the penicillins, try to achieve high, sustained blood and tissue levels by frequent dosing and/or the use of probenecid. Measure peak and trough blood levels when possible.

When choosing a third generation cephalosporin, there are several points to remember: Ceftriaxone is administered twice daily (an advantage for home therapy), but has 95% biliary excretion and can crystallize in the biliary tree with resultant colic and possible cholecystitis. GI excretion results in a large impact on gut flora. Biliary and superinfection problems with ceftriaxone can be lessened if this drug is given in interrupted courses (known commonly as "pulse therapy"- refer to chapter on this on page 20), so the current recommendation is to administer it four days in a row each week. Cefotaxime, which must be given at least every eight hours or as a continuous infusion, is less convenient, but as it has only 5% biliary excretion, it never causes biliary concretions, and may have less impact on gut flora.

ERYTHROMYCIN has been shown to be almost ineffective as monotherapy. The azalide azithromycin is somewhat more effective but only minimally so when given orally. As an IV drug, much better results are seen. Clarithromycin is more effective as an oral agent than azithromycin, but can be difficult to tolerate due to its tendency to promote yeast overgrowth, bad aftertaste, and poor GI tolerance at the high doses needed. These problems are much less severe with the ketolide telithromycin, which is generally well tolerated.

Erythromycins (and the advanced generation derivatives mentioned above) have impressively low MBCs and they do concentrate in tissues and penetrate cells, so they theoretically should be ideal agents. So why is it that erythromycin is ineffective, and why have initial clinical results with azithromycin (and to a lesser degree, clarithromycin) been disappointing? It has been suggested that when Bb is within a cell, it is held within a vacuole and bathed in fluid of low pH, and this acidity may inactivate azithromycin and clarithromycin. Therefore, they are administered concurrently with hydroxychloroquine or amantadine, which raise vacuolar pH, rendering these antibiotics more effective. It is not known whether this same technique will make erythromycin a more effective antibiotic in LB. Another alternative is to administer azithromycin parenterally. Results are excellent, but expect to see abrupt Jarisch-Herxheimer reactions.

Telithromycin, on the other hand, is stable in the intracellular acid environment, which may be why this is currently by far the most effective drug of this class, and may replace the others in the majority of patients with LB. Likewise, there is no need to co-administer amantadine or hydroxychloroquine. This antibiotic has other advantages- it has been engineered to prevent drug resistance, has almost no negative impact on E. coli in the intestinal tract (hopefully minimizing the risk for diarrhea), and it can be taken with or without food.

However, there are disadvantages:
1. May interact with a wide variety of medications because it is an inhibitor of the cytochrome CYP3A4. It is vital that this be taken into account as many Lyme patients take a variety of medications concurrently, and often from several practitioners.
2. May lengthen the QT interval. This should be measured prior to prescribing this drug, and if borderline, rechecked after it is begun.
3. Can transiently cause blurry vision, delayed accommodation, and even double vision.
4. Liver enzymes may become elevated. Blood tests should be done regularly to monitor this.
5. The usual precautions of any antibiotic also still apply- risk for allergy, stomach upset, Herxheimer reactions, etc.

QTc INTERVAL
- QTc is the QT corrected for heart rate
- Measure the precordial lead that has the best T wave (usually V-2 or V-5)
- Measure from the start of the Q wave to the end of the T wave
- QT interval is inversely related to the heart rate (slow pulse results in a longer QT)
- QTc = QT ÷ √RR interval
- Normals: Females <450 ms, Males < 470 ms
- Want K+ > 4.0, Mg++ > 2.0; avoid hypocalcemia

METRONIDAZOLE (Flagyl) When present in a hostile environment, such as growth medium lacking some nutrients, spinal fluid, or serum with certain antibiotics added, Bb can change into a cyst form. This cyst seems to be able to remain dormant, but when placed into an environment more favorable to its growth, the cyst can revert into the spirochete form. The conventional antibiotics used for Lyme, such as the penicillins, cephalosporins, etc do not kill the cystic form of Bb, yet there is laboratory evidence that metronidazole will kill it. Therefore, the trend now is to treat the chronically infected patient who has resistant disease by combining metronidazole with one or two other antibiotics to target all forms of Bb. Because there is laboratory evidence that tetracyclines may inhibit the effect of Flagyl, this class of medication should not be used in these two- and three-drug regimens. Some clinicians favor tinidazole as this may be equally effective but result in fewer side effects. However, this has yet to be documented.

Important precautions:
1. Pregnancy while on Flagyl is not advised, as there is a risk of birth defects.
2. No alcohol consumption! A severe, "Antabuse" reaction will occur, consisting of severe nausea, flushing, headache, and other symptoms.
3. Yeast overgrowth is especially common. A strict anti-yeast regimen must be followed.
4. Flagyl can be irritative to the nervous system- in the short term, it may cause irritability, "spacey" feelings, etc. Longer term, it can affect the peripheral nerves, causing tingles, numbness, etc. If mild, a change in dose may be required. Often, extra vitamin B can clear these symptoms. If the nerve symptoms persist or are strong, then metronidazole must be discontinued or these symptoms may become very long lasting.
5. Strong Herxheimer-like reactions are seen in almost everyone.

RIFAMPIN is a well-known antibiotic that has been in use for many decades. It is primarily used to treat tuberculosis, but also has been used in other conditions, such as prevention of meningitis in those exposed, for treating resistant Staph, etc. Potentially, rifampin may be effective in treating Bartonella, Ehrlichia, Mycoplasma, and Borrelia. There are as yet no formal clinical studies on the use of this medication in these illnesses, but many patients have been treated with rifampin and have had favorable results. When used, regular blood tests (CBC, liver enzymes) are usually performed to monitor for side effects. Rifampin can also discolor urine, tears and sweat (brownish-orange). It may also stain some types of water-permeable contact lenses. Taking rifampin during pregnancy is not advised. Finally, because this drug is an inducer of cytochromes (CYP3A4), co-administration with other medications may result in lower and more brief blood levels of the co-administered drug. Thus, be aware of these potential drug interactions.

BENZATHINE PENICILLIN Comparative studies published by Fallon et. al. at Columbia University have shown that parenteral therapy is superior to oral therapy in chronic patients. Options include intramuscular long acting penicillin G (benzathine penicillin, or "Bicillin-LA") or intravenous antibiotics.

For an antibiotic in the penicillin class to be effective, time-killing curves show that significant levels of antibiotic must be sustained for 72 hours. Bicillin LA is a sustained release formulation that meets these criteria.

Published studies in children and adults, combined with over a decade of experience with this therapy by front line, Lyme-treating physicians have established the efficacy, safety and usefulness of this medication. In many patients it is more effective than oral antibiotics for treating Lyme, and compares closely to intravenous therapy in terms of efficacy if the dose is high enough.

It is usually administered three or four times weekly for six to twelve months. It has the advantage of being relatively inexpensive, free of gastrointestinal side effects, unlikely to promote the overgrowth of yeast, and has an excellent safety record spanning many decades.

Finally, an added plus is that family members can be trained to administer this treatment at home.

CEFTRIAXONE TREATMENT A subset of patients who have severe, longstanding illness due to Borrelia burgdorferi carry persistent infection despite having previously received antibiotic treatments which have eliminated the disease in less ill individuals. The mechanism for such persistence has been the subject of many peer reviewed articles. They include persistence of B. burgdorferi in protective niches, inhibition and lysis of lymphocytes, survival in phagocytic vacuoles, antigenic shifts, slow growth, shifting into alternate forms, and dormancy and latency.

One successful approach in the more ill patient, published in the early 1990s, is to use higher doses of ceftriaxone in a pulsed-dose regimen. Since then, clinical experience has expanded upon this concept, and at the MLDA Lyme Congress in September, 2002, Cichon presented data on a pulsed, high dose regimen which supports and refines this concept. This regimen is now considered the current standard of care in the use of ceftriaxone.

Treatment with ceftriaxone is dosed at 4 grams daily- given either as 2 grams IV twice daily, or 4 grams slowly once a day, four days in a row each week, usually for 14 or more weeks. Such a regimen is not only more effective in the Chronic Lyme patient, but regular interruptions in treatment lessen the potential complications of intensive antibiotic therapy with ceftriaxone, such as biliary sludging and colitis. Hence a more effective, safer regimen that by virtue of the treatment breaks, is less costly and affords the patient a more acceptable lifestyle. IV access with a heparin lock becomes possible (and preferred).

COURSE DURING THERAPY
As the spirochete has a very long generation time (12 to 24 hours *in vitro* and possibly much longer in living systems) and may have periods of dormancy, during which time antibiotics will not kill the organism, treatment has to be continued for a long period of time to eradicate all the active symptoms and prevent a relapse, especially in late infections. If treatment is discontinued before all symptoms of active infection have cleared, the patient will remain ill and possibly relapse further. In general, early LB is treated for four to six weeks, and late LB usually requires a minimum of four to six months of continuous treatment. All patients respond differently and therapy must be individualized. It is not uncommon for a patient who has been ill for many years to require open ended treatment regimens; indeed, some patients will require ongoing maintenance therapy for years to remain well.

Several days after the onset of appropriate antibiotic therapy, symptoms often flare due to lysis of the spirochetes with release of increased amount of antigenic material and possibly bacterial toxins. This is referred to as a Jarisch Herxheimer-like reaction. Because it takes 48 to 72 hours of therapy to initiate bacterial killing, the Herxheimer reaction is therefore delayed. This is unlike syphilis, in which these reactions can occur within hours.

It has been observed that symptoms will flare in cycles every four weeks. It is thought that this reflects the organism's cell cycle, with the growth phase occurring once per month (intermittent growth is common in Borrelia species). As antibiotics will only kill bacteria during their growth phase, therapy is designed to bracket at least one whole generation cycle. This is why the minimum treatment duration should be at least four weeks. If the antibiotics are working, over time these flares will lessen in severity and duration. The very occurrence of ongoing monthly cycles indicates that living organisms are still present and that antibiotics should be continued.

With treatment, these monthly symptom flares are exaggerated and presumably represent recurrent Herxheimer-like reactions as Bb enters its vulnerable growth phase and then are lysed. For unknown reasons, the worst occurs at the fourth week of treatment. Observation suggest that the more severe this reaction, the higher the germ load, and the more ill the patient. In those with long-standing highly symptomatic disease who are on I.V. therapy, the week-four flare can be very severe, similar to a serum sickness reaction, and be associated with transient leucopenia and/or elevations in liver enzymes. If this happens, decrease the dose temporarily, or interrupt treatment for several days, then resume with a lower dose. If you are able to continue or resume therapy, then patients continue to improve. Those whose treatment is stopped and not restarted at this point usually will need retreatment in the future due to ongoing or recurrent symptoms because the infection was not eradicated. Patients on I.V. therapy who have a strong reaction at the fourth week will need to continue parenteral antibiotics for several months, for when this monthly reaction finally lessens in severity, then oral or IM medications can be substituted. Indeed, it is just this observation that guides the clinician in determining the endpoint of I.V. treatment. In general, I.V. therapy is given until there is a clear positive response, and then treatment is changed to IM or po until free of signs of active infection for 4 to 8 weeks. Some patients, however, will not respond to IM or po treatment and I.V. therapy will have to be used throughout. As mentioned earlier, leucopenia may be a sign of persistent Ehrlichiosis, so be sure to look into this.

Repeated treatment failures should alert the clinician to the possibility of an otherwise inapparent immune deficiency, and a workup for this may be advised. Obviously, evaluation for co-infection should be performed, and a search for other or concurrent diagnoses needs to be entertained.

There are three things that will predict treatment failure regardless of which regimen is chosen: Non-compliance, alcohol use, and sleep deprivation. Advise them to take a break when (or ideally _before_) the inevitable mid afternoon fatigue sets in (napping is encouraged).

All patients must keep a carefully detailed daily diary of their symptoms to help us document the presence of the classic four week cycle, judge the effects of treatment, and determine treatment endpoint. One must follow such diaries, temperature readings in late afternoon, physical findings, notes from physical therapists, and cognitive testing to best judge when to change or end antibiotics.

Remember- there currently is no test for cure, so this clinical follow-up assumes a major role in Lyme Disease care.

ANTIBIOTIC CHOICES AND DOSES

ORAL THERAPY: Always check blood levels when using agents marked with an *, and adjust dose to achieve a peak level above ten and a trough greater than three. Because of this, the doses listed below may have to be raised. Consider Doxycycline first in early Lyme due to concern for Ehrlichia co-infections.

*Amoxicillin- Adults: 1g q8h plus probenecid 500mg q8h; doses up to 6 grams daily are
often needed

Pregnancy: 1g q6h and adjust.
Children: 50 mg/kg/day divided into q8h doses.
*Doxycycline- Adults: 200 mg bid with food; doses of up to 600 mg daily are often needed, as doxycycline is only effective at high blood levels. Not for children or in pregnancy.
If levels are too low at tolerated doses, give parenterally or change to another drug.
*Cefuroxime axetil- Oral alternative that may be effective in amoxicillin and doxycycline failures. Useful in EM rashes co-infected with common skin pathogens.
Adults and pregnancy: 1g q12h and adjust. Children: 125 to 500 mg q12h based on weight.
Tetracycline- Adults only, and not in pregnancy. 500 mg tid to qid
Erythromycin- Poor response and not recommended.
Azithromycin- Adults: 500 to 1200 mg/d. Adolescents: 250 to 500 mg/d
Add hydroxychloroquine, 200-400 mg/d, or amantadine 100-200 mg/d
Cannot be used in pregnancy or in younger children.
Overall, poor results when administered orally
Clarithromycin- Adults: 250 to 500 mg q6h plus hydroxychloroquine, 200-400 mg/d, or amantadine 100-200 mg/d. Cannot be used in pregnancy or in younger children.
Clinically more effective than azithromycin
Telithromycin- Adolescents and adults: 800 mg once daily
Do not need to use amantadine or hydroxychloroquine
So far, the most effective drug of this class, and possibly the best oral agent if tolerated. Expect strong and quite prolonged Herxheimer reactions.
Must watch for drug interactions (CYP3A-4 inhibitor), check the QTc interval, and monitor liver enzymes.
Not to be used in pregnancy.
*Augmentin- Standard Augmentin cannot exceed three tablets daily due to the clavulanate, thus is given with amoxicillin, so that the total dose of the amoxicillin component is as listed above for amoxicillin. This combination can be effective when Bb beta lactamase is felt to be significant.
*Augmentin XR 1000- This is a time-release formulation and thus is a better choice than standard Augmentin.
Dose- 1000 mg q 8 h, to 2000 mg q 12 h based on blood levels.
Chloramphenicol- Not recommended as not proven and potentially toxic.
Metronidazole: 500 to 1500 mg daily in divided doses. Non-pregnant adults only.

PARENTERAL THERAPY
Ceftriaxone- Risk of biliary sludging (therefore often Actigall is co-administered- one to three tablets daily).
Adults and pregnancy: 2g q12 h, 4 days in a row each week
Children: 75 mg/kg/day up to 2g/day
Cefotaxime- Comparable efficacy to ceftriaxone; no biliary complications.
Adults and pregnancy: 6g to 12g daily. Can be given q 8 h as divided doses, but a continuous infusion may be more efficacious. When exceeding 6 g daily, use pulsed-dose schedule
Children: 90 to 180 mg/kg/day dosed q6h (preferred) or q8h, not to exceed 12 g daily.
*Doxycycline- Requires central line as is caustic.
Surprisingly effective, probably because blood levels are higher when given parenterally and single large daily doses optimize kinetics of killing with this drug.
Always measure blood levels.
Adults: Start at 400 mg q24h and adjust based on levels.
Cannot be used in pregnancy or in younger children.
Tigecycline- requires central line as is caustic

>By far the most effective tetracycline, and very useful to also treat difficult intracellular co-infections
>Cannot be used in pregnancy and in younger children
>Dose is 50 mg IV q 12h.

Azithromycin- Requires central line as is caustic.
>Dose: 500 to 1000 mg daily in adolescents and adults.

Penicillin G- IV penicillin G is minimally effective and not recommended.

Benzathine penicillin- Surprisingly effective IM alternative to oral therapy. May need to
>begin at lower doses as strong, prolonged (6 or more week) Herxheimer-like reactions have been observed.
>Adults: 1.2 million U- three to four doses weekly.
>Adolescents: 1.2 to 3.6 million U weekly.
>May be used in pregnancy.

Vancomycin- observed to be one of the best drugs in treating Lyme, but potential toxicity limits its use.
>It is a perfect candidate for pulse therapy to minimize these concerns. Use standard doses and confirm levels.

Primaxin and Unisyn- similar in efficacy to cefotaxime, but often work when
>cephalosporins have failed.
>Must be given q6 to q8 hours.

Cefuroxime- useful but not demonstrably better than ceftriaxone or cefotaxime.

*Ampicillin IV- more effective than penicillin G. Must be given q6 hours.

TREATMENT CATEGORIES

PROPHYLAXIS of high risk groups- education and preventive measures. Antibiotics are not given.

TICK BITES - Embedded Deer Tick With No Signs or Symptoms of Lyme (see appendix):
Decide to treat based on the type of tick, whether it came from an endemic area, how it was removed, and length of attachment (anecdotally, as little as four hours of attachment can transmit pathogens). The risk of transmission is greater if the tick is engorged, or of it was removed improperly allowing the tick's contents to spill into the bite wound. High-risk bites are treated as follows (remember the possibility of co-infection!):
>1) Adults: Oral therapy for 28 days.
>2) Pregnancy: Amoxicillin 1000 mg q6h for 6 weeks. Test for Babesia, Bartonella and Ehrlichia.
>>Alternative: Cefuroxime axetil 1000 mg q12h for 6 weeks.
>3) Young Children: Oral therapy for 28 days.

EARLY LOCALIZED - Single erythema migrans with no constitutional symptoms:
>1) Adults: oral therapy- must continue until symptom and sign free for at least one month, with a 6 week minimum.
>2) Pregnancy: 1st and 2nd trimesters: I.V. X 30 days then oral X 6 weeks
>>3rd trimester: Oral therapy X 6+ weeks as above.
>>Any trimester- test for Babesia and Ehrlichia
>3) Children: oral therapy for 6+ weeks.

DISSEMINATED DISEASE - Multiple lesions, constitutional symptoms, lymphadenopathy, or any other manifestations of dissemination.

EARLY DISSEMINATED: Milder symptoms present for less than one year and not complicated by immune deficiency or prior steroid treatment:
>1) Adults: oral therapy until no active disease for 4 to 8 weeks (4-6 months typical)
>2) Pregnancy: As in localized disease, but treat throughout pregnancy.
>3) Children: Oral therapy with duration based upon clinical response.

PARENTERAL ALTERNATIVES for more ill patients and those unresponsive to or intolerant of oral medications:
>1) Adults and children: I.V. therapy until clearly improved, with a 6 week minimum. Follow with oral

therapy or IM benzathine penicillin until no active disease for 6-8 weeks. I.V. may have to be resumed if oral or IM therapy fails.
2) Pregnancy: IV then oral therapy as above.

LATE DISSEMINATED: present greater than one year, more severely ill patients, and those with prior significant steroid therapy or any other cause of impaired immunity:
1) Adults and pregnancy: extended I.V. therapy (14 or more weeks), then oral or IM, if effective, to same endpoint. Combination therapy with at least two dissimilar antibiotics almost always needed.
2) Children: IV therapy for 6 or more weeks, then oral or IM follow up as above. Combination therapy usually needed.

CHRONIC LYME DISEASE (PERSISTENT/RECURRENT INFECTION)
By definition, this category consists of patients with active infection, of a more prolonged duration, who are more likely have higher spirochete loads, weaker defense mechanisms, possibly more virulent or resistant strains, and probably are significantly co-infected. Neurotoxins may also be significant in these patients. Search for and treat for all of these, and search for concurrent infections including viruses, chlamydias, and mycoplasmas. Be sure to do an endocrine workup if indicated. These patients require a full evaluation for all of these problems, and each abnormality must be addressed.

This group will most likely need parenteral therapy, especially high dose, pulsed therapy, and antibiotic combinations, including metronidazole. Antibiotic therapy will need to continue for many months, and the antibiotics may have to be changed periodically to break plateaus in recovery. Be vigilant for treatment-related problems such as antibiotic-associated colitis, yeast overgrowth, intravenous catheter complications, and abnormalities in blood counts and chemistries.

If treatment can be continued long term, then a remarkable degree of recovery is possible. However, attention must be paid to all treatment modalities for such a recovery- not only antibiotics, but rehab and exercise programs, nutritional supplements, enforced rest, low carbohydrate, high fiber diets, attention to food sensitivities, avoidance of stress, abstinence from caffeine and alcohol, and absolutely no immunosuppressants, even local doses of steroids (intra-articular injections, for example).

Unfortunately, not all patients with chronic Lyme disease will fully recover and treatment may not eradicate the active Borrelia infection. Such individuals may have to be maintained on open-ended, ongoing antibiotic therapy, for they repeatedly relapse after antibiotics are stopped. Maintenance antibiotic therapy in this select group is thus mandatory.

In patients who have chronic Lyme, who do not fully respond to antibiotics, one must search for an explanation. In many cases, these patients are found to have pituitary insufficiency of varying degrees. The abnormalities may be extremely subtle, and provocative testing must be done for full diagnosis. Persistent fatigue, limited stamina, hypotension, and loss of libido suggest this possibility.

Similarly, a small but significant number of these patients harbor toxic levels of heavy metals. Challenge testing by knowledgeable, experienced clinicians is necessary for evaluation. Treatment must be directed toward correcting the specific abnormalities found, and post-treatment retesting to assess efficacy of treatment and endpoint of therapy should be done. Suspect this when poor immune responsiveness and persistent neuropathic signs and symptoms are present.

INDICATORS FOR PARENTERAL THERAPY
(The following are guidelines only and are not meant to be absolute. It is based on retrospective study of over 600 patients with late Lyme disease.)
- Illness for greater than one year
- Prior immunosuppressive therapy while infected with Bb.
- Major neurological involvement
- Active synovitis with high sedimentation rate

- Elevated protein or cells in the CSF

ADVANCED TREATMENT OPTIONS

PULSE THERAPY consists of administering antibiotics (usually parenteral ones) two to four days in a row per week. This allows for several advantages:
* Dosages are doubled (ie: cefotaxime, 12 g daily), increasing efficacy
* More toxic medications can be used with increased safety (ie: vancomycin)
* May be effective when conventional, daily regimens have failed.
* IV access may be easier or more tolerable
* More agreeable lifestyle for the patient
* Often less costly than daily regimens

Note that this type of treatment is expected to continue for a minimum of ten weeks, and often must continue beyond twenty weeks. The efficacy of this regimen is based on the fact that it takes 48 to 72 hours of continuous bactericidal antibiotic levels to kill the spirochete, yet it will take longer than the four to five days between pulses for the spirochetes to recover. As with all Lyme treatments, specific dosing and scheduling must be tailored to the individual patient's clinical picture based upon the treating physician's best clinical judgment.

COMBINATION THERAPY (see page 12)
This consists of using two or more dissimilar antibiotics simultaneously for antibiotic synergism, to better compensate for differing killing profiles and sites of action of the individual medications, and to cover the three known forms of Bb. A typical combination is the use of a cell wall agent plus a protein inhibitor (ie: amoxicillin plus clarithromycin). Note that GI intolerance and yeast superinfections are the biggest drawbacks to this type of treatment. However, these complications can often be prevented or easily treated, and the clinically observed benefits of this type of regimen clearly have outweighed these problems in selected patients.

LYME DISEASE AND PREGNANCY
It is well known that B. burgdorferi can cross the placenta and infect the fetus. In addition, breast milk from infected mothers has been shown to harbor spirochetes that can be detected by PCR and grown in culture.

The Lyme Disease Foundation in Hartford, CT had kept a pregnancy registry for eleven years beginning in the late 1980s. They found that if patients were maintained on adequate doses of antibiotic therapy during gestation, then no babies were born with Lyme. My own experience over the last twenty years agrees with this.

The options for treating the mother include oral, intramuscular, and intravenous therapy as outlined above. It is vital that peak and trough antibiotic levels be measured if possible at the start of gestation and at least once more during treatment.

During pregnancy, symptoms generally are mild as the hormonal changes seem to mask many symptoms. However, post-partum, mothers have a rough time, with a sudden return of all their Lyme symptoms including profound fatigue. Post partum depression can be particularly severe. I always advise help in the home for at least the first month, so adequate rest and time for needed treatments are assured.

I also advise against breast feeding for obvious reasons as mentioned above.

MONITORING THERAPY
Drug levels are measured, where possible, to confirm adequate dosing. Often, the regimen may have to be modified to optimize the dose. This may have to be repeated again at any time major changes in the treatment regimen occur, and serially during pregnancy. With parenteral therapy, CBC and chem/liver panels are done at least twice each month, especially during symptom flares, with urinalysis and pro-time monitored less frequently.

SAFETY
Over two decades of experience in treating thousands of patients with Lyme has proven that therapy as described above, although intense, is generally well tolerated. The most common adverse reaction seen is allergy to probenecid. In addition, yeast superinfections are seen, but these are generally easily recognized and managed. The induction of Clostridium difficile toxin production is seen most commonly with ceftriaxone, but can occur with any of the antibiotic regimens mentioned in this document. However, pulsed dose therapy and regular use of the lactobacillus preparations seems to be helpful in controlling yeast and antibiotic related colitis, as the number of cases of C. difficile in Lyme patients is low when these guidelines are followed. Be sure to test stool for both toxin A and toxin B when evaluating for C. difficile colitis.

When using central intravenous lines including PICC lines (peripherally inserted central catheters), if ANY line problems arise, it is recommended that the line be pulled for patient safety. Salvage attempts (urokinase, repairing holes) are often ineffective and may not be safe.

Please advise all patients who take the tetracyclines of skin and eye sensitivity to sunlight and the proper precautions, and advise birth control if appropriate. When doxycycline is given parenterally, do not refreeze the solution prior to use!

Remember, years of experience with chronic antibiotic therapy in other conditions, including rheumatic fever, acne, gingivitis, recurrent otitis, recurrent cystitis, COPD, bronchiectasis, and others have not revealed any consistent dire consequences as a result of such medication use. Indeed, the very real consequences of untreated, chronic persistent infection by B. burgdorferi can be far worse than the potential consequences of this treatment.

CO-INFECTIONS IN LYME

PIROPLASMOSIS (Babesiosis)
GENERAL INFORMATION
It had been thought that Babesia microti is the only significant piroplasm affecting humans. Now it is believed that many of the over two dozen known species of piroplasms can be carried by ticks and potentially be transmitted to the human. Unfortunately, we have no widely available tests for these non-microti species. That is why, again, a clinical diagnosis is required.

Piroplasms are not bacteria, they are protozoans. Therefore, they will not be eradicated by any of the currently used Lyme treatment regimens. Therein lies the significance of co-infections- if a Lyme patient has been extensively treated yet is still ill, and especially if they are experiencing atypical symptoms, suspect a co-infection. From the literature:
- "Co-infection generally results in more intense acute illness, a greater array of symptoms, and a more prolonged convalescence than accompany either infection alone."
- "Spirochete DNA was evident more often and remained in the circulation longer in co-infected subjects than in those experiencing either infection alone."
- "Co-infection might also synergize spirochete-induced lesions in human joints, heart and nerves."
- "Babesia infections may impair human host defense mechanisms…"
- "The possibility of concomitant Babesia infection should be considered when moderate to severe Lyme Disease has been diagnosed."

Babesia infection is becoming more commonly recognized, especially in patients who already have Lyme Disease. It has been published that as many as 66% of Lyme patients show serologic evidence of co-infection with Babesia microti. It has also been reported that Babesia infections can range in severity from mild, subclinical infection, to fulminant, potentially life threatening illness. Subclinical infection is often missed because the symptoms are incorrectly ascribed to Lyme. Babesia infections, even mild ones, may recur even after treatment and cause severe illness. This phenomenon has been reported to occur at any time, including up to several years after the initial infection! Furthermore, such Babesia carriers pose a risk to the blood supply as this infection has been reported to be passed on by blood transfusion.

SYMPTOMS
Clues to the presence of Babesiosis include a more acute initial illness- patients often recall a high fever and chills at the onset of their Lyme. Over time, they can note night sweats, air hunger, an occasional cough, persistent migraine-like headache, a vague sense of imbalance without true vertigo, encephalopathy and fatigue. The fulminant presentations are seen in those who are immunosuppressed, especially if asplenic, and in advanced ages. They include high fevers, shaking chills and hemolysis, and can be fatal.

DIAGNOSTIC TESTS
Diagnostic tests are insensitive and problematic. There are at least thirteen, and possibly as many as two dozen Babesia forms found in ticks, yet we can currently only test for B. microti and WA-1 with our serologic and nuclear tests. Standard blood smears reportedly are reliable for only the first two weeks of infection, thus are not useful for diagnosing later infections and milder ones including carrier states where the germ load is too low to be detected. Therefore, multiple diagnostic test methods are available and each have their own benefits and limitations and often several tests must be done. Be prepared to treat based on clinical presentation, even with negative tests.

- SEROLOGY- Unlike Lyme, Babesia titers can reflect infection status. Thus, persistently positive titers or western blots suggest persistent infection.
- PCR- This is more sensitive than smears for B. microti, but will not detect other species.
- ENHANCED SMEAR- This utilizes buffy coat, prolonged scanning (up to three hours per sample!) and digital photography through custom-made microscopes. Although more sensitive than standard smears, infections can still be missed. The big advantage is that it will display multiple species, not just B. microti.
- FLUORESCENT IN-SITU HYBRIDIZATION ASSAY (FISH)- This technique is also a form of blood smear. It is said to be 100-fold more sensitive than standard smears for B. microti, because instead of utilizing standard, ink-based stains, it uses a fluorescent-linked RNA probe and ultraviolet light. The Babesia organisms are then much easier to spot when the slides are scanned. The disadvantage is that currently only B. microti is detected.

TREATMENT
Treating Babesia infections had always been difficult, because the therapy that had been recommended until 1998 consisted of a combination of clindamycin plus quinine. Published reports and clinical experience have shown this regimen to be unacceptable, as nearly half of patients so treated have had to abandon treatment due to serious side effects, many of which were disabling. Furthermore, even in patients who could tolerate these drugs, there was a failure rate approaching 50%.

Because of these dismal statistics, the current regimen of choice for Babesiosis is the combination of atovaquone (Mepron, Malarone), 750 mg bid, plus an erythromycin-type drug, such as azithromycin (Zithromax), clarithromycin (Biaxin), or telithromycin (Ketek) in standard doses. This combination was initially studied in animals, and then applied to Humans with good success. Fewer than 5% of patients have to halt treatment due to side effects, and the success rate is clearly better than that of clindamycin plus quinine.

The duration of treatment with atovaquone combinations for Babesiosis varies depending on the degree of infection, duration of illness before diagnosis, the health and immune status of the patient, and whether the patient is co-infected with Borrelia burgdorferi. Typically, a three-week course is prescribed for acute cases, while chronic, longstanding infections with significant morbidity and co-infection will require a minimum of four months of therapy. Relapses have occurred, and retreatment is occasionally needed.

Problems during therapy include diarrhea, mild nausea, the expense of atovaquone (over $600.00 per bottle- enough for three weeks of treatment), and rarely, a temporary yellowish discoloration of the vision. Blood counts, liver panels and amylase levels are recommended every three weeks during any prolonged course of therapy as liver enzymes may elevate. Treatment failures usually are related to inadequate atovaquone levels. Therefore, patients who are not cured with this regimen can be retreated with higher doses (and atovaquone blood levels can be checked), as this has proven effective in many of my patients. Artemesia (a non-prescription herb) should be added in all cases. Metronidazole or Bactrim can also be added to increase efficacy, but there is minimal clinical data on how much more effective this will be.

BARTONELLA-LIKE ORGANISMS

It has been said that Bartonella is the most common of all tick-borne pathogens. Indeed, there seems to be a fairly distinct clinical syndrome when this type of organism is present in the chronic Lyme patient. However, several aspects of this infection seem to indicate that this tick-associated strain of Bartonella is different from that described as "cat scratch disease". For example, in patients who fit the clinical picture, standard Bartonella blood testing is commonly non-reactive. Furthermore, the usual Bartonella medications do not work for this- they suppress the symptoms but do not permanently clear them. For these reasons I like to refer to this as a "Bartonella-like organism" (BLO), rather than assume it is a more common species.

Indicators of BLO infection include CNS symptoms out of proportion to the other systemic symptoms of chronic Lyme. There seems to be an increased irritability to the CNS, with agitation, anxiety, insomnia, and even seizures, in addition to other unusually strong symptoms of encephalitis, such as cognitive deficits and confusion. Other key symptoms may include gastritis, lower abdominal pain (mesenteric adenitis), sore soles, especially in the AM, tender subcutaneous nodules along the extremities, and red rashes. These rashes may have the appearance of red streaks like stretch marks that do not follow skin planes, spider veins, or red papular eruptions. Lymph nodes may be enlarged and the throat can be sore.

Because standard Bartonella testing, either by serology or PCR, may not pick up this BLO, the blood test is very insensitive. Therefore, the diagnosis is a clinical one, based on the above points. Also, suspect infection with BLO in extensively treated Lyme patients who still are encephalitic, and who never had been treated with a significant course of specific treatment.

The drug of choice to treat BLO is levofloxacin. Levofloxacin is usually never used for Lyme or Babesia, so many patients who have tick-borne diseases, and who have been treated for them but remain ill, may in fact be infected with BLO. Treatment consist of 500 mg daily (may be adjusted based on body weight) for at least one month. Treat for three months or longer in the more ill patient. It has been suggested that levofloxacin may be more effective in treating this infection if a proton pump inhibitor is added in standard doses.

Another subtlety is that certain antibiotic combinations seem to inhibit the action of levofloxacin, while others seem to be neutral. I advise against using an erythromycin-like drug, as clinically such patients do poorly. On the other hand, combinations with cephalosporins, penicillins and tetracyclines are okay. Alternatives to levofloxacin include rifampin, gentamicin and possibly streptomycin. A very recent article suggests that prior use of quinine-like drugs including atovaquone (Mepron, Malarone) may render Levaquin less effective. Therefore, in a co-infected patient, treat the BLO before you address Babesia species.

Levofloxacin is generally well tolerated, with almost no stomach upset. Very rarely, it can cause confusion- this is temporary (clears in a few days) and may be relieved by lowering the dose. There is, however, one side effect that would require it to be stopped- it may cause a painful tendonitis, usually of the largest tendons. If this happens, then the levofloxacin must be stopped or tendon rupture may occur. It has been suggested that loading the patient with magnesium may prevent this problem, and if the tendons do become affected, parenteral high dose vitamin C (plus parenteral magnesium) may afford rapid relief.

Unfortunately, levofloxacin and drugs in this family cannot be given to those under the age of 18, so other alternatives, such as azithromycin, are used in children.

Incidentally, animal studies show that Bartonella may be transmitted across the placenta. No human studies have been done.

EHRLICHIA (AND ANAPLASMA)
GENERAL INFORMATION

While it is true that this illness can have a fulminant presentation, and may even become fatal if not treated, milder forms do exist, as does chronic low-grade infection, especially when other tick-borne organisms are present. The potential transmission of Ehrlichia during tick bites is the main reason why doxycycline is now the first choice in treating tick bites and early Lyme, before serologies can become positive. When present alone or co-infecting with B. burgdorferi, persistent leukopenia is an important clue. Thrombocytopenia and elevated liver enzymes, common in acute infection, are less often seen in those who are chronically infected, but likewise should not be ignored. Headaches, myalgias, and ongoing fatigue suggest this illness, but are extremely difficult to separate from symptoms caused by Bb.

DIAGNOSTIC TESTING
Testing is problematic with Ehrlichia, similar to the situation with Babesiosis. More species are known to be present in ticks than can be tested for with clinically available serologies and PCRs. In addition, serologies and PCRs are of unknown sensitivity and specificity. Standard blood smears for direct visualization of organisms in leukocytes are of low yield. Enhanced smears using buffy coats significantly raise sensitivity and can detect a wider variety of species. Despite this, infection can be missed, so clinical diagnosis remains the primary diagnostic tool. Again, consider this diagnosis in a Lyme Borreliosis (LB) patient not responding well to Lyme therapy who has symptoms suggestive of Ehrlichia.

TREATMENT
Standard treatment consists of Doxycycline, 200 mg daily for two to four weeks. Higher doses, parenteral therapy, and longer treatment durations may be needed based on the duration and severity of illness, and whether immune defects or extreme age is present. However, there are reports of treatment failure even when higher doses and long duration treatment with doxycycline is given. In such cases, consideration may be given for adding rifampin, 600 mg daily, to the regimen.

SORTING OUT THE CO-INFECTIONS
In addition to *Borrelia burgdorferi* (Bb), ticks may carry and transmit other infections. Furthermore, patients with disseminated Lyme complicated by these co-infections are usually immunocompromized and may also manifest signs and symptoms of reactivated latent infections and opportunists. All can add to morbidity and may need to be treated.

Because of the large number of these other infections, the cost of reliably testing for all of them as a matter of routine is prohibitive. Also, as in the case with Bb infection, laboratory tests for them are often insensitive. Thus there is a need to sort it all out clinically to provide guidance in testing and treatment. Here are some clues:

CLASSIC LYME (Bb infection)-
- Gradual onset of initial (viral-like) symptoms- this often makes it difficult to pinpoint when the infection began.
- Multisystem- almost always, in disseminated stages, involves more than one part or system (i.e. joint pain plus cognitive dysfunction).
- Migratory- first a knee will hurt, then over time this may lessen and the elbow or shoulder acts up, and later the joints calm down but headaches worsen.
- Stiff joints and loud joint crepitus, especially the neck ("Lyme shrug").
- Headaches are often nuchal and associated with stiff, painful and crepitant neck.
- Afternoon fevers, often unnoticed- most Lyme patients have subnormal temperatures in the AM but rise to 99+ by early to mid-afternoon. No obvious sweats.
- Tiredness and limited stamina- often is a strong need to rest or even nap in the afternoon, especially when the flushed face and elevated temperature appears.
- 4-week cycles- Bb activity, and thus symptoms, wax and wane in a cycle that repeats roughly every four weeks. This cycle, if clear, can guide your treatments.
- Slow response to treatment, with an initial symptom flare in most ("Herxheimer-like reaction") then improvement over weeks, punctuated by the monthly symptom flares. Likewise, if treatment is ended too soon, an initial period of well-being will gradually, over a few weeks, be replaced by a return of symptoms.
- EM rash in 25% to 50%

BARTONELLA & "BARTONELLA-LIKE ORGANISMS"-

- Gradual onset of initial illness.
- CNS symptoms are out of proportion to the musculoskeletal ones- if a patient has no or minimal joint complaints but is severely encephalopathic (see below), then think of Bartonella/BLO.
- Obvious signs of CNS irritability can include muscle twitches, tremors, insomnia, seizures, agitation, anxiety, severe mood swings, outbursts and antisocial behavior.
- GI involvement may present as gastritis or abdominal pain (mesenteric adenitis).
- Sore soles, especially in the morning.
- Tender sub-cutaneous nodules along the extremities, especially outer thigh, shins, and occasionally along the triceps.
- Occasional lymphadenopathy.
- Morning fevers, usually around 99. Occasionally light sweats are noted.
- Elevated vascular endothelial growth factor (VEGF) occurs in a minority, but the degree of elevation correlates with activity of the infection and may be used to monitor treatment.
- Rapid response to treatment changes- often symptoms improve within days after antibiotics are begun, but relapses occur also within days if medication is withdrawn early.
- May have papular or linear red rashes (like stretch marks that do not always follow skin planes), especially in those with GI involvement.

BABESIA SPECIES-
- Rapid onset of initial illness, often with sudden onset of high fever, severe headaches, sweats and fatigue, thus it is easy to know when infection began.
- Obvious sweats, usually at night, but can be day sweats as well.
- Air hunger, need to sigh and take a deep breath; dry cough without apparent reason.
- Headaches can be severe - dull, global (involves the whole head, described like the head is in a vise).
- Fatigue is prominent, does not clear with rest, and is made worse with exercise.
- Mental dullness and slowing of reactions and responses.
- Dizziness- more like a tippy feeling, and not vertigo or purely orthostasis.
- Symptoms cycle rapidly, with flares every four to six days.
- Hypercoaguable states are often associated with *Babesia* infections.
- Rarely, splenomegaly
- Very severe Lyme Disease can be a clue to *Babesia* infection, as it will make Lyme symptoms worse and Lyme treatments less effective.

EHRLICHIA/ANAPLASMA-
- Rapid onset of initial illness with fever, headache, prostration.
- Headaches are sharp, knife-like, and often behind the eyes.
- Muscle pain, not joint pain, and can be mild or severe.
- Low WBC count, elevated liver enzymes, and (rarely) inclusions seen in the WBCs.
- Rarely see diffuse vasculitic rash, including palms and soles (less than 10%).
- Rapid response to treatment.

DNA VIRUSES (HHV-6, EBV, CMV)
- Persistent fatigue, made worse with exercise.
- Sore throat, lymphadenopathy, and other viral-like complaints.
- May see elevated liver enzymes and low WBC counts.
- Autonomic dysfunction.

<u>**SUPPORTIVE THERAPY**</u>

CERTAIN **ABSOLUTE RULES** MUST BE FOLLOWED IF LYME SYMPTOMS ARE TO BE PERMANENTLY CLEARED:
1. Not allowed to get behind in sleep, or become overtired.
2. No caffeine or other stimulants that may affect depth or duration of sleep, or reduce or eliminate naps.

3. Absolutely no alcohol!
4. No smoking at all.
5. Aggressive exercises are required and should be initiated as soon as possible.
6. Diet must contain generous quantities of high quality protein and be high in fiber and low in fat and carbohydrates- no simple carbohydrates are allowed. Instead, use those with low glycemic index.
7. Certain key nutritional supplements should be added.
8. COMPLIANCE!

NUTRITIONAL SUPPLEMENTS IN DISSEMINATED LYME DISEASE

BACKGROUND INFORMATION
Studies on patients with chronic illnesses such as Lyme and Chronic Fatigue have demonstrated that some of the late symptoms are related to cellular damage and deficiencies in certain essential nutrients. Double blinded, placebo controlled studies, and in one case direct assay of biopsy specimens have proven the value of some of the supplements listed. Some are required, while others are optional -see below. They are listed in order of importance.
I suggest patients use a pill organizer. These are multi-compartment boxes that you pre-fill with your pills once a week. This makes the task of taking a large number of tablets much, much simpler and can markedly minimize missed doses. The Vitamin Shop sells a variety of good organizers.

I have found that the quality of supplements used is often more important than the dose. In fact, I do not recommend "mega doses". Instead, seek out, if possible, pharmaceutical grade products, especially if USP certified. I recommend, among others, Pharmanex, Researched Nutritionals and Nature Made products because they fit these criteria. In the list below, it is indicated whether the products should be gotten from Pharmanex, Researched Nutritionals, a different specific manufacturer, or even if a generic substitute is OK.

-To order products from Pharmanex, users need to register as a customer with a referral from another registered customer. You may use my referral number (US9256681) to get started. Call 1-800-487-1000.
-Researched Nutritionals generally markets its products only through physician's offices. If you physician does not do this, he or she can still call the company to order the items for you. The number is 1-800-755-3402.
-Nature Made products are widely available in vitamin stores and pharmacies.

BASIC DAILY REGIMEN (in order of importance)

1. PROBIOTICS (required when on antibiotics)
Kefir: This is a yogurt-like drink that is said to more permanently replenish beneficial flora. It is only necessary to drink 2 to 4 ounces a day.
Acidophilus: the best kinds are frozen or refrigerated to ensure potency. Usual dose is two with each meal. Plan to mix together several different brands to broaden the spectrum. Acidophilus can be gotten from most vitamin stores but some generic brands are of unknown freshness and potency. An alternative that does not need refrigeration and can be taken only once a day is a high potency, patented product called "**Pro Bio**" from Pharmanex. The ultimate mix of pre- and probiotics with soil based organisms is a product called "**Prescript-Assist Pro**" from Researched Nutritionals. This too does not need refrigeration.
In addition, have 4 ounces of sugar-free **yogurt** on occasion.

2. MULTI-VITAMIN (required)
I recommend the **Life Pack** family of multivitamins available through Pharmanex. These are unique supplements- pharmaceutical grade and USP certified, they are the only products clinically proven in double blinded, placebo controlled crossover studies to quench free radicals and raise antioxidant levels in the blood and lipids. Choose LifePak for males under 40, LifePak Women for hormonally active women, LifePak Prenatal when pregnant, and LifePak Prime for postmenopausal women and for men over 40. LifePak Teen is also available. Continue long term.

3. CO-Q10- *required, but do not use while taking the prescription drug atovaquone (Mepron, Malarone).*
Deficiencies have been related to poor function of the heart, limitations of stamina, gum disease, and poor resistance to infections. Heart biopsy studies in Lyme patients indicated that they should take between 300 and 400mg daily. I recommend the Co Q-10 from Researched Nutritionals. One caplet contains 400 mg, so the dose is one a day with food.

4. ALPHA LIPOIC ACID (required)
This facilitates entry of CoQ-10 into mitochondria. Dose is 300 mg twice daily. Generic is OK.

5. VITAMIN B (required).
Clinical studies demonstrated the need for supplemental vitamin B in infections with Borrelia, to help clear neurological symptoms. Take one 50 mg B-complex capsule daily. If neuropathy is severe, an additional 50 mg of B-6 can be added. Generics are OK.

6. MAGNESIUM (required)
Magnesium supplementation is very helpful for the tremors, twitches, cramps, muscle soreness, heart skips and weakness. It may also help in energy level and cognition. The best source is magnesium L-lactate dehydrate ("**Mag-tab SR**", sold by Niche Pharmaceuticals: 1-800-677-0355, and available at Wal-Mart). DO NOT rely on "cal-mag", calcium plus magnesium combination tablets, as they are not well absorbed. Take at least one tablet twice daily. Higher doses increase the benefit and should be tried, but may cause diarrhea. In some cases, intramuscular or intravenous doses may be necessary.

7. ESSENTIAL FATTY ACIDS: (required)
Studies show that when EFAs are taken regularly, statistically significant improvements in fatigue, aches weakness, vertigo, dizziness, memory, concentration and depression are likely. There are two broad classes: GLA (omega-6 oils) and EPA (omega-3 oils), derived respectively from plant and fish oils. This is what to take:
Plant Oil: Use a refrigerated liquid product of mixed omega oils obtained from the local health food store (always avoid capsules as the plant oils within may be rancid and you would never know). Take one to two tablespoons of the liquid oil daily. May be mixed with food, put on salads, etc.
Fish Oil: Use "**Marine Omega**" by Pharmanex. Use four daily, taken on a full stomach (this brand is required because it is made not from fish, but from Krill and is certified to be free of any measurable amounts of heavy metals and organic toxins).

8. NT-FACTOR
This product addresses the mitochondrial damage thought to underlie the metabolic dysfunction associated with chronic diseases which, in patients with tick-borne illnesses, is manifest by fatigue and neurologic dysfunction. *It is the single most reliable agent I have found that can give noticeably increased energy levels.* When supplements known to support neurological function are added (see below), improved cognition and memory often result. Effects will be noted in two to three weeks. It also contains high quality prebiotics and probiotics. Available from Researched Nutritionals.

OPTIONAL SUPPLEMENTS FOR SPECIAL CIRCUMSTANCES

FOR NEUROLOGIC SYMPTOMS- here, the goal is three-fold- supply the metabolic needs, replenish what has become depleted, and protect the neurons and their supportive cells. The "required" supplements, above, must be taken, and the items that follow below are considered "add-ons".

ACETYL-L-CARNITINE- this is taken along with **SAM-e**. This combination can result in noticeable gains in short term memory, mood and cognition. The Acetyl Carnitine also is said to help heart and muscle function. Doses: Acetyl-L-carnitine- 1500-2000 mg daily on empty stomach; SAM-e- 400 mg daily with the acetyl carnitine. Positive results may appear as early as 3 weeks; use for 2 to 3 months, but repeat or extend this course if needed. Available in most vitamin stores; Generic acetyl carnitine is okay, but I recommend "Nature Made" brand SAM-e (also available at most vitamin stores).

METHYLCOBALAMIN (Methyl B12)
Methylcobalamin is a prescription drug derived from vitamin B12. This can help to heal problems with the central and peripheral nervous system, improve depressed immune function, and help to restore more normal sleeping patterns. Many patients note improved energy as well. Because the oral form is not absorbed when swallowed or dissolved under the tongue, Methyl B12 must be taken by injection. Dose is generally 25 mg. (1 c.c.) daily for 3 to 6 months. Long term studies have never demonstrated any side effects from this drug. However, *the urine is expected to turn red shortly after each dose*- if the urine is not red, a higher dose may be needed or the present supply may have lost potency. The injectable form of this is not available in regular drug stores. It must be manufactured (compounded) by specialty pharmacies on order.

GREEN TEA
Green, but not black or white tea contains some of the most potent antioxidants around (80-100 times more effective than vitamin C). I strongly recommend this to any patient with degenerative changes to the central nervous system. At least four cups daily are needed to reap this benefit, and the tea must be decaffeinated. A nice alternative is **"TeGreen"** capsules by Pharmanex. They contain 97% pure tea polyphenols and each capsule is the equivalent of four cups of decaffeinated green tea. Take one to three daily.

CORDYMAX
Cordyceps is a well-known herb from Tibet that has been shown in clinical studies to improve stamina, fatigue, and enhance lung and antioxidant function. It also raises superoxide dismutase levels, important to prevent lesions in the central nervous system, which is why *this (along with green tea) is essential if neurodegeneration is part of your illness.* The positive effects can be dramatic; should be used long term. USP- certified cordyceps is available from Pharmanex as "**CordyMax**".

CITICHOLINE
Many studies have shown benefits to cognition, *especially memory*. Benefits are slow to notice, so plan to use this long-term. Dose is 500 to 1000 mg twice a day.

FOR IMMUNE SUPPORT
"REISHI MAX "
This enhanced extract from cracked spores of the Reishi mushroom has been shown in clinical studies to augment function of the Natural Killer Cells as well as macrophages. Recommended in all patients who have a CD-57 count below 60. Take four a day. Available only from Pharmanex.

TRANSFER FACTORS are the body's natural signals meant to activate the pathogen-killing effects of the cellular immune system. Therapy with these agents consists of taking both a general stimulator, plus specific transfer factors for the infection you have. Personal experience made me a believer in transfer factor therapy. For Lyme patients, use **Transfer Factor Multi-Immune** as the general stimulant, and **Transfer Factor Lyme-Plus** as the specific agent. Both are exclusives from Researched Nutritionals, and I have found them to be surprisingly effective in making the very ill respond better to treatment. Take as directed on the label.

FOR JOINT SYMPTOMS
GLUCOSAMINE
Glucosamine can be of long term benefit to the joints. Do not be misled into buying a product that also contains chondroitin, as this chemical does not add anything, but it can make the product more expensive. Look for a product that contains the herb Boswellia serrata- this is a non-irritative anti-inflammatory. Although many generics exist, the Pharmanex product, "**Cartilage Formula**" has the right ingredients and is of proven efficacy. Expect improvement only over time (several weeks), but plan to use this indefinitely to maintain joint health.

VITAMIN C
Vitamin C is important to aid in maintaining healthy connective tissues. High doses are recommended- 1000 to 6000 mg a day as tolerated (if the dose is too high for you it may cause acid stomach, gas and loose

stools, so therefore dose titration is necessary). Consider using **"Ester-C"** (non-acid and longer acting), or **"C-Salts"** (very well tolerated). Start with a low dose and increase slowly to find your tolerance level.

FLEX CREAM
This is an amazing liniment-like product that really works and has a money back guarantee. Use for any type of body pain- spread on a thick layer and do not rub in. It takes 30 to 60 minutes to work, then lasts many hours. A Pharmanex exclusive.

OTHER OPTIONAL SUPPLEMENTS
VITAMIN D
Surprisingly, most people in America are vitamin D deficient. In the Lyme patient, low vitamin D levels can cause diffuse body aches and cramps that are not responsive to magnesium or calcium supplements. Some also believe that vitamin D is essential for normal immune and hormone function. I strongly urge you to have a fasting blood level drawn. It is recommended that the blood levels be in the upper half or the normal range. If it is not, then 2000 to 4000 units daily are needed for several weeks to make up for the deficit, and then a lower maintenance dose may be necessary, based on results from repeated blood level monitoring. If vitamin D is needed, improvements take 2 to 3 weeks to note, but are well worth the wait.

CREATINE
Creatine has been shown to be of benefit in neuromuscular degenerative diseases such as Lou Gherig's Disease (ALS) and can be very helpful in supporting low blood pressure, as in NMH. It may also benefit strength, stamina, and heart function. Important: To use this safely, you must have an adequate fluid intake. The creatine product should contain taurine, an amino acid needed to enhance creatine absorption, plus some carbohydrate to aid creatine entry into muscle. You will need a 20 gram daily loading dose for the first five days, then 4 to 10 grams daily maintenance. Try "**Cell Tech**" from the Vitamin Shop, and follow label directions.

MILK THISTLE
Useful to support liver function. Take 175 mg daily- use an 80% Silymarin extract. Available from many vitamin stores.

LYME DISEASE REHABILITATION

Despite antibiotic treatments, patients will NOT return to normal unless they exercise, so therefore an aggressive rehab program is absolutely necessary. It is a fact that a properly executed exercise program can actually go beyond the antibiotics in helping to clear the symptoms and to maintain a remission.

Although the scientific basis for the benefits of exercises is not known, there are several reasonable theories. It is known that Bb will die if exposed to all but the tiniest oxygen concentrations. If an aggressive exercise program can increase tissue perfusion and oxygen levels, then this may play a role in what is being seen. Also, during aggressive exercise, the core body temperature can rise above 102 degrees; it is known that B. burgdorferi is very heat sensitive. Perhaps it is the added tissue oxygenation, or higher body temperature, or the combination that weakens the Lyme Borrelia, and allows the antibiotics and our defenses to be more effective. Regular exercise-related movements can help mobilize lymph and enhance circulation. In addition, there is now evidence that a carefully structured exercise program may benefit T-cell function: this function will depress for 12 to 24+ hours after exercise, but then rebound. This T-cell depression is more pronounced after aerobics which is why aerobics are not allowed. The goal is to exercise intermittently, with exercise days separated by days of total rest, including an effort to have plenty of quality sleep. The trick is to time the exercise days to take advantage of these rebounds. For an example, begin with an exercise day followed by 3 to 5 rest days; as stamina improves, then fewer rest days will be needed in between workouts. However, because T-cell functions do fall for at least one day after aggressive exercises, be sure to never exercise two days in a row. Finally, an in intermittent exercise program, properly executed, may help to reset the HPA axis more towards normal. On the following page is an exercise prescription that details these recommendations.

This program may begin with classical physical therapy if necessary. The physical therapy should involve massage, heat, ultrasound and simple range of motion exercises to relieve discomfort and promote better sleep and flexibility. Ice (vasoconstriction) and electrical stimulation (muscle spasm and trauma) should not be used!

The program must evolve into a graded, ultimately strenuous exercise program that consists of a specific regimen of *non-aerobic* conditioning- see below. Have the patient complete a gentle hour of prescribed exercise, then go home, have a hot bath or shower, than try to take a nap. Initially, patients will need this sleep, but as they recover, the exercise will energize them and then a nap will no longer be needed. NOTE: a cardiac stress test may be necessary prior to exercising to ensure safety.

LYME REHAB-PHYSICAL THERAPY PRESCRIPTION

NAME_____

D.O.B._____ DATE_____

Please enroll this patient in a program of therapy to rehabilitate him/her from the effects of chronic tick-borne diseases. If necessary, begin with classic physical therapy, then progress when appropriate to a **whole body conditioning program.**

THERAPEUTIC GOALS (to be achieved <u>in order</u> as the patient's ability allows):

PHYSICAL THERAPY (if needed):
1. **The role of physical therapy here is to prepare the patient for the required, preferably gym-based exercise program outlined below. Plan on several weeks of classic PT then transition to the gym.**
2. Relieve pain and muscle spasms utilizing multiple modalities as available and as indicated: massage, heat, ultrasound, and passive and active range of motion. DO NOT use ice or electrical stim unless specifically ordered by our office. Paraffin baths can be quite useful.
3. Increase mobility, tone and strength while protecting damaged and weakened joints, tendons, and ligaments, and teach these techniques to the patient. Use minimal resistance but a lot of repetitions in any exercises prescribed. At the start of the exercise program, especially if the patient is weak, avoid free weights, bands and large exercise balls, and favor machines (especially hydraulics) that can guide limbs through a prescribed arc; free weights, etc. can risk hyperextension and uncontrolled movements that may cause or add to injuries. Transition the patient slowly to the gym-based program outlined below. **Note- aerobics are not permitted.**
4. Please see the patient two or three days per week- but do not schedule two days in a row!

EXERCISE Begin with a private trainer for careful direction and education.

PATIENT EDUCATION AND MANAGEMENT (to be done during the initial one-on-one sessions and reinforced at all visits thereafter):
1. Instruct patients on **correct exercise technique**, including proper warm-up, breathing, joint protection, proper body positioning during the exercise, and how to cool-down and stretch afterwards.
2. Please work one muscle group at a time and perform extensive and extended **stretching** to each muscle group immediately after each one is exercised, before moving on to the next muscle group.
3. A careful **interview** should be performed at the start of each session to make apparent the effects, both good and bad, from the prior visit's therapy, and adjust therapy accordingly.

PROGRAM:
1. **Aerobic exercises are NOT allowed**, not even low impact variety, until the patient has recovered.
2. **Conditioning**: work to improve strength and reverse the poor conditioning that results from Lyme, through a whole-body exercise program, consisting of light calisthenics and/or resistance training, using light resistance and many repetitions. This can be accomplished in exercise classes called "stretch and tone", or "body sculpture", or can be achieved in the gym with exercise machines or carefully with free weights (see cautions above).
3. **Each session should last one hour.** A gentle hour is preferable to a strenuous half-hour. If the patient is unable to continue for the whole hour, then decrease the intensity to allow him/her to do so.
4. **Exercise no more often than every other day**. The patient may need to start by exercising every 4th or 5th day initially, and as abilities improve, work out more often, but NEVER two days in a row. The non-exercise days should be spent resting.
5. This whole-body conditioning program is what is required to achieve wellness. A simple walking program will not work, and simply placing the patient on a treadmill or an exercise bike is not acceptable (except very briefly, as part of a warm-up), as aerobics can be damaging and must be avoided.

PHYSICIAN'S SIGNATURE_____

MANAGING YEAST OVERGROWTH

Many patients with weakened defenses, such as from chronic illnesses, including Lyme Disease, develop an overgrowth of yeast. This begins in the mouth and then spreads to the intestinal tract. Therefore the primary line of defense is careful oral hygiene, replenishing the beneficial bacteria by daily intake of yogurt, Kefir, and/or acidophilus, and by following a strict low carbohydrate diet.

ORAL HYGEINE:
   CLEANSING
   Brush the teeth, tongue, gums, inner cheeks and palate first with toothpaste, then again for 30 seconds while holding an antiseptic mouthwash in the mouth Then, rinse by scrubbing while holding plain water in the mouth.
   TOOTHPASTE
   Use "AP-24" toothpaste, sold by NuSkin Enterprises. Unlike conventional toothpastes that may contain alcohols, formaldehydes and abrasives, this product cleans in a unique way. It contains two "surfactants" (detergent-like cleansers) that are very effective without being harsh. This product is available in two forms- regular and whitening (both contain fluoride). Choose either one.
   In addition, get from them their patented toothbrush that is designed to work with this toothpaste. It cleans better and is far gentler than regular or electric toothbrushes.
   Order AP-24 products by calling 1-800-487-1000. The U.S. reference # is 9256681-R
   MOUTHWASHES
   Use an antiseptic mouthwash (Scope, Listerine, etc.), and brush the teeth, tongue, gums, cheeks and the roof of the mouth while holding the mouthwash in the mouth. Do this for 30 seconds, then rinse repeatedly with water.

For especially thick or resistant thrush, the most effective (and drastic) treatment, employed as a last resort, consists of using "Dakin's Solution" as a mouth rinse. Make this by mixing one teaspoon of household liquid bleach (Clorox) in four ounces of water. A small amount is held in the mouth while brushing, then spit out, and repeated until the thrush has cleared. This is usually a one-time treatment, but may have to be repeated every few weeks.
After using an antiseptic, it is necessary to immediately eat yogurt or chew an acidophilus capsule to replenish the beneficial flora in the mouth. Because the germ count, both harmful and beneficial, will be artificially reduced after such a cleaning, and because yeasts are opportunists, the yeast infection can come back. By having the yogurt or acidophilus then, the yeast will be crowded out and a more normal oral flora will result.

INTESTINAL TRACT: An overgrowth of yeast here will ferment dietary sugars and starches, forming acids, gas, alcohols and a variety of organic chemicals. Symptoms include gas, bloat, heartburn and/or pain in the stomach area, and because of the organic chemicals, there can be headaches, dizziness, lightheadedness, wooziness and post-meal fatigue. To clear intestinal yeast, first the tongue and mouth must be cleansed so yeast does not reenter the system with every swallow. Next, since yeast germs feed on sugars and starches, follow the low carbohydrate diet outlined below. Finally, to replenish the normal, beneficial microbes, eat PLAIN yogurt daily, drink Kefir, 4 ounces daily, and/or take acidophilus, 2 capsules three times daily after meals.

YEAST CONTROL DIET- restricted carbohydrate regimen

UNRESTRICTED FOODS
All protein foods, such as meat, fish, fowl, cheese, eggs, dairy, tofu

RESTRICTED FOODS
FRUITS
Fruits may be a problem because they contain a large amount of sugars. However, if the fruit contains a lot of fiber, this may make up for the sugars to some degree. Thus:
- Fruits are only allowed at the end of a meal, and never on an empty stomach
- Only high fiber fruits are allowed
- Only very small amounts!

EXAMPLES:
ALLOWED IN GENEROUS AMOUNTS
Grapefruit, lemons, limes, tomatoes, avocado
ALLOWED IN SMALL AMOUNTS ONLY! (The high fiber content in these hard, crunchy fruits partially makes up for the carbohydrates)
    Pears, apples, strawberries, cantaloupe, etc.
NOT ALLOWED (These soft fruits do not have enough fiber)
Oranges, watermelons, bananas, grapes, etc.
No fruit juices either!

VEGETABLES
Green vegetables and salads are O.K. Avoid or limit starchy vegetables (potato, rice, beans, etc.) and avoid pasta.

STARCHES
None!! If it is made from flour- any kind of flour- it is not allowed. (No breads, cereals, cake, pasta, etc.)

SWEETENERS
    NOT ALLOWED
    No sugars at all, and no fructose or corn syrup
    ALLOWED (if tolerated)
    Stevia (safest), honey, and Splenda (if tolerated)
    Aspartame (NutraSweet, Equal) may not be tolerated by some patients
    Saccharin products are not recommended

DRINKS
ALLOWED
    Water, seltzer, caffeine-free diet sodas, coffee and tea without sugar or caffeine, vegetable juices
NOT ALLOWED
    Fruit juices, regular sodas, and any drinks sweetened with sugars or syrups
    No Alcohol at all

OTHERS
Do not skip any meals. At least three regular meals daily are needed; a better option is to eat very small portions but have between meal snacks to maintain blood sugar and insulin levels. Bedtime snacks, if taken, must be totally carbohydrate free!

PATIENT INSTRUCTIONS ON TICK BITE PREVENTION AND TICK REMOVAL

HOW TO PROTECT YOURSELF FROM TICK BITES

PROPERTY Remove wood piles, rock walls, and bird feeders as these attract tick-carrying small animals and can increase the risk of acquiring Lyme.
INSECTICIDES: Property should be treated with a product designed to target the rodents that carry ticks- bait boxes and a product called "Damminix" can be used. Use these products in conjunction with liquid or granular insecticides.
LIQUID & GRANULAR PESTICIDES: Products meant for widespread application such as permethrin and its derivatives are preferred. They are available as a liquid concentrate and as granules. If liquid insecticides are used, application should be by fogging, not by coarse sprays. Apply these products in a strip a few feet wide at the perimeter of the lawn at any areas adjacent to woods and underbrush. Also treat any ornamental shrubs near the house that may serve as a habitat for small animals. The best time to apply these products is in late Spring and early Fall. In every case, professional application is recommended.

CLOTHING When wearing long pants, tuck the cuffs into the socks so any ticks that get on shoes or socks will crawl on the outside of the pants and be less likely to bite. Also, light colored clothing should be worn so the ticks will be easier to spot. Smooth materials such as windbreakers are harder for ticks to grab onto and are preferable to knits, etc.

Tick repellents that contain "permethrin" (Permanone, Permakill) are meant to be sprayed onto clothing. Spray the clothes before they're put on, and let them dry first. Do not apply this chemical directly to the skin.

Ticks are very intolerant of being dried out. After being outdoors in an infested area, place clothes in the dryer for a few minutes to kill any ticks that may still be present.

SKIN: Insect repellents that contain "DEET" are somewhat effective when applied to the arms, legs, and around the neck. Do not use any repellent over wide areas of the body as they can be absorbed causing toxicity. Also, it is inadvisable to use a product that contains more than 50% DEET, and 25% concentrations are preferred. Use repellents cautiously on small children, as they are more susceptible to their toxic effects. Be aware that this repellent evaporates quickly and must be reapplied frequently.

Check carefully for ticks not only when you get home but frequently while still outside!

HOW TO REMOVE AN ATTACHED TICK
Using a tweezer (not fingers!), grasp the tick as close to the skin as possible and pull straight out. Then apply an antiseptic. Do not try to irritate them with heat or chemicals, or grasp them by the body, as this may cause the tick to inject <u>more</u> germs into your skin. Tape the tick to a card and record the date and location of the bite. Remember, the sooner the tick is removed, the less likely an infection will result.

APPENDIX
RATIONALE FOR TREATING TICK BITES
Prophylactic antibiotic treatment upon a known tick bite is recommended for those who fit the following categories:
1. People at higher health risk bitten by an unknown type of tick or tick capable of transmitting Borrelia burgdorferi, e.g., pregnant women, babies and young children, people with serious health problems, and those who are immunodeficient.
2. Persons bitten in an area highly endemic for Lyme Borreliosis by an unidentified tick or tick capable of transmitting B. burgdorferi.
3. Persons bitten by a tick capable of transmitting B. burgdorferi, where the tick is engorged, or the attachment duration of the tick is greater than four hours, and/or the tick was improperly removed. This means when the body of the tick is squeezed upon removal, irritated with toxic chemicals in an effort to get it to back out, or disrupted in such a way that its contents were allowed to contact the bite wound. Such practices increase the risk of disease transmission.

4. A patient, when bitten by a known tick, clearly requests oral prophylaxis and understands the risks. This is a case-by-case decision.

The physician cannot rely on a laboratory test or clinical finding at the time of the bite to definitely rule in or rule out Lyme Disease infection, so must use clinical judgment as to whether to use antibiotic prophylaxis. Testing the tick itself for the presence of the spirochete, even with PCR technology, is helpful but not 100% reliable.

An established infection by B. burgdorferi can have serious, long-standing or permanent, and painful medical consequences, and be expensive to treat. Since the likelihood of harm arising from prophylactically applied anti-spirochetal antibiotics is low, and since treatment is inexpensive and painless, it follows that the risk-benefit ratio favors tick bite prophylaxis.

SUGGESTED ADDITIONAL READING

Evidence Based Guidelines for the Management of Lyme Disease. The International Lyme and Associated Diseases Society. Expert Rev. Anti-infect. Ther.2(1), Suppl. (2004)

Lyme Disease: Point/Counterpoint. Stricker, Raphael B. Lautin, Andrew. Burrascano, Joseph J. Expert Rev. Anti-infect. Ther, April 2005. 3(2), 155-165

An Understanding of Laboratory Testing for Lyme Disease. Harris, Nick S. J. Spiro. and Tick-Borne Dis. Vol 5, 1998. 16-26

Gestational Lyme Borreliosis. MacDonald, Alan B. Rheumatic Diseases Clinics of North America 15 (4), Nov. 1989. 657-678

Cerebral Malaria. Newton, Charles R.et al. J. Neurol. Neurosurg. Psychiatry. 2000. Vol 69, 433-441.

RESOURCES

International Lyme and Associated Diseases Society
www.ILADS.org
P.O. Box 341461
Bethesda, MD 20827-1461

Lyme Disease Association, Inc.
P.O. Box 1438, Jackson, NJ 08527
(888) 366-6611
www.lymediseaseassociation.org

APPENDIX B

Summary of IGeneX Australian Panels

Australian Tick Borne Disease Panel 1

Test Code	Test
188	Lyme IgM Western blot
189	Lyme IgG Western blot
200	Babesia microti IgG & IgM antibody
720	Babesia duncani IgG & IgM antibody
206	HGE (Anaplasma phagocytophila) IgG & IgM antibody
203	HME (Human monocytic ehrlichia) IgG & IgM antibody
285	Bartonella henselae IgG & IgM
965	Rickettesi rickettsi/typhi IgG antibody

Australian Tick Borne Disease Panel 2

Test Code	Test
188	Lyme IgM Western blot
189	Lyme IgG Western blot
200	Babesia microti IgG & IgM antibody
720	Babesia duncani IgG & IgM antibody
206	HGE (Anaplasma phagocytophila) IgG & IgM antibody
203	HME (Human monocytic ehrlichia) IgG & IgM antibody
285	Bartonella henselae IgG & IgM
965	Rickettesi rickettsi/typhi IgG antibody
453 & 456	Lyme Multiplex PCR - serum & whole blood

Australian Tick Borne Disease Panel 3

Test Code	Test
188	Lyme IgM Western blot
189	Lyme IgG Western blot
200	Babesia microti IgG & IgM antibody
720	Babesia duncani IgG & IgM antibody
206	HGE (Anaplasma phagocytophila) IgG & IgM antibody
203	HME (Human monocytic ehrlichia) IgG & IgM antibody
285	Bartonella henselae IgG & IgM
965	Rickettesi rickettsi/typhi IgG antibody
453 & 456	Lyme Multiplex PCR - serum & whole blood
640	Babesia FISH
289	Bartonella FISH

APPENDIX C

Healthy Fats to Take With Mepron and Malarone

Mepron and malarone are special cases as they absorb best when taken with fatty food. But before you rush out for a helping of French fries, think first of the healthy ways you can get those fats!

Research shows that 20-25 grams of fat is ideal; absorption studies have been done using 23 grams. Here are some amounts of fat contained in various foods.

Food	Amount	Fat
Eggs	1 medium	5 grams
Cashew/ almond butter	1 tablespoon	10 grams
Tahini (sesame butter)	1 tablespoon	8 grams
Avocado	1 medium	30 grams
Coconut oil	1 tablespoon	14 grams
Kefir	1 cup (250ml)	8.75 grams
Almonds (raw)	1/4 cup	11.5 grams
Chicken breast	single (1/2 breast)	3.2 grams
Sausage (pork)	1 link	7 grams
Sausage (chicken)	1 link	10 grams
Cheese (cheddar)	1 oz slice	9 grams

Fat content of fish and flax oil supplements

Omega-3 supplements are definitely healthy fats but in gelcap form will not meet the amount of fat required for the absorption of Mepron. Fatty acids in liquid form are better bets.

Fish oil (gelcaps)	1 gelcap	5 grams
Fish oil (liquid)	1 tablespoon	15 grams
Flax oil (Omega Swirl)	1 tablespoon	5 grams
Flax oil (liquid)	1 tablespoon	15 grams

So, here are some suggestions for what to eat along with each dose of Mepron –

2 1/2 tablespoons cashew or almond butter
1 ½ tablespoons coconut oil
1 ¼ tablespoons fish or flax oil
4 tablespoons Omega Swirl
2 ½ tablespoons tahini
½ cup almonds
3 large eggs

APPENDIX D

Summary of Medications and Common Dosages

Form of Borrelia	Medication Class	Commonly Used Examples
Spirochetes	Penicillins	Amoxicillin, Bicillin LA
	Cephalosporins	Cefuroxime, Ceftriaxone
Cell-wall deficient	Macrolides	Azithromycin, Clarithromycin
	Tetracyclines	Doxycycine, Minocycline
Cyst forms		Tinidazole, Metronidazole Hydroxychloroquine (Plaqunil), Alinia

The ultimate goal of therapy for Borrelia –

- ▶ 1 cell-wall active medication (for spirochetes)
- ▶ 2 intracellular medications (for cell-wall deficient forms)
- ▶ 1 cyst form medication (for cysts)

Plus medications added for relevant co-infections.

COMMON DOSAGES

Penicillins:

Amoxicillin	1000mg	3-6 daily
Augmentin XR	2000mg	2x daily
Bicillin LA	0.9 mill units	2 vials injected IM 3x weekly

Cephalosporins:

Cefuroxime	500mg	3x daily
Ceftriaxone	2 gram	2 gram twice daily IV 4 days/week

LYME DISEASE in Australia

Macrolides:

Azithromycin	500mg	1x daily
Clarithromycin	500mg	2x daily
Telithromycin	800mg	1x daily

Tetracyclines:

Minocycline	100mg	3-4x daily
Doxycycline	100mg	2 twice daily
Tetracycline	500mg	3-4x daily

Cyst-form medications:

Metronidazole	500mg	2x daily; 2 weeks on/ 2 weeks off
Tinidazole	500mg	2x daily; 2 weeks on/ 2 weeks off
Hydroxychloroquine	200mg	2x daily

Babesia medications:

Atovaquone (wellvone)	750mg/ 5mL	1-2 teaspoons twice daily
Malarone	250/ 100mg	2 twice daily
Mefloquine	250mg	1 every five days
Alinia	500mg	2x daily

Bartonella, Erlichia, Anaplasma, Rickettsia medications:

Rifampin	300mg	2x daily
Ciprofloxacin	500mg	1x daily
Bactrim DS	800/160mg	2x daily

APPENDIX E

Coping With Herx Reactions

A herx reaction is caused by neurotoxins released by microbes when they are being killed off. A Herx usually starts a few days into treatment - starting a new medication or supplement that is killing bugs. Herx reactions can last anywhere from a few hours to days or even weeks.

To minimize Herx reactions here are some things that can be helpful:

- Drink fresh squeezed lemon or lime juice in warm water, 2-3 times daily. Clean your teeth afterwards to protect tooth enamel as lemon and lime juice are acidic.
- Drink ionized, alkaline water – 2 litres per day.
- Eat a clean diet of lean proteins, healthy uncooked oils and vegetables. Juice greens if possible or drink wheatgrass juice.
- Take Epsom salts baths as the magnesium sulfate assists with detox. Magnesium is also relaxing for sore aching muscles.
- Alka-Seltzer Gold (must be gold, not regular) can be helpful.
- Try to rest and sleep as much as possible.
- Use far infrared sauna if possible, but only for short durations as tolerated.
- Do coffee enemas to help the liver and bowels flush out toxins.

Supplements to take or increase during a Herx:

- Dr Nicola's Smilax – this herbal tincture helps to neutralize neurotoxins. 1-2 droppersful twice daily in water.
- Dr Nicola's Detox Formula (#1 or #2) – herbs to assist the function of the liver and to cleanse the blood. 1-2 droppersful twice daily in water.
- TriFortify Liposomal Glutathione – 1 teaspoon in water once or twice daily.

- Dr Nicola's Nerve Pain Formula – for symptomatic relief of nerve pain such as burning and stabbing pain, and headache/ migraine.
- Activated Charcoal – 1-2 capsules twice daily 2 hours apart from other meds/ supplements. Acts as a binding agent in the gut to bind up the neurotoxins.
- Fibre blend containing soluble and insoluble fibre (such as Dr. Nicola's Fibre Plus) – to help bind and sweep out bowels to get toxins out.

APPENDIX F

Castor Oil Pack Instructions

Castor oil packs aid in elimination and detoxification processes in the body and have been used for a variety of conditions ranging from cholecystitis (inflammation of the gall bladder) to sluggish liver, poor elimination, headaches and toxaemia.

A castor oil pack is an external application of castor oil. A piece of wool flannel is saturated in castor oil and applied to the upper right quadrant of the abdomen (over the liver) with a heating pad. The purpose is to increase detoxification via the liver and lymphatic system, to reduce inflammation through cytokine modulation, and to improve the function of the colon. This can have a positive impact on systemic inflammation improving symptoms such as joint pain, headache, constipation and abdominal pain.

Castor oil packs should be used with caution or avoided if one has bleeding disorders and active ulcers or is pregnant. Individuals with chemical sensitivity disorders may have an increase in symptoms after using the castor oil pack, especially at the beginning of treatment, as it aids (and stimulates) the process of elimination and detoxification. Initially, it may be best to shorten the length of time of the castor oil pack treatment.

What You Will Need

- Flannel Cloth (cotton or wool, washed and dried, 20" to 40" x 24" to 48")
- Plastic wrap (clear kitchen plastic wrap or plastic bag without printing)
- Glass dish (Pyrex or similar dish large enough to warm the flannel castor oil pack prior to use)
- Old bath towel

- Hot water bottle or hot gel pack
- Castor oil
- Large zip-lock bag

Directions

1. Fold the washed and dried flannel cloth so that it is 2-3 layers thick and fits over most of your abdomen.
2. Soak the flannel cloth in castor oil. Strip or loosely wring out the excess oil. There will be excess oil for the first few applications. After that the castor oil pack should not drip excess oil.
3. Put the castor oil pack in a heat-safe glass dish and place in the oven or in the microwave to heat to a comfortable temperature.
4. Lie down in a comfortable position. You may want to place a plastic sheet or an old towel under you during the initial applications to avoid oil stains from getting on your bedding, upholstery or carpeting. Place the castor oil pack directly on your abdomen.
5. Cover the pack with a sheet of plastic, again to avoid staining.
6. Wrap an old towel around your abdomen to hold the castor oil pack in place and secure. Place a hot water bottle or gel pack over the towel. Wrap yourself in a warm blanket.
7. Leave the castor oil pack on for 45-60 minutes or overnight.
8. It is fine to fall asleep with the castor oil pack on, as long as you are not using an electrical heating source.
9. When you are done, store the pack in a large zip-lock bag in the refrigerator. The pack can be used repeatedly, adding more castor oil as needed. The castor oil pack can be used for several months.

APPENDIX G

Dry Skin Brushing Instructions

The skin is the largest organ of the body and is responsible for a significant amount of the body's elimination processes (approximately one quarter each day). The skin and the lungs are often forgotten when we discuss detoxification, with the liver and kidneys receiving most of the attention. Granted, most medications clear through the liver and/or kidneys, however the skin, with its porous structure and vast surface area, should not be forgotten.

Skin brushing is a technique that assists in clearing the lymphatic system, improving the surface circulation on the skin, keeping the pores open, encouraging the body's discharge of metabolic wastes, and boosting immune function. The lymphatic system is the waste management system of the body, transporting the waste products that have been filtered from the blood back to the large vessels for proper excretion. The lymph system often gets sluggish and backed up with wastes, so clearing it is important.

Benefits of skin brushing –

- Tightens skin
- Removes dead skin cells
- "Sweeps" the lymphatic fluid back towards the heart for proper elimination
- Encourages healthy cell renewal and exchange of wastes and nutrients between cells
- Strengthens the immune system
- Stimulates the glands, encouraging optimal function

The key to effective skin brushing is selecting the right brush. The brush should have natural fibres, not synthetic, as synthetic bristles will scratch the skin and create irritation. Natural fibres should feel soft on the skin.

At first the skin may feel a little itchy after brushing as the circulation is stimulated, but this will subside after the first few times. I like the boar hair brushes by Bass. They are available online or in many health food stores. Purchase one with a long handle so you can brush all parts of your body, even your back and legs.

The second key is brushing towards the heart. Imagine that your lymphatic system is carrying waste material towards the heart to dump into the large veins of the body. We are trying to assist by "sweeping" that material towards the heart, so always use strokes that go in one direction only, towards the heart. The only exception to this is around the chest area itself, where you can brush towards the armpits.

The third key is always brushing dry skin, before a shower is ideal as then you rinse away any dead skin cells that you have sloughed during brushing. Brushing wet skin will not have the same effect. Try to brush once or twice daily.

APPENDIX H

Summary of Biofilm Protocols

Biofilm protocols have five main goals:

1. Eat through the goo-like matrix using enzymes and thinning agents
2. Break the bonds between the goo using Ca-EDTA
3. Kill the now-exposed bugs using antimicrobials
4. Sweep the whole mess out using fibres and binders
5. Rebuild the gut lining with happy, healthy critters

Breaking Down the Biofilm Structure

Boulouke Lumbrokinase – this is a substance that acts as a fibrinolytic and anti-coagulant agent. In other words, it can thin out blood that is too thick and "sticky", and reduce the density of the biofilm. 1-2 capsules 30 minutes before meals, 3x daily.

InflaQuell – these are proteolytic enzymes that were discussed under the anti-inflammatory category. Because of their ability to break down proteins they are also useful in breaking down the biofilm matrix. 3 capsules twice daily on an empty stomach.

Breaking Bonds Between the Goo Structure

Ca-EDTA has classically been used as a heavy metal chelator with an affinity for lead. In the context of biofilm, it can be effective in complexing with the ions that hold the matrix together, thus reducing the ability of the matrix to hold together.

Killing the Bugs that are Now Exposed and Not Hiding/Stuck in the Goo

This can be antibiotics, natural antimicrobials, or a combination of both. Care must be taken as killing these newly exposed bugs can cause a Herx.

Sweeping Out the Residues
(both the polysaccharide matrix residues and the die-off products from the bugs themselves)

Toxi HMF (BioGenesis) is a good option for this as it contains apple pectin, sodium alginate and bentonite clay which all serve to bind and facilitate excretion. Psyllium husk and ground up flax seeds in a 1:4 ratio also accelerate this process. This mix can be blended into a smoothie or mixed with kefir. If a lot of endotoxins have been released, then cholestyramine may be a good option, but that can bind with many medications and supplements so care must be taken with timing.

Rebuilding the Gut Lining
Emphasis on probiotics such as Inner Health Plus and/or Prescript-Assist Pro to recolonize the gut with healthy flora. Sometimes intensive recolonization with high potency products such as RestorProbiotic Powder may be needed (these two contain upwards of 100 billion organisms per dose.

APPENDIX I

Sample Naturopathic Protocols

* RestorMedicine products

** Researched Nutritionals

More information and ordering at www.restormedicine.com.

Detoxification Support

Smilax*	40 drops twice daily
Detox Support Formula*	40 drops twice daily
Tri-Fortify Glutathione **	1 teaspoon in the morning in water
Dr. Nicola's Detox Plus Powder*	2 scoops daily

Immune Support

Transfer Factor Multi-Immune **	2 capsules before bed
Transfer Factor LymPlus **	2 capsules before bed

Digestive Support

RestorProbiotic Powder *	½ - 1 scoop before bed
(or) Inner Health Plus	2 capsules at night before bed
Dr. Nicola's Fibre Plus*	4 capsules at night
Anti-Parasite Formula *	40 drops three times daily
Anti-Fungal Formula *	40 drops three times daily

Pain and Inflammation

Soothe and Relaxx **	3 capsules twice daily
InflaQuell **	3 capsules twice daily between meals
Nerve Pain Formula *	40 drops three or four times daily

Mood and Sleep

Soothe and Relaxx **	3 capsules twice daily

Sleep Support Formula *	2 to 4 capsules before bed
200mg of Zen (ARG)	2 capsules twice daily
5-HTP	50mg 1 twice daily for mood; up to 4 before bed for sleep

Cognitive Function

Tri-Fortify Glutathione **	1 teaspoon in the morning in water
Cognicare **	2 twice daily

Adrenal Support (Energy)

Energy Multiplex **	3 capsules in the morning
Liquorice Plus (Metagenics)	2 tablets twice daily
Adreset (Metagenics)	1 capsule twice daily
DHEA Plus (Douglas Labs)	1 capsule daily in the morning

Mitochondrial Support (Energy)

ATP Fuel **	5 capsules twice daily
CoQ10 400mg **	1 capsule daily
Ribos-Cardio **	1 scoop daily

Antimicrobial

Teasel Root *	5 drops twice daily
Lyme Support Formula*	10 drops twice daily
Artemisinin SOD **	2 capsules twice daily
HH2 Formula (Zhang)	1 capsule three times daily

Biofilm

Boulouke Lumbrokinase **	1 capsule twice daily between meals
InflaQuell **	3 capsules twice daily between meals
Interfase Plus (Klaire Labs)	2 capsules twice daily between meals

Heavy Metal Chelation

Chelex (Xymogen)	4 capsules one or two times daily
DMSA 250mg (Thorne)	1 capsule three times daily, 3 days on/ 7 days off
EDTA 750mg	(compounded) 1 suppository every other night
Multiple Mineral (Klaire Labs)	2 capsules on non-DMSA/ non-EDTA days

BioMed Publishing Group
2013-2014 Product Catalog

Books & DVDs on
Lyme Disease
and Related Topics

"Empowering your ascent to health with educational resources recommended by patients and physicians worldwide."

www.LymeBook.com
Toll Free (866) 476-7637

For complete, detailed product information, please visit our website.

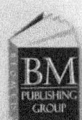

Order Online: www.LymeBook.com

The Top 10 Lyme Disease Treatments: Defeat Lyme Disease With The Best Of Conventional And Alternative Medicine

By Bryan Rosner
Foreword by James Schaller, M.D.

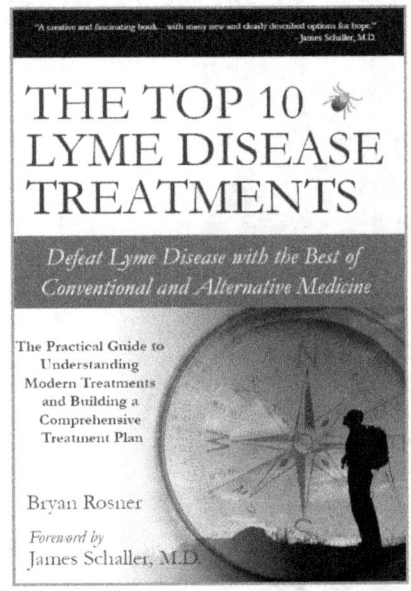

Book • $35

This information-packed book identifies ten promising conventional and alternative Lyme disease treatments and gives practical guidance on integrating them into a comprehensive treatment plan that you and your physician can customize for your individual situation and needs.

The book was not written to replace Bryan Rosner's first book (*Lyme Disease and Rife Machines*, opposing page). It was written to complement that book, offering Lyme sufferers many new foundational and supportive treatment options, based on the author's extensive research and years of personal experience. Topics include*:

- Systemic enzyme therapy, which helps detoxify tissues and blood, reduce inflammation, stimulate the immune system, and kill Lyme disease bacteria.
- Lithium orotate, a powerful yet all-natural mineral (belonging to the same mineral group as sodium and potassium) capable of profound neuroprotective activity.
- Thorough and extensive coverage of a complete Lyme disease detoxification program, including discussion of both liver and skin detoxification pathways. Specific detoxification therapies such as liver cleanses, bowel cleanses, the Shoemaker Neurotoxin Elimination Protocol, sauna therapy, mineral baths, mineral supplementation, milk thistle, and many others. Ideas to reduce and control herx reactions.
- Tips and clinical research from James Schaller, M.D.
- A detailed look at one method for utilizing antibiotics during a rife machine treatment campaign.
- Wide coverage of the Marshall Protocol, including an in-depth discussion of its mechanism of action in relation to Lyme disease pathology. Also, the author's personal experience with the Marshall Protocol over 3 years.
- An explanation of and new information about the Salt / Vitamin C protocol.
- Hot-off-the-press information on mangosteen fruit (not to be confused with mango) and its many benefits, including antibacterial, anti-inflammatory, and anti-cancer properties.
- New guidelines for combining all the therapies discussed in both of Rosner's books into a complete treatment plan. Brief and articulate for consideration by you and your doctor.
- Also includes updates on rife therapy, cutting-edge supplements, political challenges, an exclusive interview with Willy Burgdorfer, Ph.D. (discoverer of Lyme), and much more!

"Bryan Rosner thinks big and this new book offers big solutions."
- James Schaller, M.D.

"Another ground-breaking Lyme Disease book."
- Jeff Mittelman, moderator of the Lyme-and-rife group

"Brilliant and thorough."
- Nenah Sylver, Ph.D.

Do not miss this top Lyme disease resource. Discover new healing tools today! Bring this book to your doctor's appointment to help with forming a treatment plan.

Paperback book, 7 x 10", 367 pages, $35

Order by Phone: (866) 476-7637

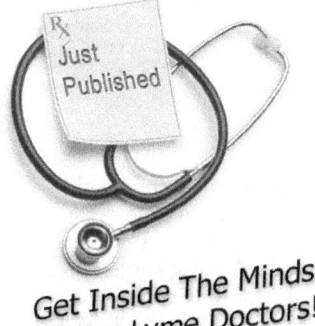

Get Inside The Minds Of Top Lyme Doctors!

13 Lyme Doctors Share Treatment Strategies!

In this new book, not one, but thirteen Lyme-literate healthcare practitioners describe the tools they use in their practices to heal patients from chronic Lyme disease. Never before available in book format!

Insights Into Lyme Disease Treatment: 13 Lyme Literate Health Care Practitioners Share Their Healing Strategies

By Connie Strasheim
Foreword by Maureen Mcshane, M.D.

If you traveled the country for appointments with 13 Lyme-literate health care practitioners, you would discover many cutting-edge therapies used to combat chronic Lyme disease. You would also spend thousands of dollars on hotels, plane tickets, and medical appointment fees—not to mention the time it would take to embark on such a journey.

Even if you had the time and money to travel, would the physicians have enough time to answer all of your questions? Would you even know which questions to ask?

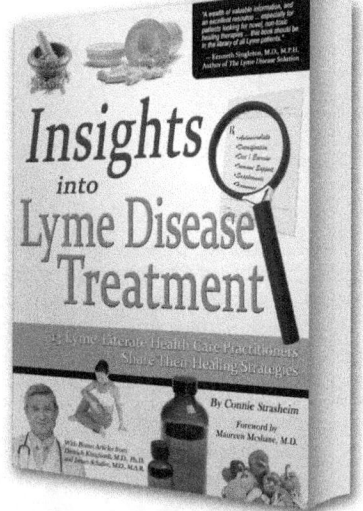

Paperback • 443 Pages • $39.95

In this long-awaited book, health care journalist and Lyme patient Connie Strasheim has done all the work for you. She conducted intensive interviews with 13 of the world's most competent Lyme disease healers, asking them thoughtful, important questions, and then spent months compiling their information into 13 organized, user-friendly chapters that contain the core principles upon which they base their medical treatment of chronic Lyme disease. The practitioners' backgrounds span a variety of disciplines, including allopathic, naturopathic, complementary, chiropractic, homeopathic, and energy medicine. All aspects of treatment are covered, from anti-microbial remedies and immune system support, to hormonal restoration, detoxification, and dietary/lifestyle choices. **PHYSICIANS INTERVIEWED:**

- Steven Bock, M.D.
- Ginger Savely, DNP
- Ronald Whitmont, M.D.
- Nicola McFadzean, N.D.
- Jeffrey Morrison, M.D.
- Steven J. Harris, M.D.
- Peter J. Muran, M.D., M.B.A.

- Ingo D. E. Woitzel, M.D.
- Susan L. Marra, M.S., N.D.
- W. Lee Cowden, M.D., M.D. (H)
- Deborah Metzger, Ph.D., M.D.
- Marlene Kunold, "Heilpraktiker"
- Elizabeth Hesse-Sheehan, DC, CCN
- Visit our website to read a FREE CHAPTER!

Paperback book, 7 x 10", 443 pages, $39.95

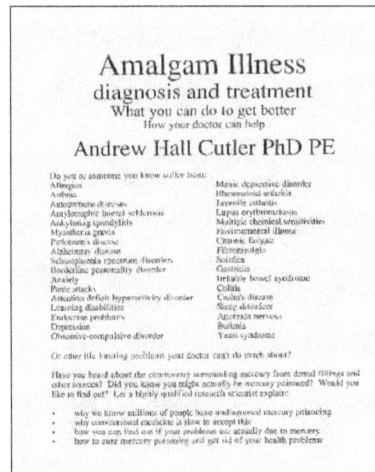

Book • $35

Amalgam Illness, Diagnosis and Treatment: What You Can Do to Get Better, How Your Doctor Can Help

By Andrew Cutler, PhD

This book was written by a chemical engineer who himself got mercury poisoning from his amalgam dental fillings. He found that there was no suitable educational material for either the patient or the physician. Knowing how much people can suffer from this condition, he wrote this book to help them get well. With a PhD in chemistry from Princeton University and extensive study in biochemistry and medicine, Andrew Cutler uses layman's terms to explain how people become mercury poisoned and what to do about it. The author's research shows that mercury poisoning can easily be cured at home with over-the-counter oral chelators – this book explains how.

In the book you will find practical guidance on how to tell if you really have chronic mercury poisoning or some other problem. Proper diagnostic procedures are provided so that sick people can decide what is wrong rather than trying random treatments. If mercury poisoning is your problem, the book tells you how to get the mercury out of your body, and how to feel good while you do that. The treatment section gives step-by-step directions to figure out exactly what mercury is doing to you and how to fix it.

> "Dr. Cutler uses his background in chemistry to explain the safest approach to treat mercury poisoning. I am a physician and am personally using his protocol on myself."
>
> - Melissa Myers, M.D.

Sections also explain how the scientific literature shows many people must be getting poisoned by their amalgam fillings, why such a regulatory blunder occurred, and how the debate between "mainstream" and "alternative" medicine makes it more difficult for you to get the medical help you need.

This down-to-earth book lets patients take care of themselves. It also lets doctors who are not familiar with chronic mercury intoxication treat it. The book is a practical guide to getting well. Sections from the book include:

- Why worry about mercury poisoning?
- What mercury does to you – symptoms, laboratory test irregularities, diagnostic checklist.
- How to treat mercury poisoning easily with oral chelators.
- Dealing with other metals including copper, arsenic, lead, cadmium.
- Dietary and supplement guidelines.
- Balancing hormones during the recovery process.
- How to feel good while you are chelating the metals out.
- How heavy metals cause infections to thrive in the body.
- Politics and mercury.

This is the world's most authoritative, accurate book on mercury poisoning.

Paperback book, 8.5 x 11", 226 pages, $35

Order by Phone: (866) 476-7637

Hair Test Interpretation: Finding Hidden Toxicities

By Andrew Cutler, PhD

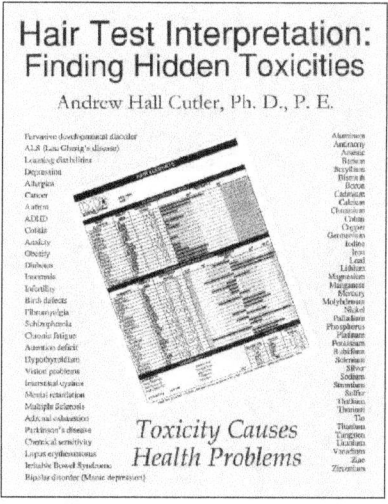

Book • $35

Hair tests are worth doing because a surprising number of people diagnosed with incurable chronic health conditions actually turn out to have a heavy metal problem; quite often, mercury poisoning. Heavy metal problems can be corrected. Hair testing allows the underlying problem to be identified – and the chronic health condition often disappears with proper detoxification.

Hair Test Interpretation: Finding Hidden Toxicities is a practical book that explains how to interpret **Doctor's Data, Inc.** and **Great Plains Laboratory** hair tests. A step-by-step discussion is provided, with figures to illustrate the process and make it easy. The book gives examples using actual hair test results from real people.

One of the problems with hair testing is that both conventional and alternative health care providers do not know how to interpret these tests. Interpretation is not as simple as looking at the results and assuming that any mineral out of the reference range is a problem mineral.

Interpretation is complicated because heavy metal toxicity, especially mercury poisoning, interferes with mineral transport throughout the body. Ironically, if someone is mercury poisoned, hair test mercury is often low and other minerals may be elevated or take on unusual values. For example, mercury often causes retention of arsenic, antimony, tin, titanium, zirconium, and aluminum. An inexperienced health care provider may wrongfully assume that one of these other minerals is the culprit, when in reality mercury is the true toxicity.

"This new book of Andrew's is the definitive guide in the confusing world of heavy metal poisoning diagnosis and treatment. I'm a practicing physician, 20 years now, specializing in detoxification programs for treatment of resistant conditions. It was fairly difficult to diagnose these heavy metal conditions before I met Andrew Cutler and developed a close relationship with him while reading his books. In this book I found his usual painful attention to detail gave a solid framework for understanding the complexity of mercury toxicity as well as the less common exposures. You really couldn't ask for a better reference book on a subject most researchers and physicians are still fumbling in the dark about."
- Dr. Rick Marschall

So, as you can see, getting a hair test is only the first step. The second step is figuring out what the hair test means. Andrew Cutler, PhD, is a registered professional chemical engineer with years of experience in biochemical and healthcare research. This clear and concise book makes hair test interpretation easy, so that you know which toxicities are causing your health problems.

Paperback book, 8.5 x 11", 298 pages, $35

Order Online: www.LymeBook.com

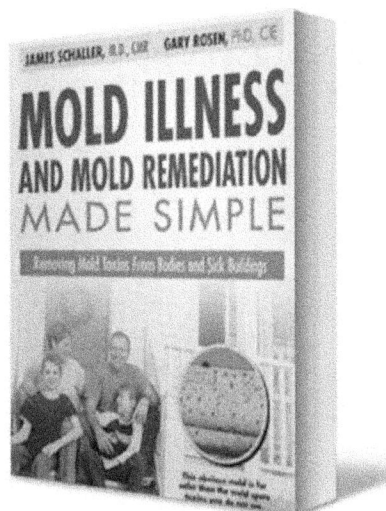

Book • $32.95

Mold Illness and Mold Remediation Made Simple: Removing Mold Toxins from Bodies and Sick Buildings

By James Schaller, M.D. and Gary Rosen, Ph.D.

Indoor mold toxins are much more dangerous and prevalent than most people realize. Visible mold in and around your house is far less dangerous than the mold you cannot see. Indoor mold toxicity, in addition to causing its own unique set of health problems and symptoms, also greatly contributes to the severity of most chronic illnesses.

In this book, a top physician and experienced contractor team up to help you quickly recover from indoor mold exposure. This book is easy to read with many color photographs and illustrations.

Dr. Schaller is a practicing physician in Florida who has written more than 15 books. He is one of the few physicians in the United States successfully treating mold toxin illness in children and adults.

Dr. Rosen is a biochemist with training under a Nobel Prize winning researcher at UCLA. He has written several books and is an expert in the mold remediation of homes. Dr. Rosen and his family are sensitive to mold toxins so he writes not only from professional experience, but also from personal experience.

Together, the two authors have certification in mold testing, mold remediation, and indoor environmental health. This book is one of the most complete on the subject, and includes discussion of the following topics:

- Potential mold problems encountered in new homes, schools, and jobs.
- Diagnosing mold illness.
- Mold as it relates to dryness and humidity.
- Mold toxins and cancer treatment.
- Mold toxins and relationships.
- Crawlspaces, basements, attics, home cleaning techniques, and vacuums.
- Training your eyes to discern indoor mold.
- Leptin and obesity.
- Appropriate/inappropriate air filters and cleaners.
- How to handle old, musty products, materials and books, and how to safely sterilize them.
- A description of various types of molds, images of them, and their relative toxicity.
- Blood testing and how to use it to find hidden health problems.
- The book is written in a friendly, casual tone that allows easy comprehension and information retention.

> "A concise, practical guide on dealing with mold toxins and their effects."
>
> - Bryan Rosner

Many people are affected by mold toxins. Are you? If you can find a smarter or clearer book on this subject, buy it!

Paperback book, 8.5 x 11", 140 pages, $32.95
Also available on our website as an eBook!

Order by Phone: (866) 476-7637

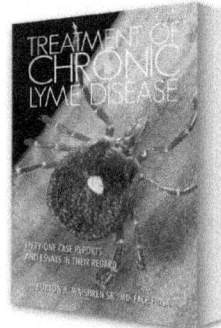

Book • $24.95

Treatment of Chronic Lyme Disease: 51 Case Reports and Essays In Their Regard
By Burton Waisbren Sr., MD, FACP, FIDSA

DON'T MISS THIS BOOK! A MUST-HAVE RESOURCE. What sets this Lyme disease book apart are the credentials of its author: he is not only a Fellow of the Infectious Diseases Society of America (IDSA), he is also one of its Founders! With 57+ years experience in medicine, Dr. Waisbren passionately argues for the validity of chronic Lyme disease and presents useful information about 51 cases of the disease which he has personally treated. His position is in stark contrast to that of the IDSA, which is a very powerful organization. **Quite possibly the most important book ever published on Lyme disease, as a result of the author's experience and credentials.**

Paperback book, 6x9", 169 pages, $24.95

Bartonella: Diagnosis and Treatment
By James Schaller, M.D.

2 Book Set • $99.95

As an addition to his growing collection of informative books, Dr. James Schaller penned this excellent 2-part volume on Bartonella, a Lyme disease co-infection. The set is an ideal complementary resource to his Babesia textbook (next page).

Bartonella infections occur throughout the entire world, in cities, suburbs, and rural locations. It is found in fleas, dust mites, ticks, lice, flies, cat and dog saliva, and insect feces.

This 2-book set provides advanced treatment strategies as well as detailed diagnostic criteria, with dozens of full-color illustrations and photographs.

Both books in this 2-part set are included with your order.

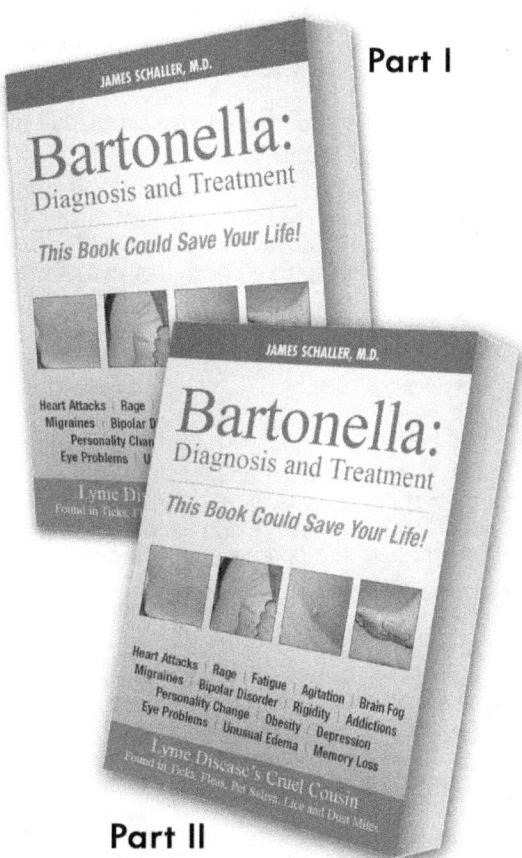

Part I

Part II

2 paperback books included, 7 x 10", 500 pages, $99.95

351

The Diagnosis and Treatment of Babesia: Lyme's Cruel Cousin – The Other Tick-Borne Infection

By James Schaller, M.D.

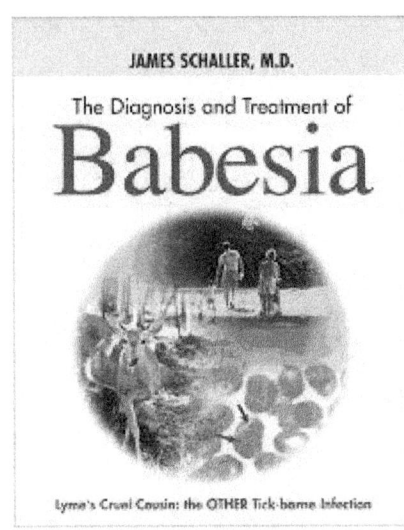

Book • $55

Do you or a loved one experience excess fatigue? Have you ever had unusually high fevers, chills, or sweats? You may have Babesia, a very common tick-borne infection. Babesia is often found with Lyme disease and, like all tick-borne infections, is rarely diagnosed and reported accurately.

The deer tick which carries Lyme disease and Babesia may be as small as a poppy seed and injects a painkiller, an antihistamine, and an anticoagulant to avoid detection. As a result, many people have Babesia and do not know it. Numerous forms of Babesia are carried by ticks. This book introduces patients and health care workers to the various species that infect humans and are not routinely tested for by sincere physicians.

Dr. Schaller, who practices medicine in Florida, first became interested in Babesia after one of his own children was infected with it. None of the elite pediatricians or child specialists could help. No one tested for Babesia or considered it a possible diagnosis. His child suffered from just two of these typical Babesia symptoms:

- Significant Fatigue
- Coughing
- Dizziness
- Trouble Thinking
- Fevers
- Memory Loss

- Chills
- Air Hunger
- Headache
- Sweats
- Unresponsiveness to Lyme Treatment

With 374 pages, this book is the most current and comprehensive book on Babesia in the English language. It reviews thousands of articles and presents the results of interviews with world experts on the subject. It offers you top information and broad treatment options, presented in a clear and simple manner. All treatments are explained thoroughly, including their possible side effects, drug interactions, various dosing strategies, pros/cons, and physician experiences.

"Once again Dr. Schaller has provided us with a much-needed and practical resource. This book gave me exactly what I was looking for."

- Thomas W., Patient

Finally, the book also addresses many other aspects of practical medical care often overlooked in this infection, such as treatment options for managing fatigue. Plainly stated, this book is a must-have for patients and health care providers who deal with Lyme disease and its co-infections. Dr. Schaller's many years in clinical practice give the book a practical angle that many other similar books lack. Don't miss this user-friendly resource!

Paperback book, 7 x 10", 374 pages, $55
Also available on our website as an eBook!

Order by Phone: (866) 476-7637

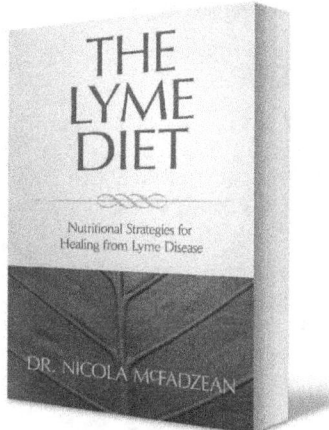

Book • $24.95

The Lyme Diet: Nutritional Strategies for Healing from Lyme Disease

By Nicola McFadzean, N.D.

We know about antibiotics and herbs. But what is the right diet for Lyme sufferers? Now you can read about the experience of Dr. Nicola McFadzean, N.D., in treating Lyme patients using proper diet.

The author is a Naturopathic Doctor and graduate of Bastyr University in Seattle, Washington. She is currently in private practice at her clinic, RestorMedicine, located in San Diego, California.

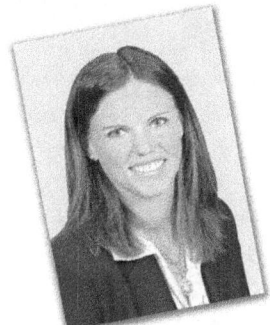

Nicola McFadzean, N.D.

This book covers numerous topics (not just diet-related):

- Reducing and controlling inflammation
- Maximizing immune function via dietary choices
- Restoring the gut & regaining healthy digestion
- Detoxification with food
- Hormone imbalances
- Biofilms
- Kefir vs. yogurt vs. probiotics
- Candida, liver support, and much more!

Paperback book, 6x9", 214 Pages, $24.95
Also available as an eBook on our website!

The Stealth Killer: Is Oral Spirochetosis the Missing Link in the Dental & Heart Disease Labyrinth? By William D. Nordquist, BS, DMD, MS

Can oral spirochete infections cause heart attacks? In today's cosmopolitan urban population, more than 51 percent of those with root canal–treated teeth probably have infection at the apex of their root. Dr. Nordquist, an oral surgeon practicing in Southern California, believes that any source of bacteria with resulting chronic infection (including periodontal disease) in the mouth may potentially lead to heart disease and other systemic diseases. With more than 40 illustrations and x-ray reproductions, this book takes you behind the scenes in Dr. Nordquist's research laboratory, and provides many tips on dealing with Lyme-related dental problems. A breakthrough book in dentistry & infectious disease!

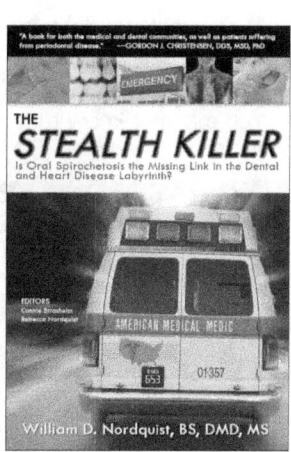

Paperback Book • $25.95

Paperback book, 6x9", 161 pages, $25.95

Sauna Therapy for Detoxification and Healing

By Lawrence Wilson, MD

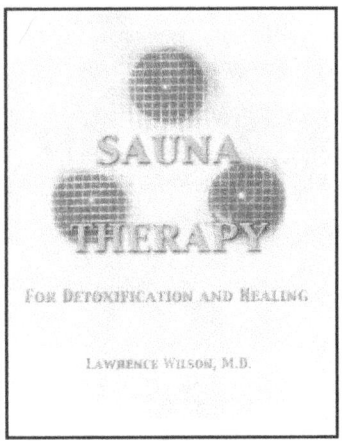

Book • $22.95

This book provides a thorough yet articulate education on sauna therapy. It includes construction plans for a low-cost electric light sauna. The book is well referenced with an extensive bibliography.

Sauna therapy, especially with an electric light sauna, is one of the most powerful, safe and cost-effective methods of natural healing. It is especially important today due to extensive exposure to toxic metals and chemicals.

Fifteen chapters cover sauna benefits, physiological effects, protocols, cautions, healing reactions, and many other aspects of sauna therapy.

Dr. Wilson is an instructor of Biochemistry, Hair Mineral Analysis, Sauna Therapy and Jurisprudence at various colleges and universities including Yamuni Institute of the Healing Arts (Maurice, LA), University of Natural Medicine (Santa Fe, NM), Natural Healers Academy (Morristown, NJ), and Westbrook University (West Virginia). His books are used as textbooks at East-West School of Herbology and Ohio College of Natural Health. Go to www.LymeBook.com for free book excerpts!.

Paperback book, 8.5 x 11", 167 pages, $22.95

Physicians' Desk Reference (PDR) Books (opposing page)

Most people have heard of *Physicians' Desk Reference* (PDR) books because, for over 60 years, physicians and researchers have turned to PDR for the latest word on prescription drugs.

You may not know that Thomson Healthcare, publisher of PDR, offers PDR reference books not only for drugs, but also for herbal and nutritional supplements. No available books come even close to the amount of information provided in these PDRs—*PDR for Herbal Medicines* weighs 5 lbs and has over 1300 pages, and *PDR for Nutritional Supplements* weighs over 3 lbs and has more than 800 pages.

> "I relied heavily on the PDRs during the research phase of writing my books. Without them, my projects would have greatly suffered."
> - Bryan Rosner

We carry all three PDRs. Although PDR books are typically used by physicians, we feel that these resources are also essential for people interested in or recovering from chronic disease. For the supplements, herbs, and drugs included in the books, you will find the following information: Pharmacology, description and method of action, available trade names and brands, indications and usage, research summaries, dosage options, history of use, pharmacokinetics, and much more! Worth the money for years of faithful use.

Order by Phone: (866) 476-7637

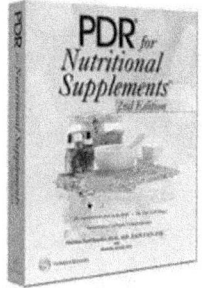

PDR for Nutritional Supplements 2nd Edition!

This PDR focuses on the following types of supplements:

- Vitamins
- Minerals
- Amino acids
- Hormones
- Lipids
- Glyconutrients
- Probiotics
- Proteins
- Many more!

Book • $69.50

> "In a part of the health field not known for its devotion to rigorous science, [this book] brings to the practitioner and the curious patient a wealth of hard facts."
>
> - Roger Guillemin, M.D., Ph.D., Nobel Laureate in Physiology and Medicine

The book also suggests supplements that can help reduce prescription drug side effects, has full-color photographs of various popular commercial formulations (and contact information for the associated suppliers), and so much more! Become educated instead of guessing which supplements to take.

Hardcover book, 11 x 9.3", 800 pages, $69.50

PDR for Herbal Medicines 4th Edition!

PDR for Herbal Medicines is very well organized and presents information on hundreds of common and uncommon herbs and herbal preparations. Indications and usage are examined with regard to homeopathy, Indian and Chinese medicine, and unproven (yet popular) applications.

In an area of healthcare so unstudied and vulnerable to hearsay and hype, this scientifically referenced book allows you to find out the real story behind the herbs lining the walls of your local health food store.

Use this reference before spending money on herbal products!

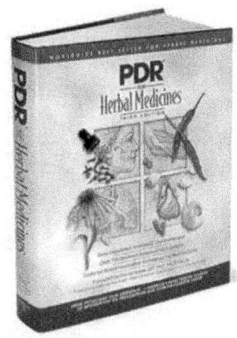

Book • $69.50

Hardcover book, 11 x 9.3", 1300 pages, $69.50

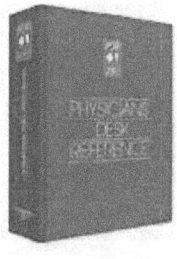

PDR for Prescription Drugs Current Year's Edition!

With more than 3,000 pages, this is the most comprehensive and respected book in the world on over 4,000 drugs. Drugs are indexed by both brand and generic name (in the same convenient index) and also by manufacturer and product category. This PDR provides usage information and warnings, drug interactions, plus a detailed, full-color directory with descriptions and cross references for the drugs. A new format allows dramatically improved readability and easier access to the information you need now.

Book • $99.50

Hardcover book, 12.5 x 9.5", 3533 pages, $99.50

Order Online: www.LymeBook.com

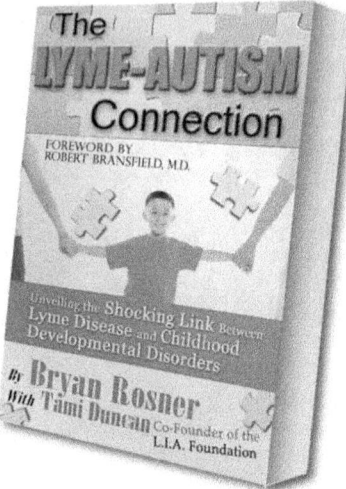

Book • $25.95

The Lyme-Autism Connection: Unveiling the Shocking Link Between Lyme Disease and Childhood Developmental Disorders
By Bryan Rosner & Tami Duncan

Did you know that Lyme disease may contribute to the onset of autism?

This book is an investigative report written by Bryan Rosner and Tami Duncan. Duncan is the co-founder of the *Lyme Induced Autism (LIA) Foundation*, and her son has an autism diagnosis.

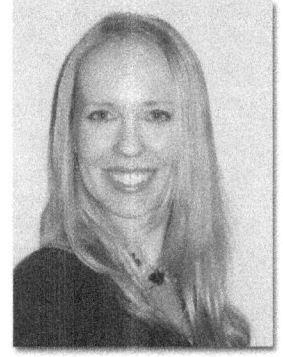

Tami Duncan, Co-Founder of the Lyme Induced Autism (LIA) Foundation

Awareness of the Lyme-autism connection is spreading rapidly, among both parents and practitioners. *Medical Hypothesis*, a scientific, peer-reviewed journal published by Elsevier, recently released an influential study entitled *The Association Between Tick-Borne Infections, Lyme Borreliosis and Autism Spectrum Disorders*. Here is an excerpt from the study:

> "Chronic infectious diseases, including tick-borne infections such as Borrelia burgdorferi, may have direct effects, promote other infections, and create a weakened, sensitized and immunologically vulnerable state during fetal development and infancy, leading to increased vulnerability for developing autism spectrum disorders. An association between Lyme disease and other tick-borne infections and autistic symptoms has been noted by numerous clinicians and parents."

—Medical Hypothesis Journal.
Article Authors: Robert C. Bransfield, M.D., Jeffrey S. Wulfman, M.D., William T. Harvey, M.D., Anju I. Usman, M.D.

Nationwide, 1 out of 150 children are diagnosed with Autism Spectrum Disorder (ASD), and the LIA Foundation has discovered that many of these children test positive for Lyme disease/Borrelia related complex—yet most children in this scenario never receive appropriate medical attention. This book answers many difficult questions: How can infants contract Lyme disease if autism begins before birth, precluding the opportunity for a tick bite? Is there a statistical correlation between the incidences of Lyme disease and autism worldwide? Do autistic children respond to Lyme disease treatment? What does the medical community say about this connection? Do the mothers of affected children exhibit symptoms? **Find out in this book.**

Paperback book, 6x9", 287 pages, $25.95

Order by Phone: (866) 476-7637

**Dietrich Klinghardt, M.D., Ph.D.
"Fundamental Teachings"
5-DVD Set**

Includes Disc Exclusively For Lyme Disease!

Dietrich Klinghardt, M.D., Ph.D. is a legendary healer known for discovering and refining many of the cutting-edge treatment protocols used for a variety of chronic health problems including Lyme disease, autism and mercury poisoning.

Now you can find out all about this doctor's treatment methods from the privacy of your own home! This 5-DVD set includes the following DVDs:

- **DISC 1**: The Five Levels of Healing and the Seven Factors
- **DISC 2**: Autonomic Response Testing and Demonstration
- **DISC 3**: Heavy Metal Toxicity and Neurotoxin Elimination / Electrosmog
- **DISC 4**: Lyme disease and Chronic Illness
- **DISC 5**: Psycho-Emotional Issues in Chronic Illness & Addressing Underlying Causes

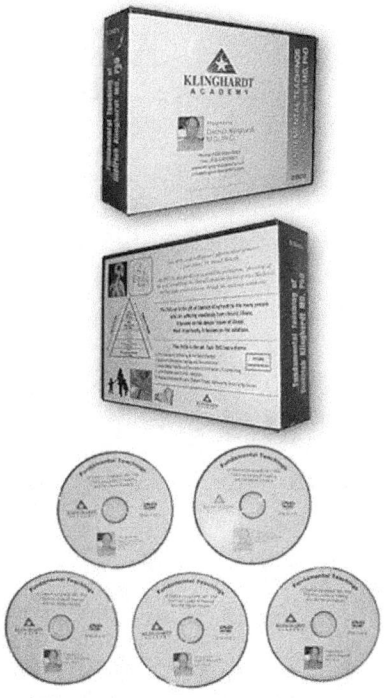

5-DVD Set • $125

Dr. Dietrich Klinghardt is one of the most important contributors to modern integrative treatment for Lyme disease and related medical conditions. This comprehensive DVD set is a must-have addition to your educational library.

5-DVD Set, $125

Our catalog has space limitations, but our website does not! Visit www.LymeBook.com to see even more exciting products.

Don't Miss These New Books & DVDs, Available Online:
- Babesia Update 2009, by James Schaller, M.D.
- Marshall Protocol 5-DVD Set
- Cure Unknown, by Pamela Weintraub
- The Experts of Lyme Disease, by Sue Vogan
- The Lyme Disease Solution, by Ken Singleton, M.D.
- **Lots of Free Chapters and Excerpts Online!**

Don't use the internet? No problem, just call (530) 573-0190.

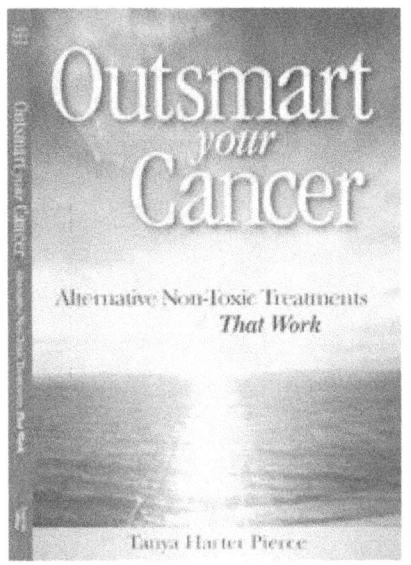

Book and Audio CD • $24.50

Outsmart Your Cancer: Alternative Non-Toxic Treatments That Work   By Tanya Harter Pierce

Why BLUDGEON cancer to death with common conventional treatments that can be toxic and harmful to your entire body?

When you OUTSMART your cancer, only the cancer cells die — NOT your healthy cells! *OUTSMART YOUR CANCER: Alternative Non-Toxic Treatments That Work* is an easy guide to successful non-toxic treatments for cancer that you can obtain right now! In it, you will read real-life stories of people who have completely recovered from their advanced or late-stage lung cancer, breast cancer, prostate cancer, kidney cancer, brain cancer, childhood leukemia, and other types of cancer using effective non-toxic approaches.

Plus, *OUTSMART YOUR CANCER* is one of the few books in print today that gives a complete description of the amazing formula called "Protocel," which has produced incredible cancer recoveries over the past 20 years. **A supporting audio CD is included with this book.** Pricing = $19.95 book + $5.00 CD.

Paperback book, 6 x 9", 437 pages, with audio CD, $24.95

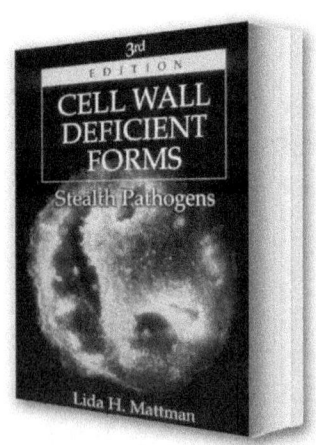

Hardcover Book • $169.95

Cell Wall Deficient Forms: Stealth Pathogens

By Lida Mattman, Ph.D.

This is one of the most influential infectious disease textbook of the century. Dr. Mattman, who earned a Ph.D. in immunology from Yale University, describes her discovery that a certain type of pathogen lacking a cell wall is the root cause of many of today's "incurable" and mysterious chronic diseases. Dr. Mattman's research is the foundation of our current understanding of Lyme disease, and her work led to many of the Lyme protocols used today (such as the Marshall Protocol, as well as modern LLMD antibiotic treatment strategy). Color illustrations and meticulously referenced breakthrough principles cover the pages of this book. A must have for all serious students of chronic, elusive infectious disease.

Hardcover book, 7.5 x 10.5", 416 pages, $169.95

Order by Phone: (866) 476-7637

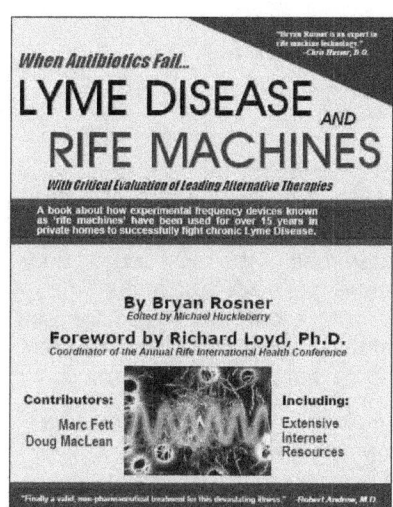

Book • $35

When Antibiotics Fail: Lyme Disease And Rife Machines, With Critical Evaluation Of Leading Alternative Therapies

By Bryan Rosner
Foreword by Richard Loyd, Ph.D.

There are enough books and websites about what Lyme disease is and which ticks carry it. But there is very little useful information for people who actually have a case of Lyme disease that is not responding to conventional antibiotic treatment. Lyme disease sufferers need to know their options, not how to identify a tick.

This book describes how experimental electromagnetic frequency devices known as rife machines have been used for over 15 years in private homes to fight Lyme disease. Also included are evaluations of more than 25 conventional and alternative Lyme disease therapies, including:

- Homeopathy
- IV and oral antibiotics
- Mercury detox.
- Hyperthermia / saunas
- Ozone and oxygen
- Samento®
- Colloidal Silver
- Bacterial die-off detox.
- Colostrum
- Magnesium supplementation
- Hyperbaric oxygen chamber (HBOC)
- ICHT Italian treatment
- Non-pharmaceutical antibiotics
- Exercise, diet and candida protocols
- Cyst-targeting antibiotics
- The Marshall Protocol®

Many Lyme disease sufferers have heard of rife machines, some have used them. But until now, there has not been a concise and organized source to explain how and why they have been used by Lyme patients. In fact, this is the first book ever published on this important topic.

The Foreword for the book is by Richard Loyd, Ph.D., coordinator of the annual Rife International Health Conference. The book takes a practical, down-to-earth approach which allows you to learn about*:

"This book provides life-saving insights for Lyme disease patients."

- Richard Loyd, Ph.D.

- Antibiotic treatment problems and shortcomings—why some people choose to use rife machines after other therapies fail.
- Hypothetical treatment schedules and sessions, based on the author's experience.
- The experimental machines with the longest track record: High Power Magnetic Pulser, EMEM Machine, Coil Machine, and AC Contact Machine.
- Explanation of the "herx reaction" and why it may indicate progress.
- The intriguing story that led to the use of rife machines to fight Lyme disease 20 years ago.
- Antibiotic categories and classifications, with pros and cons of each type of drug.
- Visit our website to read FREE EXCERPTS from the book!

__Disclaimer:__ Your treatment decisions must be made under the care of a licensed physician. Rife machines are not FDA approved and the FDA has not reviewed or approved of these books. The author is a layperson, not a doctor, and much of the content of these books is a statement of opinion based on the author's personal experience and research.

Paperback book, 8.5 x 11", 203 pages, $35

Order Online: www.LymeBook.com

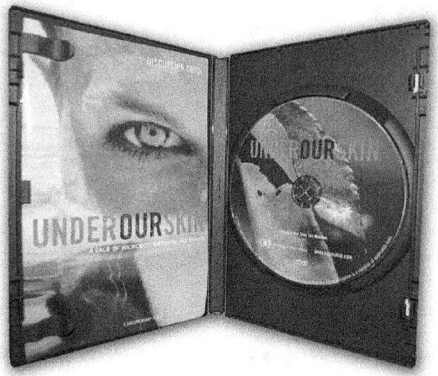

DVD • $34.95

**Under Our Skin:
Lyme Disease Documentary Film**

A gripping tale of microbes, medicine & money, UNDER OUR SKIN exposes the hidden story of Lyme disease, one of the most serious and controversial epidemics of our time. Each year, thousands go undiagnosed or misdiagnosed, often told that their symptoms are all in their head.

Following the stories of patients and physicians fighting for their lives and livelihoods, the film brings into focus a haunting picture of the health care system and a medical establishment all too willing to put profits ahead of patients.

Bonus Features: 32-page discussion guidebook, one hour of bonus footage, director's commentary, and much more! **FOR HOME USE ONLY**

DVD with bonus features, 104 minutes, $34.95 *MUST SEE!*

Ordering is Easy!

Phone: Toll Free (866) 476-7637
Online: www.LymeBook.com

Detailed product information and secure online ordering is available on our website. Bulk orders to bookstores, health food stores, or Lyme disease support groups – call us for wholesale terms.

Do you have a book inside you? Submit your book proposal online at: www.lymebook.com/submit-book-proposal.

Join Lyme Community Forums at: www.lymecommunity.com.

Get paid to help us place our books in your local health food store. Learn more: www.lymebook.com/local-store-offer.

DISCLAIMER

This disclaimer is in reference to all books, DVDs, websites, flyers, and catalogs published by Bryan Rosner, DBA BioMed Publishing Group.

Our materials are for informational and educational purposes only. They are not intended to prevent, diagnose, treat, or cure disease. Some of the treatments described are not FDA-Approved. Bryan Rosner is a layperson, not a medical professional, and he is not qualified to dispense medical advice.

These books and DVDs are not intended to substitute for professional medical care. Do not postpone receiving care from a licensed physician. Please read our full disclaimer online at: www.lymebook.com/homepage-disclaimer.pdf.

INDEX

5-HTP 199-200, 207, 342
5-methyl-tetrahydrafolate 176

A

Abdominal pain 106, 189, 313, 335
Acetazolamide 295
Acetyl carnitine 317
Aches 27, 104, 177, 259, 261, 263
    dull 258
    muscles 108, 197, 231, 241, 333
    weakness 317
Achilles tendon 157
Acidity 148, 186, 219, 303, 333
Acidophilus 175, 322
Acids 186, 211, 322
    alpha-ketoglutaric 194, 225
    alpha-lipoic 205, 270
    amino 193, 200, 215, 319
    caprylic 186, 220
    hydrochloric 188
    lactic 225
    lauric 220
    malic 198, 225
    nucleic 35, 297
    pantothenic 193
    salicylic 179
Acrodermatitis Chronica Atrophicans 300
Actigall 307
Acupuncture 279
Adaptogens 192
Adolescents 307-8

Adrenal glands 83, 160, 191-6, 221, 223-5, 227, 281
    animal 192
    hormones 193
    insufficiency 192
Aerobics 319, 321
Africa 14-15, 185, 255, 265
Aggressiveness 164
Agitation 106, 313, 315
Air hunger 100, 107, 253, 299, 312, 315
Alcohol 102, 150-1, 223, 267, 299, 306, 309, 316, 322-3
Algae 181, 204
Alinia 152, 155, 164, 277, 331-2
Alka-seltzer Gold 333
Allergens 214
Allergies 102, 136, 146, 155, 157, 190, 214, 254, 311
    sulfa 295
Almond butter 330
Alzheimers 256
Amalgam fillings 201-2
Amantadine 25, 148-9, 303-4, 307
American strains 50-1, 128
Amoxicillin 25, 145-6, 162-3, 165-6, 303, 306-8, 310, 331
Ampicillin IV 308
Anaesthesia 160
Anaplasma 10, 58, 80, 107, 120, 126, 129-30, 157, 165, 293-4, 313, 327-8, 332

Anti-anxiety medications 240, 246
Anti-fungals 185-7, 207, 341
Anti-inflammatory 150-1, 171, 174, 180, 182, 184, 187, 198, 212, 255-6, 279, 339
   natural 191
   non-irritative 318
   pharmaceutical 179
Anti-inflammatory oils 220
Antibodies 35, 50-1, 114-16, 120, 125, 128, 130, 181-2, 195, 236, 297
   anti-thyroglobulin 195
   complex anti-Borrelia 35
   complexed 293
   high thyroid 274
   positive 122
   rabbit 113
   trapping Bb 293
   typhi 120
   very high 137
Antibody tests 31, 36, 59, 113, 115, 120, 125, 128, 293
Antigen detection tests 112, 294
Antigenic material 305
Antigenic shifts 305
Antigens 31, 35, 51, 112, 115, 117, 119, 294, 296-7
Antioxidants 171, 174, 182, 184, 215, 318
Antiseptic mouthwash 322, 324
Antisocial behavior 106, 315
Anxiety 77, 101, 106, 138, 141, 154-5, 199-200, 240, 246, 253, 262, 264-5, 267, 269, 271-2
AP-24 322
Appetite 108, 262
Apple pectin 172, 178, 190, 205, 340
Aromatherapy 279
Artemesia 313
Artemisinin 184-5, 208, 261, 342
Arthritis 18, 22, 31, 35, 47, 255, 257

Ashwaghanda 192
Asia 44, 58
Aspartame 323
Aspergillus 185
Asthma 214, 258
Atherosclerosis 202
Atopic eczema 209
Atovaquone 153-5, 312-13, 317, 332
Attention Deficit Disorder 97
Augmentin 145, 165, 303, 307, 331
Australian Biologics 122, 128, 132, 215
Australian health authorities 43
Australian Lyme support groups 253
Australian media 70
Australian ticks 44-5, 48-9, 55, 129-30, 328
Autism 97, 292
Autoantibodies 295
Autoimmunity 98, 151, 180, 195-6, 198, 213
Autopsy 18, 20, 82
Avocado 219-20, 222, 323, 330
Azithromycin 141, 144, 147-8, 151, 154, 156-8, 160, 162-6, 276, 301, 303, 307-8, 312-13, 331

B

B-complex capsule 317
Babesia duncani 59, 67-8, 120-1, 129-30, 154, 327-8
Babesia microti 59, 120, 129-30, 154, 311, 327-8
Babesia species 58-9, 293
Babesia titers 312
Babesia vogeli and Babesia gibsoni 60
Baby spinach 220
Bactrim 154-7, 165-7, 269, 313, 332
Baking soda 177
Bananas 214, 323
Banderol 94, 184-5

Index

Bandicoots 46, 80
Barley 181, 213
Bartonella antibodies 137
Bartonella cases 200
Bartonella henselae 59, 89, 129-30, 327-8
Baths
   epsom salt 253, 279
   hot 177, 270, 320
Beans 220, 323
Bedding 227, 336
Bedroom 227, 241
Beets 219-20, 222
Bell's palsy 22, 77, 90, 99, 107, 137, 273
Bentonite clay 172, 205, 340
Benzathine 25, 305, 308
Beta glucans 181-2
Beta lactamases 301
Biaxin 253, 312
Bicillin 146, 161-2, 164-7, 258, 261, 263, 268-70, 303, 305, 331
Bifido bacteria 175
Bile 173-4, 177-8, 205, 302
Biliary concretions 303
Biliary sludging 305, 307
Biliary tree 303
Binders 172, 178, 187, 190, 205, 334, 339
Bio-identical hormones 196-7
Biodynamic Cranial Osteopathy 279
Biofilm 93-5, 124-5, 130, 184, 187-8, 208, 252, 287, 339, 342
Biomed Publishing Group 15, 41, 249
Biopsies 52, 60, 110, 112, 294, 297, 300, 316
Bipolar disorder 98, 101, 155, 298
Bird feeders 324
Birds 9-10, 15, 52, 80, 84, 218
Birth control 161, 311
Black cohosh 197
Black walnut 189

Bloating 65, 175, 189, 217, 302
Blood-brain barrier 89, 171
Blood pressure 192, 266, 319
Blumenthal, Richard 37-9, 41
Body weight 313
Bone marrow 82
Boswellia 318
Boulouke 208, 252, 339, 342
Brain fog 22, 77, 146, 159, 171, 175-6, 253, 257, 267, 269
Brazil 15
Brazil nuts 219
Bread maker 273
Breads 213, 221, 264, 323
Breastfeeding 84, 146-7, 149, 162-3, 243, 310
Breasts 107, 330
British Columbia 13
Broccoli 219-20
Bronchiectasis 311
Bull's eye rash 24, 71, 76, 90, 252
BUN 161
Burrascano, Joseph 70, 77-8, 142, 160, 162, 236, 269, 278, 287, 289-90, 325

C

Cadmium 201, 205
Caffeine 267, 272, 309, 315, 323
Calcium 94, 150, 317
Calcium EDTA 187
California Lyme Disease Association 70
California poppy 199
Calories 67-8
Camping 76, 114
Canada 12-13, 62, 84, 88, 99, 265
Candida albicans 92, 138, 148, 158, 161, 175, 182, 186, 217, 221, 225
Cape Cod 17
Capillary angiomas 107, 137

363

Carbohydrates 213, 217, 219, 221, 309, 316, 319, 323
Cardiac involvement 78, 106, 140, 149, 259, 266, 295
Carrots 220, 222
Casein 222
Cashew 330
Castor oil packs 177, 287, 335-6
Cat scratch disease 313
Caterpillar 89-90
Cats 251
  feral 80
Cats claw 229
Cattle 60, 220
Cauliflower 220
CD-57 Test 123-5, 131, 181, 260, 267, 275, 282, 291-2, 296-7, 318
Cefotaxime 301, 303, 307-8, 310
Ceftin 252, 261, 303
Ceftriaxone 25, 32, 34, 36, 147, 161, 164-5, 273, 303, 305, 307-8, 311, 331
Cefuroxime 25, 144, 147, 162, 165-7, 261, 303, 307-8, 331
Cellulitis 76
Cephalosporins 25, 145, 147, 165, 301, 303-4, 308, 313, 331
Cereals 264, 323
Cerebral Malaria 325
Cerebrolvascular insufficiency 295
Chaste tree 197
Cheese 213-14, 264, 322, 330
Chelator, heavy metal 187, 202-3, 205, 339
Chelex 205, 208, 343
Chemical sensitivities 102, 335
Chemotherapy 32, 241
Chest pain 100, 267
Chicken 215, 220, 330
Chicken pox 281
Chiggers 80, 84-5
Children 11, 18, 65, 82, 146-7, 149-50, 163, 204, 243, 297, 305, 307-9, 313, 324
Chills 108, 312
Chinese sarsaparilla 171
Chiropractor 253
Chlamydia pneumonia 92, 122, 126, 128, 275, 309
Chlamydia trachomatis 126
Chloramphenicol 46, 307
Chlorella 172, 177-8, 204-5, 222
Chlorophyll 177
Chlortetracycline 46
Chocolate 197, 217, 264
Cholesterol 178, 186, 256
Cholestyramine 26, 302, 340
Cilantro 204-5
Ciprofloxacin 157-8, 165, 184, 332
Circadian rhythm 191
Circulation 302, 311, 319, 338
Clarithromycin 141, 144, 148, 151, 154, 156, 164-6, 257, 260-1, 268, 276, 303, 307, 310, 312
Clindamycin 149, 153, 161, 252, 312
Clostridia difficile 189, 311
Clover, red 197
Co Q-10 154, 194, 208, 225, 270, 317, 342
Coartem 155
Coconut oil 186-7, 220, 222, 253, 330
Coffee 174, 223, 264, 323, 333
Colitis 149, 161, 257, 305, 309, 311
Colloidal silver 253-5, 278
Colostrum 181-2
Connective tissues 32, 157, 179, 318
Constipation 100, 189-90, 198, 216-17, 299, 302, 335
Cordyceps 318
Corn 214, 253
Corn syrup 221, 323
Cortisol 191-3, 196, 224, 226
Costa Rica 15
Cough 65, 312, 315

Cox-2 pathways 179
Cramps 100, 269, 298-9, 317, 319
Creatine 319
Crohn's Disease 97
Cryptolepis 184
Cryptosporidium 152, 189
Cumanda 185
Curcumin 198-9
Cyanocobalamin 195
CYP3A4 304-5, 307
Cytochromes 305
Cytokines 139, 179, 335
Cytomegalovirus 92, 186
Czech Republic 30, 80, 85

D

Dairy 212-14, 218, 222, 283, 322
    avoiding 182
    cow 214
    goat 214
    proteins 213
    sheep 214
Dakin's Solution 322
Dandelion Root 173-4, 219
Deer 9, 19, 80, 84, 251
DEET 324
Deglycyrrhizinated liquorice 188, 190
Dental pain 99, 299
DHEA 193, 208, 342
Diarrhea 100, 149, 152, 161, 178, 189-90, 217, 267, 299, 304, 312
Diflucan 252
Digestion 172-3, 186, 188, 198, 207, 213, 216-17, 229, 341
Digital clock radios 227
Dimethylglycine (DMG) 176
DMSA 202-3, 205, 208, 343
DNA 10-11, 18, 27, 84, 88, 94, 111-12, 121, 171, 194
Douglas Douglas 208, 342
Doxycycline 25, 35, 48, 135, 137, 141, 144, 148-50, 156-8, 165-7, 260-1, 268-9, 302-3, 306-7, 314
Dream 248
    remembering 257
    violent 107
    vivid 154
Drenching sweats 241
Drug allergies 183
Drug companies 39
Drug interactions 305, 307
Dry chronic cough 107
Dry skin brushing 179, 287, 337
Dyslipidemia 295

E

Ear pain 298
EDTA 205, 208, 343
Eggs 214-15, 218, 220, 222, 264, 322, 330
Ehrlichia 58, 75, 92-3, 105, 107, 126-7, 130, 137, 144, 149, 153, 157, 293-4, 308, 313-15
Ehrlichia chaffeensis 59, 120
EKG 149, 299
Elbows 157, 298, 314
    tennis 100
Electric toothbrushes 322
Electrical heating source 336
Electrical stimulation 320-1
Electromagnetic fields 227
Electron microscopy 31-2
Eleuthrococcus 192
Elevated temperature 314
ELISA Test 22-3, 51, 67, 110, 113-17, 126, 236, 296
Embedded Deer Tick 308
Emotional Freedom Technique (EFT) 242, 246, 254
Emotional issues 27, 29, 192, 242, 245-6, 248-9, 254
Encephalitis 12, 22, 77, 97, 292, 313, 315

Encephalopathy 34, 295, 297, 302, 312
Endemic region 13, 58, 300, 324
Endocarditis 101
Endocrine dyscrasias 295
Endorphins 198, 226
Endotoxins 139-40, 170, 340
Enula 185
Enzymes 94, 187, 215, 339
   digestive 179, 198
   proteolytic 179-80, 187, 198, 339
EPA 317
Epidemiology 43
Epinephrine 200
Epsom salts 177, 197, 199, 227, 333
Epstein-Barr 92
Equivocal 117-18
Erythema migrans (EM) 12, 18, 22, 24-5, 31, 50, 63, 76, 78, 83, 132, 291, 296, 298, 303
Erythema migrans, recurrent 31
Erythromycin 303, 307
European strains 50-1, 53, 88, 128
Exercise 179, 223-6, 262, 264-5, 270-2, 283, 315, 319-21
   aerobic 270
   aggressive 316, 319
   anaerobic 269
Exhaustion 223, 225
   emotional 191
   perpetual 226
Eye exam 100, 151

F

F-scan 277
Facial flushing 99
Factive 157
Faith 265, 268, 280, 284
 personal 280
   strong 249
Fasigyn 223
Fat cells 177

Fat content of fish 330
Fat soluble toxins 173
Fats
   bad 212
   good 180, 212
   saturated 212, 220-1
   unsaturated 212
Fatty acid profile 220
Fevers 14, 48, 76, 108, 255, 298, 315
   glandular 242
   high 48, 312, 315
   including rheumatic 311
   low-grade 52, 137
Fibre 172, 174, 178, 188, 190, 205, 216-17, 222, 316, 322-3, 334, 337, 339
Fibre nerve degeneration 112
Fibrinolytic 339
Fibromyalgia 97-8, 100, 105, 198, 224, 274
Fingers 66, 256, 298, 324
FIR Sauna 177, 253
Fish 180, 215, 218, 220, 294, 312, 317, 322, 330
Fish oil 213, 220, 264, 270, 317, 330
FISH tests 120-2, 128, 130, 236
Fishing gear 247
Flagellin antibodies 51
Flagyl / Metronidazole 25, 150-1, 160, 162, 164-5, 223, 252-3, 302, 304, 307, 309, 313, 331-2
Flax seeds 180, 190, 213, 216, 220-1, 264, 270, 330, 340
Fleas 60, 63, 80, 85, 89
Floaters 100, 298
Flora 158, 160, 187-8, 322, 340
Florinef 295
Flu 67-8, 259, 261, 266
Fluconazole 25, 159
Fluorescent-linked RNA probe 312
Folic acid 176
Food allergies and intolerances 214, 217, 222, 231, 309

Food particles 190, 218
Formaldehydes 322
Free T3 195, 295
French fries 329
Frozen mango 222
Fructose 217, 279, 323
Fruit juices 323
Fruits 217, 219, 221-2, 322
    crunchy 323
    frozen 222
    high fiber 322
    organic 218
    soft 323
Fry Laboratories 124-5, 130

G

GABA 200
Gall bladder 160, 335
Garlic 186, 189, 205, 214, 222
Gastritis 106, 313
Gastroenterologist 239
Gastroesophageal reflux disease 100
Gel pack, hot 336
Gemifloxacin 157
Germany 11, 17, 31, 62, 67, 125, 138, 274-6
Gestational Lyme Borreliosis 85, 325
Giardia 152
Ginger 189, 222
Ginkgo biloba 295
Glucosamine 318
Glutamine 190
Glutathione 171-3, 227, 264, 270
Gluten 213-14, 218, 221, 231, 279, 283
Granulocytic ehrlichiosis 63
Grapefruit 163, 175, 184-5
Green leafy veggies 215, 323
Green tea 269, 318
Guar gum 178
Gym 258, 266, 270, 321

H

Hair 203-4, 241
Hair analysis 203-4
Hair dyes 204
Hallucinations 155, 298
HBOT (Hyperbaric Oxygen Therapy) 140, 230
Health insurance 23, 37, 39, 113, 244, 300
Heart beat, rapid 106
Heart biopsy studies in Lyme patients 317
Heart block 101, 299
Heart murmur 299
Heart palpitations 77, 101, 259, 299
Heart racing 259
Heart rate 47, 224, 241
Heart rhythm 161
Heartburn 188, 299, 322
Heat intolerance 295
Heating pads 146, 335
Heavy metals 172-3, 178, 201, 203-5, 208, 219, 309, 317, 343
Helicobacter pylori 188
Hemobartonella muris 46
Herbal teas 219, 221
Herbal tinctures 150, 174, 223, 254, 276-7, 333
Herbs
    adaptogenic 193
    anti-parasitic 184
    wildcrafted 206
Herpes simplex 186
Herxheimer reactions 67, 99, 106, 131, 138-42, 146, 151, 155-6, 163-4, 169-73, 177-9, 183-4, 269-71, 306-7, 333
HH2 185, 208, 342
HHV-6 186, 294
HIV infection 297
Holocyclus, ixodes 45, 51, 58
Holy basil 198

Homeopathics 230, 277
Hopeless 200, 249, 283
Hormone health 94, 107, 137, 156, 195, 224, 227, 231, 293, 302
Hormone levels 295
Hormone resistance 302
Horowitz, Richard 92, 144
Hot Flashes 261
Houttuynia 185
HPA axis 319
Hydroxychloroquine 144, 148-9, 158, 303-4, 307, 332
Hyperbilirubinemia 83
Hypercholesterolemia 61
Hyperreflexia 294
Hyperthyroidism 195
Hypochondria 103
Hypoglycemia 295
Hypotension 268, 293, 309
Hypothalamic-pituitary dysregulation 196, 291, 293
Hypothalamus 195
Hypothyroidism 195, 295
Hypovolemia 295
Hypoxia 198, 224

I

Ice cream 217
IGeneX testing 59-60, 67, 113, 117-18, 120, 124, 127-8, 130-1, 236, 252, 267, 282, 287, 327
IgG 22, 110, 114-16, 118, 120-1, 129-30, 181, 214, 252, 296, 327-8
    antibodies 114-15, 117, 119, 181
    food sensitivities 214
    negative 119
    posi-tive 59
IgM 22, 59, 110, 114-20, 122, 129-31, 181, 252, 327-8
Immigration patterns 19
Immunosuppressants 293, 301, 309

Infant 82-3
InflaQuell 207-8, 339, 341-2
Insects 9, 80, 84
Insomnia 101, 106, 226-7, 253, 299, 313, 315
Insulin 216, 224, 295
Interstitial Cystitis 97, 100
Intestinal gas 175
Intestinal tract 152, 158, 174, 178, 216, 302, 304, 322
Intestine 190, 217
Intravenous hydrogen peroxide 26
Intravenous immu-noglobulin (IgG) 26
Iodine 196
Ions 187, 339
Irritability 77, 101, 199, 295, 298
    increased 313
    neuromuscular 295
Irritable bladder 100, 197, 299
Irritation 337
    vaginal 175
Isocort 192
Italy 32
Itchy skin rashes 65, 159, 175, 338
IV ceftriaxone 147, 160
IV treatment 25, 147, 159-60, 165, 273, 275, 303, 305, 308-10, 331
Ixodes 71
Ixodes pacificus 37
Ixodes persulcatus 10-11
Ixodes ricinus 58
Ixodes ticks 19, 47, 58
    adult 37

J

Jaw pain 99
Jones, Charles Ray 84, 162, 325
Juice 177, 219, 222, 333
    aloe vera 190, 270
    lime 333
    vegetable 323

wheatgrass 333
Juvenile arthritis 97

K

Kefir 316, 322, 330, 340
Ketek 312
Kindergarten 11
Knees 157, 256, 298, 314

L

L-carnitine 194, 225
L-glutamine 172, 190
Lactobacillus 311
Lactose intolerance 279
Larium 154, 165, 253, 262, 269
Lauricidin 187
Leaky Gut 189-90, 217
Leaky mitral value 259
Legs 103, 225, 324, 338
    lower 267
Leishmaniasis 11
Lemon 177, 219, 269, 323, 333
    fresh squeezed 333
Lemon balm 199
Lemon juice 219, 221
Lemon water 253
Lesions 47, 296, 318
    expanding 296
    ring-like 17
    spirochete-induced 311
    white 99, 103
Lethargy 48, 106, 224
Leucopenia 306
Leukocytes 35, 314
Leukoencephalitis 34
Levaquin 157, 313
Levofloxacin 313
Libido 102, 196, 293, 299, 309
Lice 37, 80
Lignans 216, 222
Liquorice root 174, 192, 197, 208, 219, 342

Listerine 322
Lou Gherig's Disease 319
Low body temperature 102
Low carbohydrate diet 322
Low Dose Naltrexone (LDN) 198
Low glycemic index 316
Lumbrokinase 94, 187
Lump 47, 99
Lungs 177-8, 318, 337
Lupus 97-8
Lymph nodes 106, 108, 313
Lymphadenopathy 106, 308
Lymphatic drainage 179, 253
Lymphocyte transformation test 125
Lymphocytes 305
Lysis 32, 305

M

Macrolides 141, 154-5, 165, 332
Macrophages 181, 318
Malaise 48, 52, 76
Malaria 11, 14, 154-5, 184
Malarone 154, 156, 165, 174, 194, 287, 312-13, 317, 329
Mastic gum 188
Meats 220, 322
    free-range 218
Medical bills 65
Medical boards 24
Medium chain triglycerides 220
Mefloquine 154-5, 166
Melatonin 199
Melbourne 260, 273
Memory 255, 317-18
    issues 22, 47, 77, 101, 146, 171
    short-term 29, 201
Meningitis 18, 22, 31, 77, 97, 273, 292, 297, 304
Menstrual Cycle 196-7
Mepron 148, 153, 166, 253, 262-3, 269-70, 287, 312-13, 317, 329-30
Mercury 138, 178, 200-2, 205, 218

Metabolism 149, 156
Metabolites 177
Metagenics 208, 342
Methionine 195
Methyl B12 318
Methylation 176, 191, 194-5
Methylcobalamin 176, 294, 318
Mice 9, 251
Milk 181-2, 213-14
    breast 81, 84-5, 163, 310
    mammal's 182
    mother's 84
    skim 264
Milk proteins 182
Milk thistle 154, 174, 319
Minocycline 137, 148, 150, 158, 165-6, 302-3
Mites 80, 85
Mitochondria 191, 194, 208, 317, 342
Monoarthritis 300
Monoclonal immunofluorescence 300
Monotherapy 303
Mosquitoes 80, 84
Moxi-floxacin 157
Multiple Sclerosis 67, 90, 97, 105, 123
Muscle pain 18, 76, 100, 107, 138, 148, 171, 197-8, 201, 203, 225, 298, 315, 317
Muscle twitches 66, 106, 294, 315
Muscle weakness 196, 225, 273
Mushrooms 182
Mycoplasma 92, 127-8, 137, 149, 158, 230, 293-4, 304, 309
Mycoplasma fermentans 260
Mycoplasma pneumonia 122

N

Narcolepsy 101
Natural killer cells 181, 292, 297, 318

Nausea 65, 100, 107-8, 140-1, 148, 189, 299, 303, 312
Neck symptoms 99-100, 106, 137, 253, 255, 257, 266-7, 299, 324
Nematodes 293
Netherlands 62
Neurotoxins 138, 171, 218, 302, 309, 333-4
Neurotransmitters 200
New Zealand 53, 61
Newcastle University 48-9
Nodules 99, 313
Norway 10
Nose 99
Nova Scotia 13
NT Factor 194, 317
Numbness 101, 137, 171, 201, 299, 304
Nutramedix 185
Nuts 74, 215, 220
Nymph Tick 79
Nystatin 158-9

O

Oats 181, 213
Obsessive-Compulsive Disorder 77, 97-8, 101, 106, 199-200
Oesophageal 188
Oestrogen 192-3, 197
Oils
    castor 335-6
    healthy uncooked 333
    preferred 220
Olive Oil 220
Omega fatty acids 180, 213, 220, 317, 330
Ondamed 279, 281
Onion 137, 142, 219
Opioid receptors 198
Oral bacteria 94
Oral hygiene 322
Oranges 323

Index

Oregano 186
Organ damage 293
Osteopath 277, 279, 281
Over-methylator 195
Oxygen 224-6, 230
   hyperbaric 26, 230
   increasing 226
   levels 224-5, 319
   low 224
   pumps 224

P

Paediatrician 84, 105, 162
Pain 27, 29, 100, 102, 106-7, 177, 179, 191, 197, 206-7, 248-9, 259-61, 263, 266-7, 298-9
   agonizing 138
   arthritic 53
   bone 100
   breast 299
   chest wall 299
   joint 47, 52, 100, 106-7, 140, 176, 198, 201, 241, 298, 314-15, 335
   kidney 266
   musculoskeletal 29
   nerve 171, 198-9, 334
   pelvic 102
   shooting 53, 77, 107, 241, 299
   stabbing 334
   tendon 76, 107, 157
   tooth 99
Pain management 29, 171, 197
Palpitations 267, 295
Panax Ginseng 192
Panic attacks 101, 267, 298
Papain 198
Paralysis 10, 68, 90, 101
Paranoia 199, 256, 298
Parasites 58, 61, 67, 92, 120-1, 135, 137, 170, 181, 185-6, 188-9
   blood-sucking 10

   intestinal 152, 189
   intracellular 93, 137, 184
Parenteral therapy 25, 61, 83, 291, 294-5, 303, 305, 307-10, 313-14
Parkinson's Disease 98, 171
Passionflower 199
Pastas 213, 221, 323
PCR tests 11, 32, 35-6, 45, 52, 60, 80-1, 84-5, 88, 110-12, 121-2, 127-8, 294, 296-7, 313-14
Pears 323
Penicillin allergy 141, 146, 161, 166
Penicillin G-IV 308
Penicillins
   benzathine 32, 301, 303, 305
   long-acting 146
Peppermint 189, 219
Peppermint tea 189
Peptides 36
Permakill 324
Petrol 176, 200
PH 126-8, 130, 148, 151, 303
Phagocytic vacuoles 305
Phantom smells 102
Pharmanex 316-19
Phospholipids 194
Phosphorylated serine 193
Photophobia 106
Pilates 224, 279, 281
Pins-and-needles 256
Piroplasmosis 291, 311
Pituitary gland 195, 216, 293, 295, 309
Placebo 316
Placenta 83, 310, 313
Plaquenil 144, 148, 151, 164-6, 276, 331
Plum island 19
Poke Root 179
Poland 11
Polyneuropathy 34
Polysaccharides 182
Portugal 11

Potato 220-1, 323
  sweet 221
Poultry 218
Prayer 249, 280
Prednisone 151, 193
Pregnancy 82-5, 146-7, 149-51, 162-3, 189, 243, 291, 295, 305-10
Pregnenolone 193
Primaxin 308
Probiotics 149, 162, 175-6, 188-9, 252, 257, 270, 317, 340
Progesterone 193, 196-7
Proguanil 154
Prophylaxis 143, 154, 291, 308, 325
Prostaglandins 212
Protein snack 227
Proteins 186, 188, 213, 215, 220-2
  brown rice 222
  good quality 215
  lean 219-20, 333
  pea 222
  white 222
Protozoans 124, 153, 294, 311
Psychosis 155, 298
Psyllium husk 172, 178, 190, 205, 216, 340
Pulsed dosing 147, 261, 310
Purcell 41
Pyrex 335

Q

QT interval 161, 304, 307
Quinine 153, 252, 312
Quinolones 157-8, 184
Quinovic acid glycosides 183

R

Rats 46, 80
Rattus villosissimus 46, 55
Raynaud's syndrome 98
Red meat 212, 215, 220
Reishi mushroom 318

Relapses 30, 32, 34-5, 47, 136, 284, 294, 297, 301, 305, 309, 312
Relaxation 177, 225
Repellent 10, 324
Researched Nutritionals 172, 175, 206-7, 316-18, 341
Retroviruses 187
Reverse T3 195
Rhesus macaques 35, 41
Rheumatoid arthritis 97-8, 105, 123, 151, 198, 241
Rheumatologists 30, 151, 239
Rhodiola 192
Riamet 155
Rib soreness 100
Ribose 225
Rice 221-2, 323
  bran 190
  brown 221
  milk 222
Rickettsia 18, 58-9, 75, 92-3, 105, 108, 120, 122, 127, 129-30, 137, 157, 165, 327-8, 332
Rifampicin 156-8, 165, 167, 223, 257-8, 269, 304-5, 313-14, 332
Rife machine therapy 139, 169, 230, 253-5, 277
Ringing, ear 100, 107, 137, 256, 299
Rocky Mountain Biological Laboratory 18
Rocky Mountain Spotted Fever 294
Rodents 9, 80, 85, 324
Room temperature 146, 220
Root vegetables 220
Rosner, Bryan 9, 15, 30, 41, 230
Russia 10-11

S

Saccharomyces boulardii 149, 175
Salads 213, 216, 317, 323
Salt 169, 224, 255
SAM-e 317

Index

Samento 94, 175, 183-4
Sapi, eva 94, 145, 151-2
Sauna 177, 264, 279
   infrared 270, 333
Sausage 330
Scapularis, ixodes 12-13, 18, 37, 57
Schistosomiasis 11
Schizophrenia 155
Scleroderma 98
Seafood 178, 201, 218, 264
Seizures 99, 106-7, 298, 313, 315
Semen 81
Septra 154-8
Sero-negativity 71, 119, 294, 296-7, 300
Seroconversion 300
Serotonin 176, 199-200, 226, 295
Serum 22, 51, 111, 129-30, 296, 301, 304, 327-8
Sesame butter 330
Sex Hormone Binding Globulin (SHBG) 156
Sexuality 81, 102, 196
Shoulders 298
Siberian Ginseng 192
Sida acuta 185
Silymarin extract 319
Skin
   dry 338
   red 107
   wet 338
Skullcap 199
Sleep 101, 177, 191, 199, 207, 226-7, 254, 258, 279, 283, 315, 320, 333, 341-2
   apnoea 101, 256
   deprivation 306
   hours of 226, 259
   interruption 78, 170, 196, 198-9, 226
   refreshing 104
Sleep, remedies 207, 279, 342
Slippery elm 190

Smilax 171-2, 207, 227, 257, 341
Smoothie 178, 190, 213, 221, 340
   green 222
   protein 215-16, 220-1
Socio-economic status 9
Sodium alginate 340
Soil-based probiotics 175
Soles of feet 106, 138, 298, 313
Soluble fibres 190, 217
Sound treatment 267
Spaciness 107, 137, 304
SPECT and MRI brain scans 293, 295
Speech 101, 273, 298
   stammering 101
Spheroplast 301
Spider veins 313
Spiders 37
Spinach 219, 222
Spinal fluid 35, 295, 297, 301, 304
Spiritual beliefs 249, 284
Splenda 323
Splotches, white 107
Spotted Fever 11, 18
Spouses 241
St John's Wort 199
Stamina 196, 293, 295, 299, 309, 317-19
Starches 253, 322-3
Steroids 104, 293, 301, 309
Stevia 189, 323
Stiff neck 77
Stimulants 223, 225, 315, 318
Strasheim, Connie 245, 249, 277-8
Strawberries 323
Streptomycin 46, 313
Stress 109, 131, 158, 161, 191, 205, 240, 242, 251, 259-60, 293, 309
   chronic 192
   emotional 191
   kidney 160, 170, 173, 254
   oxidative 171
   physical 191
Stress test, cardiac 266, 320

Striae 99, 106
Sugar 181, 215-17, 221-2, 225, 253, 283, 322-3
Suicidal ideation 155
Sulfa Drugs 155, 157
Sun sensitivity 141, 149-50
Sunlight 256, 311
Superinfection 303
Suppository 205, 208, 343
Surfactants 322
Surgery 61, 157, 160
Surveillance criteria   21-3, 300
Swallowing difficulties 140
Sweats 48, 66, 100, 103, 107, 137, 140, 156, 197, 261, 299, 304, 312, 315
Sweden 10
Switzerland 12
Swollen glands/lymph nodes 102
Sydney 48-9, 52, 55, 59, 61, 63, 66, 68, 128, 251-2, 260, 267, 277, 282, 286
Syphilis 20, 81-3, 138, 184, 306

T

T cells 125, 183, 319
Tachycardia 47, 106, 141
Tahini 330
Tea 174, 186, 189, 219, 318, 323
　marshmallow 190
　weak black 264
　white 318
Teasel root 175, 184, 208, 229, 257, 264, 270, 342
Teeth 163, 322, 333
Telithromycin 148-9, 154, 161, 165, 303-4, 312, 332
Temperatures 137, 220
　high 220
　lower 177
　subnormal 314
Tender sub-cutaneous nodules 106

Tendon rupture 157, 313
Tendonitis 100, 157, 313
Tendons 157, 302, 313, 321
Testosterone 193, 196-7
Tetracyclines 35, 46, 148-50, 161-3, 165, 301-3, 307-8, 311, 313, 332
Therapeutic trials 99, 109, 295
Thigh 47, 106
Thomas Jefferson University 34
Throat 48, 99, 107, 298, 313
Thrombocytopenia 314
Thyroid 98, 195-6, 200, 224, 227, 231, 274, 295
　bio-identical 196
Tibet 318
Tick endemic area 10, 251
Tick repellents 324
Tigecycline 303
Tingling 77, 99, 101, 103, 137, 171, 201, 299
Tinidazole 25, 144-5, 150-1, 162-7, 223, 257, 268-9, 302, 331
Tissue biopsies 60, 296
Tissue oxygenation 319
Tissue penetration 302
Tomatoes 220, 323
Tongue 67-8, 99, 175, 318, 322
Toxaemia 83, 335
Transfer Factor LymPlus 207, 318
Transfer factors 181, 207, 229, 318, 341
Transfusion 61
Transmission
　congenital 37, 82, 85
　sexual 81-2
Treatment durations 306, 314
Treatment failures 30-1, 120, 130, 158, 295, 301-2, 306, 312, 314
Tremors 101, 106, 298, 315, 317
Tri-Fortify Glutathione 207-8, 333, 341-2
Trimesters 82-3, 308
Trimethoprim-sulfamethoxazole 25, 155

Index

Trimethylglycine 176
Tunisia 14
Turmeric 179, 198
Twitches 99, 231, 262-3, 298, 317
Tyrosine 196, 200

U

Ultrasound 266, 319, 321
Ultraviolet light 312
Urine 81, 85, 111-13, 156, 202-3, 296, 318
Urine antigen test 113
Urine metals tests 205
Urine samples 33, 113, 202, 204
Urine test
    provoked 202-3, 205
    unprovoked 202-3

V

Vaccines 114, 119, 201
Vaginal secretions 81
Vaginal yeast infections 159
Vancomycin 25, 301, 310
Vasculitis 107
Vasoconstriction 295, 320
Vasodilators 295
VCS test 302
Vectors 19, 46, 58, 75, 80, 85
Vegetables 215, 217-22, 323, 333
    coloured 215
    fresh 215, 217
    liquefy 222
    starchy 323
Vegetations 220, 301
Vegetative endocarditis 301
Vertigo 299, 312, 317
Virus 92, 179-80, 183, 186-7, 230, 242, 253, 293-4, 309
    epstein-Barr 126, 186, 242
Viruses, herpes 293
Vision 65, 100, 153, 248, 269, 271, 282, 298, 312
    blurry 100, 107, 137
    double 304
Visual contrast sensitivity test 302
Vitamin B12 176, 195, 264, 318
Vitex 197
Vulvodynia 102

W

Waisbren, Burton 40-1
Water
    alkaline 333
    filtered 219, 269, 272
Watermelons 323
Weight loss 241, 262
Weight training 270
Welchol 178, 302
Wellvone 153-4, 156, 165, 174, 194, 262, 332
Western Blot Test 22-3, 50-1, 59, 81, 110, 112, 116-19, 122, 126-32, 137, 144, 236, 293-4, 296, 327-8
Wheat (*see also:* gluten) 213, 253
Wheelchair 103, 226
Whey protein 222
White Willow 179, 198
Wormwood 184, 189

X

Xymogen 208, 343

Y

Yellow Dock 189
Yoghurt 213-14, 216, 322

Z

Zinc 215, 274
Zinc carnosine 188
Zithromax 252-3, 312

ABOUT THE AUTHOR

Dr. Nicola McFadzean is the owner and medical director of RestorMedicine, based in San Diego, CA. While she resides in the United States, Dr. Nicola holds Lyme disease clinics in Australia twice yearly - primarily in Sydney, but occasionally also in Canberra and Noosa, QLD. Although not a licensed physician in Australia, she can order IGeneX testing, give advice on herbs, supplements, and nutrition, and give recommendations as to antibiotic protocols (Dr. Nicola cannot actually prescribe medications in Australia, but she works closely with medical practitioners there who can provide the prescriptions).

Appointments for Australian patients are scheduled through RestorMedicine's office in San Diego, CA. Patients can also make appointments for long-distance consultations via Skype and telephone, but many patients enjoy and benefit from face-to-face consultations as well as long-distance appointments.

RestorMedicine can be contacted via phone at 1 (619) 546-4065, or by email: info@restormedicine.com. Patients can also schedule their own appointments online by going to www.restormedicine.com and following the "schedule a consultation" link.

www.ingramcontent.com/pod-product-compliance
Lightning Source LLC
Chambersburg PA
CBHW081756300426
44116CB00014B/2137